PSYCHOLOGICAL ASSESSMENT OF BIPOLAR SPECTRUM DISORDERS

PSYCHOLOGICAL ASSESSMENT OF BIPOLAR SPECTRUM DISORDERS

EDITED BY

JAMES H. KLEIGER
IRVING B. WEINER

 AMERICAN PSYCHOLOGICAL ASSOCIATION

Published by
American Psychological Association
750 First Street, NE
Washington, DC 20002
https://www.apa.org

Order Department
https://www.apa.org/pubs/books
order@apa.org

In the U.K., Europe, Africa, and the Middle East, copies may be ordered from Eurospan
https://www.eurospanbookstore.com/apa
info@eurospangroup.com

Typeset in Charter and Interstate by Lumina Datamatics, India

Printer: Gasch Printing, Odenton, MD
Cover Designer: Mark Karis

Library of Congress Cataloging-in-Publication Data

Names: Kleiger, James H., 1952- editor. | Weiner, Irving B., editor.
Title: Psychological assessment of bipolar spectrum disorders / edited by
  James H. Kleiger, and Irving B. Weiner.
Description: Washington, DC : American Psychological Association, [2023] |
  Includes bibliographical references and index.
Identifiers: LCCN 2022051816 (print) | LCCN 2022051817 (ebook) | ISBN
  9781433839078 (paperback) | ISBN 9781433839085 (ebook)
Subjects: LCSH: Bipolar disorder—Diagnosis. | BISAC: PSYCHOLOGY /
  Assessment, Testing & Measurement | PSYCHOLOGY / Suicide
Classification: LCC RC516.P794 2023 (print) | LCC RC516 (ebook) |
  DDC 616.89/5—dc23/eng/20230118
LC record available at https://lccn.loc.gov/2022051816
LC ebook record available at https://lccn.loc.gov/2022051817

https://doi.org/10.1037/0000356-000

Printed in the United States of America

10 9 8 7 6 5 4 3 2 1

CONTENTS

CONTRIBUTORS

Mark A. Blais, PsyD, Massachusetts General Hospital & Harvard Medical School, Boston, MA, United States

Robert F. Bornstein, PhD, Adelphi University, Garden City, NY, United States

Virginia M. Brabender, PhD, Widener University, Chester, PA, United States

Anthony D. Bram, PhD, ABAP, FABP, private practice, Lexington, MA, United States

Bethany L. Brand, PhD, Towson University, Towson, MD, United States

James P. Choca, PhD, ABAP, Roosevelt University, Chicago, IL, United States

Kate G. Edwards, PhD, private practice, Houston, TX, United States

F. Barton Evans, PhD, East Tennessee State University College of Medicine, Johnson City, TN, United States (ret.)

Kim J. Görner, University of Toledo, Toledo, OH, United States

Christopher J. Hopwood, PhD, University of Zurich, Zurich, Switzerland

Odile Husain, PhD, private practice and l'Institut de Psychologie Projective, Montreal, QC, Canada

Sharon Rae Jenkins, PhD, University of North Texas, Denton, TX, United States

Nancy Kaser-Boyd, PhD, Geffen School of Medicine at UCLA, Los Angeles, CA, United States

Ali Khadivi, PhD, ABAP, Albert Einstein College of Medicine, New York, NY, United States

James H. Kleiger, PsyD, ABAP, ABPP, private practice, Bethesda, MD, United States

Panagiota Korenis, MD, Albert Einstein College of Medicine, New York, NY, United States

Morgan N. McCredie, MS, Texas A&M University, College Station, TX, United States

Linda Fleming McGhee, JD, PsyD, private practice, Chevy Chase, MD, United States

Joni L. Mihura, PhD, ABAP, University of Toledo, Toledo, OH, United States

Leslie C. Morey, PhD, Texas A&M University, College Station, TX, United States

Martin Sellbom, PhD, University of Otago, Dunedin, New Zealand

Samuel Justin Sinclair, PhD, Brigham and Women's Hospital & Harvard Medical School, Boston, MA, United States

Khai Tran, MD, Bronx Health Care System, New York, NY, United States

Irving B. Weiner, PhD, ABPP, University of South Florida, Tampa, FL, United States (ret.)

Megan R. Whitman, MA, Kent State University, Kent, OH, United States

Jed Yalof, PsyD, ABPP, ABAP, ABSNP, FABP, Austin Riggs Center, Stockbridge, MA, United States

PSYCHOLOGICAL ASSESSMENT OF BIPOLAR SPECTRUM DISORDERS

Introduction to Psychological Assessment of Bipolar Spectrum Disorders

Definitions and Concepts

James H. Kleiger and Irving B. Weiner

The diagnosis of bipolar disorder is a more complex, nuanced, and controversial issue than many might assume (Ghaemi et al., 2000; Malhi et al., 2012). As always, the language of diagnosis can bring clarity but also conceptual confusion. Common clinical terms, past and present, such as "manic-depressive illness" (Kraepelin, 1886/1921), "mixed states" (Weygandt, 1899), "bipolar disorder" (Leonhard, 1957/1979), "bipolar I versus bipolar II" (Dunner et al., 1976), "bipolar spectrum" or "soft signs of bipolar disorder" (Akiskal, 1983; Angst & Gamma, 2002), or the more general descriptor "bipolarity" are not simply different names for the same phenomena but have different conceptual implications for how we understand, classify, and treat these kinds of mood disorders.

Clinicians and researchers pose key questions about the nature of bipolarity, which has implications for accurate diagnosis and treatment. Essentially, from a diagnostic perspective, is bipolar disorder a categorical or a dimensional phenomena? Similarly, are bipolar disorders best conceived by a narrow set of criteria or more broadly as a spectrum of clinical conditions that shares symptoms with multiple other disorders? Relatedly, what are the boundaries between bipolar disorders and these related conditions? Furthermore, when is it necessary to establish differential diagnoses among such conditions with overlapping symptoms, and when should they be considered comorbid? Finally, how do we

https://doi.org/10.1037/0000356-001
Psychological Assessment of Bipolar Spectrum Disorders, J. H. Kleiger and I. B. Weiner (Editors)

minimize diagnostic false negatives while not risking a high rate of false positives? The dialectic between the narrow versus broader definitions of bipolarity has been heated, with each camp citing studies in support of their definition and cautioning how misdiagnosis leads to poor treatment outcomes. However, despite the current diagnostic status of bipolar disorders in the *Diagnostic and Statistical Manual of Mental Disorders* (*DSM*) and the *International Statistical Classification of Diseases and Related Health Problems* (*ICD*) systems and the criticism of the broader diagnostic conceptualization of the *Diagnostic and Statistical Manual of Mental Disorders* (5th ed.; *DSM-5*; Paris, 2009, 2012; Zimmerman et al., 2008), the widening scope of mood disorders has gained traction in how bipolar phenomena are understood and treated (Ghaemi et al., 2002; Phelps, 2016). Before examining the widening scope of what constitutes bipolarity, it is useful to review changes in diagnostic criteria introduced by the *DSM-5 Text Revision* (*DSM-5-TR*; American Psychiatric Association, 2022) and *ICD-11* (World Health Organization [WHO], 2019).

CHANGES INTRODUCED BY THE *DSM-5-TR* AND THE *ICD-11*

Both *DSM-5-TR* and *ICD-11* mark the evolving nature of the diagnostic classification of mental disorders. Compared to their predecessors, *DSM-5* (American Psychiatric Association, 2013) and *ICD-10* (WHO, 1992), changes introduced by *DSM-5-TR* and *ICD-11* are subtle but carry important clinical implications—especially in the case of *ICD-11*.

DSM-5 to DSM-5-TR

No major changes were introduced in the essential diagnostic criteria for bipolar I and II disorders. Modifications were made in the wording of Criterion B for bipolar disorders and Criterion C for bipolar II disorders, denoting the relationship between mood episodes and psychotic disorders (i.e., determining when manic or hypomanic episodes are better explained by other psychotic disorders). Additional changes were made to mood-congruent/mood-incongruent specifiers for bipolar I and II depending on the current or most recent type of mood episode. The manic specifier relies on the wording from the Bipolar and Related Disorders chapter, while the depressive specifier uses the wording from the Depressive Disorders chapter.

ICD-10 to ICD-11

Both *ICD-10* and *ICD-11* include bipolar and depressive disorders as separate categories of disturbances subsumed under a superordinate section of mood or affective disorders. Substantive changes in *ICD-11* criteria for diagnosing bipolar and related disorders are minimal, but those few changes have important implications (Angst et al., 2020). The mood disorders section of the *ICD-11* introduces uncoded mood episodes (depressive, manic, hypomanic, and mixed), which may be transient but do not reflect a pattern that exists over time (Angst et al., 2020). The most significant change has to do with the more frequent diagnosis of hypomanic episodes. The implication of lowering the threshold for identifying hypomania means that far more people will be diagnosed as hypomanic than manic, and, as a result, bipolar II will become a more common diagnosis (Angst et al., 2020). The lower threshold that the *ICD-11* sets for diagnosing hypomania and bipolar II also stands in contrast to the higher threshold established in the *DSM-5* and, by extension, the *DSM-5-TR*. Thus, when using the *ICD-11* as a guide, one is more likely to identify the presence of hypomania and possibly increase the likelihood of diagnosing a patient with bipolar II disorder.

ASSESSING BIPOLAR DISORDERS

With the increased likelihood of diagnosing hypomania and a broadening of the spectrum of bipolarity, assessment psychologists are increasingly called upon to evaluate the diagnostic nature of dysregulated and labile moods. Bipolar disorders demonstrate a range of symptoms, including alterations in mood, energy levels, speed and fluency of thinking, shifts in self-esteem, and behavioral disinhibition. These features occur across a continuum of severity, from milder manifestations to severe impairment in mood regulation, impulse control, grandiosity, thought organization, and reality testing. As such, it is important in clinical practice to assess for the presence and severity of symptom dimensions that might signal a bipolar condition and then, on the basis of this assessment, make informed decisions about an individual's current functioning capacities, possible needs for psychotherapy or hospitalization, indications to refer for medication consultation, and, if an inpatient, readiness for discharge.

Despite the importance of assessing disorders within the bipolar spectrum, the guidelines for doing so are limited. This book fills a void in the literature by presenting a broad array of evidence-based methods that can aid in diagnostic decision making. The chapters are written by assessment psychologists, all of whom are recognized for their expertise and contributions in developing and researching specific assessment instruments or clinical syndromes. Their chapters provide up-to-date information about identifying psychological and behavioral features of bipolar spectrum disorders with widely used assessment methods, including a review of their conceptual basis, psychometric properties, empirical support, and key interpretive elements. Additionally, a separate group of clinical experts provide differential diagnostic guidance for evaluating clinical conditions that need to be distinguished from or are comorbid with disorders within the bipolar spectrum.

Additionally, this book offers students, clinicians, and researchers a single resource to deepen their understanding of diagnostic issues and methods as they relate to assessing disorders within the bipolar spectrum. When bipolarity is addressed in the assessment literature, it is scattered in book chapters and articles about particular tests or assessment procedures. Psychologists seeking information about assessing bipolar spectrum disorders with their assessment methods need to search through multiple sources to find the material they need. A single, comprehensive volume will close this gap with an integrated presentation of the psychological dimensions within the bipolar spectrum that can be assessed by each of the most widely used measures. Introductory chapters are devoted to conceptual issues, with subsequent sections on self-report methods, implicit and performance-based measures, differential diagnosis, and case examples.[1]

Although this volume includes the term "spectrum," we are not imposing a strict diagnostic framework. "Spectrum" is the broadest and most inclusive term, which we mean to include both the narrow phenotype of bipolar disorder, as well as the broad phenotype of a spectrum of bipolar/mood disorders.

Before saying more about the role of psychological assessment in the diagnostic process, it is critical to examine more closely the origins of the bipolar diagnosis and the factors that gave rise to current concepts and controversies in diagnostic decision making. Understanding both the narrow or conventional definition of bipolar disorders and equally, the concept of a bipolar spectrum or, more broadly, a spectrum of mood disorders and mixed states, is crucial for diagnostic precision and clarity of communication with clinicians who refer these individuals to us.

ORIGINS, ISSUES, AND CONTROVERSIES

The history of the bipolar concept has been well-documented and traces the origins of contemporary diagnostic issues and controversies (Angst & Marneros, 2001; Mason et al., 2016). Pathological states of depression and euphoria, as well as the linkage of the two extreme mood states, were described by pre-Hippocratic philosophers and physicians. Nineteenth-century French and German psychiatrists gave life to the modern concept of bipolarity (Angst & Marneros, 2001), which integrated depression, or melancholia, and mania to form the concept of "folie circulaire" (circular madness). Emil Kraepelin, arguably the "father of modern psychiatry," developed the ideas of his predecessors to establish the concept of "manic-depressive insanity." Melancholic depression was characterized by despondency, irritability, restlessness, reduced activity and cognition, loss of appetite, sleeplessness, and suicidality. Three traditional signs and symptoms of mania included elevated affect/euphoria, racing thoughts/flight of ideas, and psychomotor excitement/hyperactivity. Depression was characterized chiefly by depressed mood, inhibition of thought, and weakness of volition (Jain et al., 2017).

Kraepelin's Model of Manic Depression

Kraepelin (1886/1921) further unified depression with mania and introduced the concept of "manic-depressive insanity," which he differentiated from the

---

[1] All clinical studies presented in this book have been disguised to protect the patient's identity.

other form of endogenous psychosis, "dementia praecox," which Eugen Bleuler later termed "schizophrenia." Kraepelin championed the concept of "circular insanity," where melancholic depression and mania were part of the same illness.

However, Kraepelin was aware of intermediate conditions that bridged manic depression and dementia praecox. Although not the first to identify schizo-affective disorders as an intermediate condition, Kraepelin viewed the boundaries between the two endogenous psychoses as elastic. Later, the soft boundary between modern-day bipolar and schizoaffective disorder led researchers to posit a closer relationship between schizoaffective and bipolar disorders than between schizoaffective disorders and schizophrenia (Angst & Marneros, 2001).

Kraepelin's model of manic-depressive illness as a unitary, dimensional concept was rejected with the advent of *DSM-III* (American Psychiatric Association, 1980), which split the mood disorder into two categorical diagnoses: major depressive disorder, on the one hand, and bipolar disorder, on the other. The dichotomy continued through subsequent iterations of the *DSM* (*IV*, *IV-TR*, *5*, and *5-TR*).

Bipolar Subtypes

Included in the current *DSM-5-TR* and *ICD-11* family of bipolar disorders are cyclothymia and bipolar II disorder. Cyclothymia is an older diagnostic concept that describes either a temperamental predisposition or a milder disorder characterized by brief fluctuating states of attenuated depression and subthreshold mania, referred to as "hypomania." Bipolar II was recognized as a bipolar subtype, which differed from the classic, cyclical form of manic-depressive insanity, called bipolar I (Dunner et al., 1976). Type I, characterized by at least one disruptive manic episode, differs from Type II, which is characterized by the occurrence of a major depressive episode (MDE) along with at least one hypomanic episode.

Angst (1978) attempted to identify bipolar subgroups that extended beyond the Type I and Type II dichotomy. He proposed classifying mood symptoms as combinations of varying degrees of severity of manic and depressive symptoms. He designated uppercase "M" for full-blown mania, "m" for hypomania, "D" for MDE, and "d" for less-severe symptoms of depression. The symptom groups could combine to form additional subgroups such as MD, Md, DM, md, and m. The permutations of mood-related states have major implications for the concepts of mixed states and a continuum of mood disorders.

Mixed States

Although the concept of mixed states dates back to antiquity, Kraepelin and his student Weygandt (1899) described states in which there were mixtures of depression and mania in the same condition. Some predominantly depressed patients exhibited manic symptoms and vice versa. Kraepelin believed that mixed states could either represent a transition between depression and mania (or, conversely between mania and depression) or that the mixed states marked the presence of a more stable disorder. More than a century later, Akiskal (1992) extended some of Kraepelin's ideas about mixed symptoms in depressive, cyclothymic, hypomanic, and manic states. Today, there is a great detail of focus on the diagnosis and treatment of individuals with mixed features (Jain et al., 2017; McIntyre et al., 2016).

DSM-5-TR (American Psychiatric Association, 2022) included mixed features as a specifier (mixed feature specifier) and lowered the threshold for making this designation. At least three depressive symptoms are required for specifying mixed features for those who meet the criteria for a manic/hypomanic episode, and the same criteria must be met in reverse for individuals who meet the criteria for an MDE. In all cases, the mixed symptoms should be observable to others and represent a departure from usual behavior. However, three "overlapping" symptoms (irritability, distractibility, and insomnia) were excluded from the *DSM-5* and *DSM-5-TR* specifier list because they are common in both manic/hypomanic and depressive conditions. Yet, research has demonstrated that these are some of the most frequently experienced symptoms in those who have mixed features (Malhi et al., 2014). Others determined that distractibility occurred in 50% of patients with mixed symptoms, whereas "nonoverlapping" symptoms such as increased activity and risk taking, decreased need for sleep, and elevated self-esteem were present in only 10% of depressed patients with mixed features (Goldberg et al., 2009). Another group of researchers (Koukopoulos et al., 2013; Sani et al., 2014) identified more clinically relevant criteria for mixed states, finding the following symptoms most characteristic of mixed states: psychic agitation/inner tension (found in 97% of mixed states), absence of retardation (82%), dramatic description of suffering and crying spells (53%), talkativeness (49%), and racing thoughts (48%). To this list, Phelps (2016) added extreme insomnia. These patients are "lying awake with racing negative ruminations. This is not a 'decreased need for sleep' (no wonder they don't endorse that)" (p. 29).

Another useful concept, which can be translated into assessment paradigms, is to think in terms of three core mood-related symptom dimensions that can vary independently. MacKinnon and Pies (2006) proposed a "waves model." The three dimensions to consider are (a) mood; (b) energy level; and (c) speed of thought and creativity, which can shift independently. Clearly, when all three go up simultaneously, we would diagnose a manic state, and when all three go down, a depressive episode. However, consider when mood goes down but energy and speed of thought increase. Here, we may find a high degree of psychomotor agitation and negative, ruminative thought. The individual may feel wound up with restlessness. They may be trapped in overthinking, trapped in negative cycles of rumination over past or future events. A high degree of anxiety may be present.

Bipolar Spectrum

The existence of mixed states lent itself to the evolving concept of a spectrum of bipolar, or more broadly, mood disorders. Over the past 40 years, the impetus to broaden the concept of bipolarity into a spectrum was based on clinical experience, where clinicians were seeing increasing numbers of patients presenting with an MDE, who simultaneously had subthreshold symptoms of mania/hypomania that eventually converted to bipolar I or II. A group of researchers concluded that bipolarity was being underdiagnosed and ineffectively treated (see Phelps, 2016).

Although the concept of a spectrum of bipolar conditions has generated contemporary interest and criticism, the notion of a continuum of manic conditions itself is not new. Klerman (1981) identified varying expressions of bipolarity, including mania, hypomania, drug-induced hypo/mania, and depression with a family history of bipolar disorders. When some speak of a bipolar spectrum, they are referring to varying degrees of severity of manic symptoms. *DSM-5* and *DSM-5-TR* bipolar disorders, with the primary subtypes of Type I, II, and cyclothymia (not including substance/medication-induced or other/unspecified variants), form a narrow grouping of related conditions, based on the severity of manic symptoms. However, technically, these subtypes are viewed as separate, but related, disorders as opposed to a continuum or spectrum. Also, it bears repeating that although the *DSM-5* attempted to establish a more dimensional, less exclusively categorical approach to diagnosis, it did classify bipolar and depressive disorders as distinct groups of disorders. This categorical separation is continued in *DSM-5-TR*.

Akiskal (1983) proposed an expanded spectrum of bipolar disorders beyond Types I and II, and proposed Type III, defined as recurrent depressive episodes without hypo/mania but a positive family history of bipolar disorder (also referred to as Type V) or as recurrent depression with antidepressant-induced hypomania. Type IV describes major depression superimposed on a hyperthymic temperament. Akiskal and Pinto (1999) further split their subtypes to develop a continuum within the broad bipolar spectrum as they identified intermediate forms, such as "bipolar I ½, bipolar II ½, and bipolar III ½." Marneros (1999) argued for a broader continuum of affectivity, which included bipolar and unipolar courses, ranging from normal fluctuations to psychotic expressions. Stahl (2013) presented an 11-point spectrum, ranging from depressive episodes that stop responding to antidepressants (bipolar ¼) all the way to bipolarity in settings of dementia (bipolar VI). Between these anchor points are bipolar I and II, in addition to various combinations of depression, associated with cyclothymic or hyperthymic temperament and antidepressant or substance-induced hypo/mania.

Mood Disorder Spectrum

A spectrum model of mood disorders assumes a continuum, not within the bipolar category of *DSM-5-TR* but across the range of mood disorders, extending from major depression to dysthymia to bipolar spectrum to other specified bipolar disorder to bipolar II to bipolar I (Phelps, 2016). Interestingly, this continuum includes the bipolar spectrum within a broader spectrum of mood disorders.

The spectrum concept has been further expanded transdiagnostically to include other mental health conditions that share common symptoms with bipolar disorders. The transdiagnostic spectrum subsumes disorders with over-lapping symptoms of depression, increased energy, mood swings, impulsivity, prolonged irritability, and "soft bipolar signs," all of which are thought to be variants of a broader bipolar spectrum. Among these related but separate disorders are highly treatment-resistant depression, impulse control disorders, substance abuse, eating disorders, personality disorders (especially borderline personality disorder), trauma-based disorders, and childhood behavioral dis-orders (attention-deficit/hyperactivity disorder, conduct and oppositional defi-ant disorders, and disruptive mood dysregulation disorders).

Nonmanic Markers

Those who advocate for the spectrum model recommend considering an underlying bipolar diathesis when individuals present with signs and symptoms that may not include a history of manic/hypomanic episodes (Phelps, 2016). Ghaemi et al. (2002) referred to these features as "nonmanic" markers and listed the following set of criteria:

- at least one MDE
- no spontaneous hypo/manic episodes
- a family history of bipolar disorder in a first-degree relative
- antidepressant-induced hypo/mania
- recurrent MDEs
- early age of onset of MDE between ages 18 and 24
- postpartum depression
- history of psychosis without drugs
- antidepressant "wear off"
- lack of response to at least three antidepressant trials

Anxiety as a Symptom of Bipolarity

The *DSM-5* does not list anxiety as a symptom of bipolar disorder; however, a review of mixed states by the International Society for Bipolar Disorders described anxiety as a "core" feature of bipolarity (Swann et al., 2013). The committee identified general hyperarousal, inner tension, irritability/impatience, and agitation as key features of mixed states. Phelps (2016) added the presence of "negative energy" or antsy-ness and ruminative overthinking as anxiety-related features found in mixed states.

Controversies

The diagnosis of bipolar disorders has been fraught with controversy, chiefly in terms of whether clinicians are underdiagnosing or overdiagnosing these dis-orders. Bipolar spectrum and mood spectrum advocates argue that too many cases have been missed in which patients present with depression. They point out that, too often, presenting symptoms of depression halt further diagnostic exploration and result in misdiagnosis and poor treatment outcomes. Thus, from their perspective, it is important to expand the spectrum to identify individuals who do not present with the standard symptoms of bipolarity. Conversely, critics point out that the expansive concept has led to overdiagnosis without a valid basis for including a broader range of conditions under the umbrella of bipolar disorders. Critics have been especially wary of a transdiagnostic extension of the bipolar spectrum, which conflates overlapping symptoms of mood instability and impulsivity with a bipolar phenotype (Kuiper et al., 2012; Zimmerman et al., 2008). In particular, critics argue that symptom overlap with borderline personality disorder and complex trauma has led to diagnostic overreach and inappropriate treatment decisions. Further muddying the already turbulent diagnostic waters is the controversial issue of pediatric bipolarity.

To complicate matters more, many of these disorders that share overlapping symptoms with bipolar disorders can also be comorbid conditions. In the real world, pure-culture cases are often the exception, not the rule. Thus, our diagnostic task is complicated not only by the need to balance false positives with false negatives but also by the need to recognize the both–and nature of clinical diagnosis. Under what set of conditions can we make an accurate differential diagnosis and, conversely, when is it appropriate to diagnose comorbid conditions?

THE IMPORTANCE OF MAKING AN EARLY AND ACCURATE DIAGNOSIS

A correct diagnosis of bipolar disorder within the first year of symptom onset is surprisingly low. More alarmingly, it may take up to 10 years for bipolar patients to receive a correct diagnosis and appropriate treatment (McIntyre & Calabrese, 2019). Additionally, the majority of patients eventually diagnosed as having bipolar II disorder are initially diagnosed with unipolar depression.

The reason for the initial misdiagnosis is that the majority of bipolar patients present when they are depressed. Furthermore, clinicians often do not ask about a history of subthreshold hypo/manic symptoms or a family history of bipolarity. Patients may not mention hypomanic experiences because they are pleasant and may be normalized. Finally, clinicians may be looking for euphoria and grandiosity and overlook irritability and flight of ideas (McIntyre & Calabrese, 2019).

The consequences of missing the presence of bipolar depression are enormous (Conus et al., 2014). Not only do misdiagnosed patients suffer a worse quality of life, but delayed diagnosis carries with it increased suicide risk. Suicide rates are twice as high in bipolar as compared with major depressive disorder. Failing to identify bipolar disorder early on can subject the individual to potentially harmful treatment and increase cycling and the risk of relapse. Finally, the longer individuals go without being correctly diagnosed, the greater the likelihood of subsequent morbidity.

THE TASK FOR ASSESSMENT PSYCHOLOGISTS

Given the complexity of bipolar disorder and the risks associated with delayed or inaccurate diagnosis, there is a clear role for assessment psychologists in the diagnostic process. With a thorough grounding in the conceptual issues relating to the traditional diagnosis of bipolar disorders and newer concepts of a bipolar and mood spectrum, psychologists can utilize multiple methods of history taking, clinical interviews, self-report inventories and rating scales, and performance-based approaches to identify cognitive and psychological features associated with bipolar conditions. However, the armamentarium of assessment methods is incomplete without an understanding of related conditions that may either masquerade as bipolar disorders or be comorbid with them. In particular, assessors need to understand medical conditions that may complicate the diagnostic picture, as well as childhood disorders, personality disorders, and trauma and dissociative disorders, all of which challenge differential diagnostic decision making. Additionally, psychologists need to understand the boundaries between bipolar and schizophrenia-spectrum disorders. Finally, understanding bipolarity within a multicultural context is necessary to remain alert to how sociocultural factors intersect with diagnostic practices.

OVERVIEW OF THE BOOK'S CONTENTS

The chapters of this book have been written for students, researchers, and seasoned practitioners alike. In a single volume, we present a collection of 20 conceptual and practice-oriented chapters that provide detailed information about the nature of the widely used clinical assessment measures and guidance in applying these measures in the assessment of bipolar spectrum disorders.

The book begins in Part I with a chapter on the value of multimethod psychological assessment and its role in assessing bipolar spectrum disorders. Part II includes six chapters on assessing bipolarity with widely used self-report methods, including the clinical interview, the Minnesota Multiphasic Personality Inventory, 3rd edition, the Personality Assessment Inventory the Millon Clinical Multiphasic Inventory–IV, the SPECTRA Indices of Psychopathology, and clinical rating scales. Assessment psychologists often include one or more of these multiscale self-report inventories to assess personality functioning for diagnostic clarification and treatment recommendations. Clinical rating scales include a range of screening measures used by researchers and clinicians to screen for the presence of bipolar spectrum disorders and to monitor patients' responses to treatment. Part III follows with four chapters on frequently used performance-based assessment measures useful in evaluating personality functioning relevant to the assessment of bipolar spectrum disorders. These methods include the Rorschach Comprehensive System, the Rorschach Performance Assessment System, the Thematic Apperception Test and other similar tests, and cognitive/neuropsychological assessment of bipolar spectrum conditions.

Performance-based methods complement self-report inventories and provide a fuller picture of personality functioning beyond what individuals are able to report directly about themselves. Separate chapters on the Rorschach Comprehensive System and Rorschach Performance Assessment System are included as both Rorschach methods continue to be used by assessment psychologists.

Part IV contains seven chapters that focus on the differential diagnosis of conditions that may overlap or co-occur with disorders with bipolar spectrum. Beginning with a chapter on childhood disorders that may be associated or conflated with bipolarity, Part IV includes a chapter on medical issues or conditions that are related to the diagnosis of bipolar disorders. Several chapters in this section examine symptom overlap, differential decision making, or comorbidity with personality disorders, trauma-related disorders, and schizophrenia. Chapters also focus on the concept of a manic-depressive personality type, as well as multicultural issues in the assessment of bipolar spectrum disorders. Highlighting multicultural issues is of critical importance in any text about the practice of psychological assessment. Although chapter authors could have briefly mentioned multicultural considerations when using specific inventories and performance methods, we decided instead to devote a separate chapter to the assessment of bipolar spectrum disorders from a multicultural perspective.

Part V concludes the book with two case illustrations. The cases were selected to demonstrate how multimethod assessment data can be utilized to describe two individuals: one an adolescent who was diagnosed with major depression with possible indications of borderline personality or bipolar disorder, the other an adult who presented with a history and symptoms of bipolarity.

Finally, with respect to current diagnostic systems for classifying bipolar disorders, when relevant, chapter authors include references to both *DSM-5-TR* and *ICD-11* criteria. In order to ground diagnostic discussions in contemporary models and to make the volume relevant to an international audience, any significant changes in diagnostic criteria in these current revisions are noted throughout the volume.

REFERENCES

Akiskal, H. S. (1983). The bipolar spectrum: New concepts in classification and diagnosis. In L. Grinspoon (Ed.), *Psychiatric update: The American Psychiatric Association annual review* (Vol. 2, pp. 271–292). American Psychiatric Association.

Akiskal, H. S. (1992). The distinctive mixed states of bipolar I, II, and III. *Clinical Neuropharmacology, 15*(Suppl. 1, Pt. A), 632A–633A. https://doi.org/10.1097/00002826-199201001-00327

Akiskal, H. S., & Pinto, O. (1999). The evolving bipolar spectrum: Prototypes I, II, III, and IV. *Psychiatric Clinics of North America, 22*(3), 517–534. https://doi.org/10.1016/S0193-953X(05)70093-9

American Psychiatric Association. (1980). *Diagnostic and statistical manual of mental disorders* (3rd ed.).

American Psychiatric Association. (2013). *Diagnostic and statistical manual of mental disorders* (5th ed.).

American Psychiatric Association. (2022). *Diagnostic and statistical manual of mental disorders: DSM-5-TR* (5th ed., text rev.).

Angst, J. (1978). The course of affective disorders. II. Typology of bipolar manic-depressive illness. *Archiv für Psychiatrie und Nervenkrankheiten, 226*(1), 65–73. https://doi.org/10.1007/BF00344125

Angst, J., Ajdacic-Gross, V., & Rössler, W. (2020). Bipolar disorders in *ICD-11*: Current status and strengths. *International Journal of Bipolar Disorders, 8*(1), Article 3. https://doi.org/10.1186/s40345-019-0165-9

Angst, J., & Gamma, A. (2002). A new bipolar spectrum concept: A brief review. *Bipolar Disorders, 4*(Suppl. 1), 11–14. https://doi.org/10.1034/j.1399-5618.4.s1.1.x

Angst, J., & Marneros, A. (2001). Bipolarity from ancient to modern times: Conception, birth and rebirth. *Journal of Affective Disorders, 67*(1–3), 3–19. https://doi.org/10.1016/S0165-0327(01)00429-3

Conus, P., Macneil, C., & McGorry, P. D. (2014). Public health significance of bipolar disorder: Implications for early intervention and prevention. *Bipolar Disorders, 16*(5), 548–556. https://doi.org/10.1111/bdi.12137

Dunner, D. L., Fleiss, J. L., & Fieve, R. R. (1976). The course of development of mania in patients with recurrent depression. *The American Journal of Psychiatry, 133*(8), 905–908. https://doi.org/10.1176/ajp.133.8.905

Ghaemi, N., Sachs, G. S., & Goodwin, F. K. (2000). What is to be done? Controversies in the diagnosis and treatment of manic-depressive illness. *World Journal of Biological Psychiatry, 1*(2), 65–74. https://doi.org/10.3109/15622970009150569

Ghaemi, S. N., Ko, J. Y., & Goodwin, F. K. (2002). "Cade's disease" and beyond: Misdiagnosis, antidepressant use, and a proposed definition for bipolar spectrum disorder. *Canadian Journal of Psychiatry, 47*(2), 125–134. https://doi.org/10.1177/070674370204700202

Goldberg, J. F., Perlis, R. H., Bowden, C. L., Thase, M. E., Miklowitz, D. J., Marangell, L. B., Calabrese, J. R., Nierenberg, A. A., & Sachs, G. S. (2009). Manic symptoms during depressive episodes in 1,380 patients with bipolar disorder: Findings from the STEP-BD. *The American Journal of Psychiatry, 166*(2), 173–181. https://doi.org/10.1176/appi.ajp.2008.08050746

Jain, R., Maletic, V., & McIntyre, R. S. (2017). Diagnosing and treating patients with mixed features. *The Journal of Clinical Psychiatry, 78*(8), 1091–1102. https://doi.org/10.4088/JCP.su17009ah1c

Klerman, G. L. (1981). The spectrum of mania. *Comprehensive Psychiatry, 22*(1), 11–20. https://doi.org/10.1016/0010-440X(81)90049-3

Koukopoulos, A., Sani, G., & Ghaemi, S. N. (2013). Mixed features of depression: Why *DSM-5* is wrong (and so was *DSM-IV*). *The British Journal of Psychiatry, 203*(1), 3–5. https://doi.org/10.1192/bjp.bp.112.124404

Kraepelin, E. (1921). *Manic-depressive insanity and paranoia* (G. M. Robertson, Ed., R. M. Barclay, Trans.). E and S Livingstone. https://doi.org/10.1097/00005053-192104000-00057 (Original work published 1886)

Kuiper, S., Curran, G., & Malhi, G. S. (2012). Why is soft bipolar disorder so hard to define? *The Australian and New Zealand Journal of Psychiatry, 46*(11), 1019–1025. https://doi.org/10.1177/0004867412464063

Leonhard, K. (1979). *The classification of endogenous psychoses* (R. Berman, Trans.; 5th ed.). Irvington. (Original work published 1957)

MacKinnon, D. F., & Pies, R. (2006). Affective instability as rapid cycling: Theoretical and clinical implications for borderline personality and bipolar spectrum disorders. *Bipolar Disorders, 8*(1), 1–14. https://doi.org/10.1111/j.1399-5618.2006.00283.x

Malhi, G. S., Bargh, D. M., Cashman, E., Frye, M. A., & Gitlin, M. (2012). The clinical management of bipolar disorder complexity using a stratified model. *Bipolar Disorders, 14*(Suppl. 2), 66–89. https://doi.org/10.1111/j.1399-5618.2012.00993.x

Malhi, G. S., Lampe, L., Coulston, C. M., Tanious, M., Bargh, D. M., Curran, G., Kuiper, S., Morgan, H., & Fritz, K. (2014). Mixed state discrimination: A *DSM* problem that won't go away? *Journal of Affective Disorders, 158*, 8–10. https://doi.org/10.1016/j.jad.2014.01.008

Marneros, A., (1999). *Handbuch der unipolaren und bipolaren Erkrankungen* [Handbook of unipolar and bipolar disorders]. Thieme.

Mason, B. L., Brown, E. S., & Croarkin, P. E. (2016). Historical underpinnings of bipolar disorder diagnostic concept. *Behavioral Sciences, 6*(3), Article E14. https://doi.org/10.3390/bs6030014

McIntyre, R. S., & Calabrese, J. R. (2019). Bipolar depression: The clinical characteristics and unmet needs of a complex disorder. *Current Medical Research and Opinion, 35*(11), 1993–2005. https://doi.org/10.1080/03007995.2019.1636017

McIntyre, R. S., Lee, Y., & Mansur, R. B. (2016). A pragmatic approach to the diagnosis and treatment of mixed features in adults with mood disorders. *CNS Spectrums, 21*(S1), 25–33. https://doi.org/10.1017/S109285291600078X

Paris, J. (2009). The bipolar spectrum: A critical perspective. *Harvard Review of Psychiatry, 17*(3), 206–213. https://doi.org/10.1080/10673220902979888

Paris, J. (2012). *The bipolar spectrum: Diagnosis or fad?* Routledge. https://doi.org/10.4324/9780203121061

Phelps, J. (2016). *A spectrum approach to mood disorders: Not fully bipolar but not unipolar– practical management.* W. W. Norton.

Sani, G., Napoletano, F., Vöhringer, P. A., Sullivan, M., Simonetti, A., Koukopoulos, A., Danese, E., Girardi, P., & Ghaemi, N. (2014). Mixed depression: Clinical features and predictors of its onset associated with antidepressant use. *Psychotherapy and Psychosomatics, 83*(4), 213–221. https://doi.org/10.1159/000358808

Stahl, S. M. (2013). *Stahl's essential psychopharmacology: Neuroscientific basis and practical applications* (4th ed.). Cambridge University Press.

Swann, A. C., Lafer, B., Perugi, G., Frye, M. A., Bauer, M., Bahk, W.-M., Scott, J., Ha, K., & Suppes, T. (2013). Bipolar mixed states: An international society for bipolar disorders task force report of symptom structure, course of illness, and diagnosis. *The American Journal of Psychiatry, 170*(1), 31–42. https://doi.org/10.1176/appi.ajp.2012.12030301

Weygandt, W. (1899). *Über die Mischzustände des manisch-depressiven Irreseins* [On the mixed states of manic-depressive insanity]. Lehmann.

World Health Organization. (1992). *The* ICD-10 *classification of mental and behavioural disorders: Clinical descriptions and diagnostic guidelines.* https://apps.who.int/iris/handle/10665/37958

World Health Organization. (2019). *International statistical classification of diseases and related health problems* (11th ed.).

Zimmerman, M., Ruggero, C. J., Chelminski, I., & Young, D. (2008). Is bipolar disorder overdiagnosed? *The Journal of Clinical Psychiatry, 69*(6), 935–940. https://doi.org/10.4088/JCP.v69n0608

A MULTIMETHOD APPROACH TO ASSESSING BIPOLAR SPECTRUM DISORDERS

1

Using the Multimethod Approach in Diagnosing Persons on the Bipolar Spectrum

Virginia M. Brabender

Thirty-five years ago, I served as a staff psychologist at a private psychiatric hospital. A major activity of psychologists at that institution was providing psychological testing with a particular focus on diagnostic issues. One of the most common questions that led to a referral for an assessment concerned bipolar disorder. Rarely was a question posed about a patient who was showing manic symptoms. Rather, the referral was most commonly made in relation to a patient with depression whose symptoms were suspected to exist within a bipolar context, even though a manic episode had not yet been documented. For these referring parties, the question of unipolar versus bipolar disorder had importance because of its implications for medication and postdischarge treatment planning (Geddes & Miklowitz, 2013). In making these referrals, members of the clinical staff (in most cases psychiatrists) were recognizing that clinical interviewing alone was insufficient to establish a diagnosis. After all, the patient had already proceeded through two diagnostic interviews—one by the admissions staff and another by the attending psychiatrist—and still, the diagnosis was uncertain. Their everyday experience taught them that many cases required the integration of data from an array of methods, including those beyond ones tapping the patient's self-report. Since that time, the accrual of empirical findings has aided assessors in using self-report tools for the diagnosis of bipolar disorder more effectively (see Miller et al., 2009). However,

https://doi.org/10.1037/0000356-002
Psychological Assessment of Bipolar Spectrum Disorders, J. H. Kleiger and I. B. Weiner (Editors)

other methods have been shown to make important contributions to the diagnosis of bipolar disorder and its differentiation from related disorders.

The purposes of this chapter are (a) to explain the multimethod approach to diagnostic assessment in general and (b) to explore its utility particularly in relation to bipolar disorder. It argues that while the use of a single diagnostic method might be attractive due to its seeming efficiency, the multimethod approach is likely to provide a more accurate diagnosis and additional information that is helpful in treatment planning.

THE MULTIMETHOD APPROACH: FIVE CATEGORIES OF ASSESSMENT TOOLS

Suppose an individual had presented for treatment six weeks prior with complaints of depression, which had greatly lessened, and was now reporting a marked elevation in intensity of goal pursuit and mood. The pattern prompted the therapist to question whether the patient's depression developed within a bipolar rather than unipolar context. To secure additional information, the clinician administered the Mood Disorder Questionnaire (Hirschfeld et al., 2000), a brief screening tool for bipolarity. This clinician's efforts can be characterized as a single approach. Note that the clinician relied on the patient's report in the session and responses to the questionnaire, both data sources reliant upon the client's self-report. This mono-method is to be contrasted with another approach in which the clinician employs multiple methods to gather data. The multimethod approach requires the assessor to employ two or more types of data gathering in the assessment of an individual.

Writers in the area of personality assessment have proffered various systems for characterizing the available methods, and these systems overlap substantially. Bornstein and Hopwood's (2014) representative system posits five categories, the first of which is the self-attribution or introspective method. This approach entails seeking from the client an appraisal of the extent to which the client possesses a given trait or experience. The practitioner described earlier, who requested that the client complete the Mood Disorder Questionnaire, was using a *self-attribution method*. All self-report instruments fall into this category, and they are tapped more than any other in training (Mihura et al., 2017), thereby setting the stage for patterns in professional practice. Data gleaned from clinical interviews, both structured and unstructured, also are self-attributional. The different forms of self-attribution techniques all reveal how the clients see themselves and how they believe others regard them (Smith & Finn, 2014).

A second category is *stimulus attribution*, entailing the client's attribution of meaning to stimulus items that are not highly defined. Two of the most representative examples of stimulus attribution tests are the Rorschach Inkblot Test (Rorschach, 1921/1942; see also Chapters 8 and 9 in this volume) and the Thematic Apperception Test (TAT; Morgan & Murray, 1935; see also Chapter 10 in this volume). In the former case, the client is asked what each inkblot might be. The responses rendered will typically be guided by the stimulus features; that is, the blots or parts of the blot will resemble some things in the world but not most others. However, the responses will also be shaped by the individual's personality traits—for example, whether the individual is dispositionally inclined to see the big picture or fine details when regarding the environment. Contextual factors and immediate experiences in the life of the person also have a role—for example, a recent traumatic event could influence how the individual perceives the inkblots. The TAT is a task in which the assessor presents the client with pictures of human figures and asks the client to create a story in relation to each picture. Both the themes of the stories and their structural characteristics (e.g., whether they are cohesive or disjointed) reveal features of the individual's personality.

Informant observations, a third category, are the earliest methods used to assess personality (McCrae & Weiss, 2007) but are among the least used in contemporary assessment, particularly with adults (Mihura & Graceffo, 2014; Vazire, 2006). Informant ratings capture how the individual is perceived by others in an individual's social world. For example, the assessment of children often entails observing them in their natural surroundings, such as the classroom or playground. These observations can be systematic or informal. Besides the assessor, other individuals in the client's life can be invited to share their observations of the client. When multiple observers are used, the assessor can obtain information about the client's variation in personality functioning across roles and characteristic adaptations in different contexts (Meyer et al., 2001).

In employing the fourth category, *constructive methods,* the assessor asks the client to engage in a constructive or creative act within a specified framework. An example of this method is the family of figure drawing techniques wherein the client is asked to draw a particular image such as a person, a house, or a tree. These expressions provide a window into the client's representations of self, others, and the world, representations that point to the individual's personality and diagnostic characteristics. Although aspects of the client's drawings are affected by the individual's drawing ability, structural features of the renderings are less sensitive to this factor (Weiner, 1997). The individual's verbal elaborations on their drawings provide further insight into the client's experiences and perceptions. Drawings are particularly useful with individuals with limited verbal abilities by virtue of their developmental status or cognitive limitations (Handler, 2014; Krishnamurthy & Meyer, 2016). A lack of adequate normative data is a weakness of this method and has limited the diagnostic value of constructive methods. However, this problem is not inherent to the method, as has been evidenced recently by the increasingly popular Crisi-Wartegg System (Crisi & Palm, 2018). It involves a task where the client is presented with a set of eight boxes with a different mark in each box and is instructed to make a drawing out of the mark in each box. What distinguishes this method from other drawing assessment techniques is the systematic collection of validity data and normative information allowing for interpretations that are not only qualitative (as in earlier techniques) but quantitative.

Behavioral techniques, the fifth category of assessment methods, entail the measurement of the individual's behaviors in naturalistic contexts, such as a psychologist's observations of how many times a child interrupts other children and the teacher at predetermined intervals in the classroom environment. Behavioral techniques also encompass physiological measures such as electro-dermal activity (Momenian-Schneider et al., 2009). As a group, these techniques have the advantage of enabling the assessor to see how the individual interacts with different types of environments, for example, a calm versus emotionally charged environment.

Certainly, tapping two or more of these categories of assessment methods will initially take more time than the adoption of a mono-method approach, but the multimethod approach in many cases will be more efficient and less expensive. If the clinician employs a formulation that is inaccurate, either because it is incomplete or simply wrong, treatment is likely to be misdirected. As is discussed in the next two sections, various factors concerning assessment in general and assessment of individuals on the bipolar spectrum specifically suggest that greater accuracy in diagnosis is more likely with the multimethod approach.

RATIONALE FOR THE MULTIMETHOD APPROACH

A consistent finding in the assessment literature is that the correlation among findings yielded by different methods is only low to moderate (Köllner & Schultheiss, 2014; Meyer et al., 2001). Initially, this fact was taken to mean that one or more of the methods was failing to yield trustworthy information about personality and features of psychopathology. Yet, this view flew in the face of another fact: Among the various methods are well-validated interpretive hypotheses. Over time, the assessment community recognized that "distinct assessment methods provide unique information" (Meyer et al., 2001, p. 145). For example, self-report methods provide the most direct communication of the individual's experience, informant ratings reveal how individuals are regarded in their social context, behavioral techniques illumine the overt manifestation of psychological trends, stimulus attribution methods show the individual's narratives about self and others, and stimulus attribution techniques indicate aspects of the personality of which the individual is minimally aware or unaware. Because each method adds a unique perspective on the individual, the fullest picture of the person can be drawn when multiple methods are used in concert with one another.

When thinking about the diagnostic enterprise, the practitioner does well to realize that each diagnostic tool operationalizes a diagnostic concept in a delimited number of ways. And yet, the concepts assessed have meanings beyond what any operational definition can capture (MacCorquodale & Meehl, 1948; Waugh, 2019). When using in aggregate the methods that vary in terms of their manner of operationalizing that concept, the assessor moves closer to the original concept itself, capturing more of its hue and texture.

In addition to varied sensitivity to different facets of a person's psychology and ways of operationalizing complex constructs, methods vary in relation to the role bias plays in the information obtained about the person. Self-report instruments relative to other methods are amenable to the individual's efforts to present in a particular fashion. This is especially true for those self-report instruments designed to measure a single construct such as depression or mania. The thematic thrust of the items is easily discernible by most test-takers, who can then alter their responses in one direction or another. Self-report instruments measuring multiple constructs are somewhat less pervious to the test-taker's self-presentational efforts, but not nearly so to the extent of other methods, such as the stimulus attribution and constructive methods. Using a multiplicity of methods enables the assessor to detect aspects of an individual's psychology even when that individual is disinclined to be transparent.

Beyond the distinctive information that these methods provide about the individual, the data points yielded by each method when viewed in relation to one another—that is, the data patterns—carry meaning. For example, on a self-report instrument, an individual might disavow experiences of ideas flowing rapidly. However, on a stimulus attribution task, the person might directly manifest flight of ideas. This disparity might suggest the presence of denial, which is commonly observed as a characteristic of bipolar disorder (Morcos et al., 2020; Ventimiglia, 2020). Conversely, if an individual attests to disorganized thinking on a self-report test and fails to show it on a stimulus attribution test, a reasonable hypothesis would be that they experience some cognitive disarray that could be due to anxiety, rumination, or some other affect-driven factor, but lack a *primary* thought disorder (i.e., a disorder that is not tied to affective stimulation). Suppose that in an adolescent or young adult, informant ratings and poorly constructed stories about social events showed pronounced social dysfunctioning, whereas self-report ratings did not. This pattern would be of importance given that the presence of social problems is a common early manifestation of bipolar disorder in adolescents and early adults (Martini et al., 2021). The fact that self-report ratings do not suggest social problems might indicate the client's obliviousness to how they are being received by others, another aspect of the individual's interpersonal difficulties.

Beyond all of the ways in which the multimethod approach can be useful in understanding and diagnosing the assessment participant is one simple empirical finding: The use of a multimethod report bolsters the incremental validity of assessment tools. Incremental validity is the extent to which the addition of variable B enhanced the accuracy of the prediction of a criterion beyond what variable A contributes (Sechrest, 1963). It requires that a given assessment method enhance the prediction of a criterion variable beyond that yielded by other easily accessible information (Hunsley & Meyer, 2003). Blais et al. (2001) explored the incremental validity of the Minnesota Multiphasic Personality Inventory (MMPI) and Rorschach test in predicting the diagnosis of *Diagnostic and Statistical Manual of Mental Disorders* (*DSM*) Cluster B disorders. They found that both the Rorschach test and the Minnesota Multiphasic Personality

Inventory–2 (MMPI-2; Butcher et al., 1989) added to the incremental validity of the prediction of borderline and narcissistic disorder diagnoses. Likewise, in the context of a meta-analytic study, the Rorschach Prognostic Rating scale (Klopfer et al., 1954), a measure of ego strength, was demonstrated to possess incremental validity in the prediction of treatment outcome beyond the MMPI Ego Strength scale and IQ testing (Meyer, 2000). Daniels (2019) found that the Rorschach and Minnesota Multiphasic Personality Inventory–2–Restructured Form (MMPI-2-RF) variables each added incremental validity to the prediction of various aspects of interpersonal dysfunctioning. Self-report ratings, information from a semistructured interview, and informant ratings each added to the prediction of lifetime occurrence of major depressive episodes (Galione & Oltmanns, 2013). For any combination of methods, incremental validity must be demonstrated rather than assumed. Although the need for cross-method incremental validity studies is great, these studies show that employing multiple methods can bolster the accuracy of predictions about psychological functioning.

Hopwood and Waugh (2020) summarized the usefulness of the multimethod approach well:

> A battery of brief, symptom-focused questionnaires or an informal diagnostic interview provides only a narrow view of the person and exposes clinicians to a heightened risk for misunderstanding and interpretive error. In contrast, a multimethod assessment provides a means for confirming and testing hypotheses generated by any single data source. Multimethod test score interpretation means making sense of test score convergences and divergences and doing so invariably enriches our understanding of the person being assessed and avoids the pitfalls of relying too much on any particular approach. (p. 229)

IMPORTANCE OF THE MULTIMETHOD APPROACH IN THE DIAGNOSIS ON THE BIPOLAR SPECTRUM

Although compelling reasons exist for the use of multiple methods in assessment practice, when a bipolar spectrum diagnosis is at issue, additional factors point to the criticality of employing methods beyond the interview or narrowband self-report instruments.

Misdiagnosis and Clinician Bias

The first reason why a multimethod approach is indicated for individuals who may lie on the bipolar spectrum is because misdiagnosis occurs with these individuals at very high rates (Bruchmüller & Meyer, 2009; Stensland et al., 2008). Wolkenstein et al. (2011) found that 60% of clinicians rendered incorrect diagnoses of individuals on the bipolar spectrum. One third of individuals with bipolar disorder received the correct diagnosis only after 10 years had passed (Hirschfeld et al., 2003). Many hypotheses have been offered for why individuals with bipolar disorder are misdiagnosed at such a high rate. One hypothesis is that clinicians are prone to heuristic biases in how they weigh different pieces of information. For example, one study (Bruchmüller & Meyer, 2009) found that clinicians arbitrarily placed a premium on clients reporting reduced need for sleep in making the diagnosis. Another hypothesis is that the diagnostic criteria of manic episodes will not be met by individuals who have only had depressive episodes in the context of a bipolar disorder (Hirschfeld & Vornik, 2004). Given the diagnostic challenge of making an accurate bipolar diagnosis, assessors need more information, and different types of information, than less.

With respect to clinician bias, one very noteworthy empirical finding is evidence of a possible racial bias in the diagnosis of bipolar disorder. In a review of the research, Akinhanmi et al. (2018) noted that in the face of comparable symptom presentations, bipolar Black individuals are far more likely to be diagnosed incorrectly (often with schizophrenia) than bipolar White individuals. Despite the underdiagnosis of bipolar disorder in particular groups, overall, it appears that currently, bipolar disorder, especially bipolar I, is overdiagnosed. Zimmerman et al. (2008) interviewed 700 individuals using the Structured Clinical Interview for *DSM-IV* (First et al., 1995), which is geared to the bipolar diagnostic criteria of the *DSM*. Within this group, 20% had been diagnosed on the bipolar spectrum. However, when the participants proceeded through a structured interview, only 43.4% of this sample were diagnosed with a bipolar disorder. Paris (2015) noted that the tendency to overdiagnose bipolar I disorder is due to the widespread attention accorded it by popular media sources as well as clinicians' preference for this diagnosis to personality disorders that might fit some clients better. Zimmerman et al. (2008) concluded, "We agree with other authors who have emphasized the importance of conducting thorough diagnostic evaluations in order to detect bipolar disorder" (p. 938).

The multimethod approach provides an antidote to clinician bias. It requires that the clinician slow down and attend to multiple types of pieces of information. It encourages more deliberate rather than automatic processing on the part of the clinician.

Personality Roots of Bipolar Disorder

In standard diagnostic manuals such as the *Diagnostic and Statistical Manual of Mental Disorders* (5th ed., text rev.; *DSM-5-TR*; American Psychiatric Association, 2022), mood disorder diagnoses are presented as if they are independent of whatever personality traits individuals bearing these diagnoses might present. However, increasingly, based upon a vast fund of research, scholars and researchers in nosology are recognizing that personality and psychopathology are inextricably tied (Krueger & Tackett, 2006). That is, particular personality traits create a vulnerability in individuals to the development of types of symptom patterns. For example, individuals who are high on the internalizing trait are prone to exhibit symptoms of anxiety and depression.

One model that has been constructed to capture relationships between personality and psychopathology is the hierarchical taxonomy of psychopathology

(HiToP; Kotov et al., 2017), developed in part to increase diagnostic accuracy. Within the hierarchy, a factor that is superordinate to all others is p, reflecting a person's degree of proneness to psychopathology. Subsumed under p are a set of six dimensions, the SPECTRA, whose variation accounts for differences among people in personality and psychopathology (see Chapter 6 in this volume). The SPECTRA are Internalizing, Thought Disorder, Externalizing Disinhibited, Externalizing Antagonistic, Detachment, and Somatoform (a provisional dimension). Embedded in the SPECTRA are Subfactors or features of personality and psychopathology that are more specific and homogeneous. Lower in the hierarchy are Syndromes, which loosely correspond to the diagnoses listed in standard diagnostic manuals such as the *DSM-5*, and lower still are Symptom components. However, unlike these traditional systems, HiToP uses dimensions rather than categories to represent the elements within it and thereby provides information about the degree of impairment. Subsumed under Mania, at the Syndrome level, are bipolar I and bipolar II disorders.

Of relevance for the diagnosis of bipolar disorder is the fact that within the hierarchy, the Subfactor Mania is positioned under Internalizing and Thought Disorder SPECTRA. The internalizing tendency represents the extent to which the individual is vulnerable to experiencing negative affective states such as anxiety, sadness, and shame and exhibiting behavioral avoidance in association with these states (D. Watson et al., 2022). Thought disorder pertains to the individual's proneness to "full-blown thought disorder symptoms such as delusions, hallucinations, and disorganization" (Cicero et al., 2022, p. 47). Reality-testing distortion is one of the symptom components embedded in the Thought Disorder Spectrum. Individuals who meet diagnostic criteria for bipolar disorder distinguish themselves by their elevated status on both dimensions. With respect to the thought disorder element in bipolar disorder, a meta-analysis of 19 studies revealed that individuals with bipolar disorder show severity of thought pathology, based on clinician ratings, comparable to that of individuals diagnosed with schizophrenia (Yalincetin et al., 2017). These manifestations extend beyond those listed in the *DSM-5* criteria of racing thoughts and pressured speech, into the realm of illogicality and circumstantial ideas and appear to be present during both manic and depressive episodes. Accordingly, it is necessary for personality assessors to consider both dimensions when a bipolar diagnosis is in question. In doing so, assessors are not only likely to increase their diagnostic accuracy but also to obtain information about the individual's personality that could be valuable in treatment planning.

METHODS FOR ASSESSING BIPOLAR SPECTRUM DISORDERS

In contemplating the design of a battery of tests when a question of bipolar disorder is present, the assessor should consider how well each of the methods described earlier captures the affective component and cognitive component of the psychopathology. As Mihura and Graceffo (2014) noted, different methods are more suited to providing information about certain types of personality information over others. In organizing a battery, the assessor must ensure that instruments are chosen that cover either or both elements well. Among the methods used in a multimethod assessment, three are particularly useful in diagnosing individuals on the bipolar spectrum.

Self-Report Instruments

Affective experiences are readily captured by wideband self-report instruments and as such are useful in the diagnosis of bipolar disorder and the differentiation of bipolar depression from unipolar depression. The Minnesota Multiphasic Personality Inventory–3 (MMPI-3), for instance, provides information about both an individual's general disposition to experience negative affects through the Emotional/Internalizing Dysfunction Scale of the Higher-order Scales, Introversion/Low Positive Emotionality of the Personality Psychopathology Five (PSY-5) scales as well as specific painful emotional states such as demoralization Restructured Clinical (RCd) and Low Positive Emotions (RC2) depression (Sellbom et al., 2021). This instrument also speaks to a person's predilection for anomalous cognitive experiences through the Thought Dysfunction Higher-Order Scale and Psychoticism of the PSY-5 scales. Other scales speaking to thought disruption are Ideas of Persecution (RC6) and Aberrant Experiences (RC8). The relevance of the information provided by the MMPI-3 to the bipolar spectrum diagnosis was suggested by a study finding that with a cutoff score of 4 on the MMPI-2-RF Activation Scale, 72% of individuals with bipolar depression and unipolar depression were correctly classified (C. Watson et al., 2011).

However, asking an individual about the presence of thinking irregularities—as occurs when self-report tools are employed—requires a capacity on the part of the client for accurate self-observation. The client's introspection can be contaminated by the very deficit on which the individual is asked to report. Indeed, Ghaemi et al. (1995) found that even when other symptoms had remitted substantially, individuals who had suffered from an acute manic episode continued to show significant difficulties with lack of insight. They concluded that impaired introspection is one of the more stable aspects of the disorder. Moreover, the diagnosis of bipolar II poses the additional problem that the mildness of the manic symptoms can lead them to go unnoticed by the client. Alternatively, some clients might see the cognitive loosening accompanying hypomanic states as desirable and therefore, not reportable (Bowden, 2001).

Stimulus Attribution Tasks

The problem of a lack of introspective ability that might impede individuals in describing and evaluating their own thought processes is bypassed by techniques that require individuals to demonstrate their thought processes. Stimulus attribution tasks such as the TAT and the Rorschach Inkblot Test provide evidence of the individual's capacity to develop a coherent narrative.

For example, in developing TAT stories, some clients will produce illogical sequences of events, such as when a client tells the story of a protagonist who is faced with insurmountable obstacles in reaching a goal only to have those obstacles magically vanish. Likewise, the Rorschach Inkblot Test that calls upon the individual to say what the inkblots look like but also explain why they look like whatever they resemble lays bare the client's reasoning abilities. As Kleiger and Mihura (2021) pointed out, Rorschach percepts can reveal two aspects of disordered thinking: (a) problems with language and speech organization and (b) errors in reasoning and understanding of causality. These thought problems reveal themselves on the Rorschach whether the individual is in a bipolar depressed or manic state (Singer & Brabender, 1993) or is euthymic (Kimura et al., 2013). A particular strength of the Rorschach is the availability of age-based norms given that children and adolescents tend to show more evidence of thought disturbance than adults (Boyette & Noordhof, 2021; Roche et al., 2015).

In the future, research should develop the potential of the Rorschach to solve common differential diagnostic problems. For example, although schizophrenic, schizoaffective, and bipolar groups all exhibit disordered thinking, the severity of the problem for each group differs based on the study (Pagel et al., 2013). Moreover, some have observed that the responses of people with bipolar disorder exhibit a playful tone that other groups lack (Bram & Peebles, 2014). The availability of information on these diagnostic groups in terms of their profiles on the thought disorder variables could assist the psychological assessor in making difficult differential diagnoses.

Analysis of Speech in Interviews and Other Linguistic Samples

The clinical interview is typically a component of a psychological assessment and, regardless of the degree of structure, provides an opportunity for the assessor to learn about the affective symptomatology associated with bipolar disorder. Although the clinician can also obtain the client's view about cognitive irregularities, attached to this approach is the same limitation of self-report techniques, namely, the patient might not recognize or be willing to acknowledge cognitive irregularities. However, the interview provides the assessor the opportunity to analyze the formal properties of the client's speech. Black and Andreasen (2021) suggested that the client be encouraged to speak for about 5 minutes without interruption. The assessor follows the client's associations to see the extent to which they follow one another on a discernible track or become derailed. Greater precision in analyzing speech for thought disturbance requires the use of a formal system such as Andreasen's (1979) Scale for the Assessment of Thought, Language and Communication, describing 18 categories of disorganized speech characteristic not only of schizophrenic individuals but all groups showing thought pathology. This system could be used with any extended narrative material including, for example, TAT stories. Like the Rorschach, the scoring requires training, skill, and time.

In sum, the fact that the bipolar spectrum engages two different realms of personality functioning—internalizing and thought disorder—creates a greater need for a multimethod approach than might be the case for less complex psychologies. Although self-report methods might seem more economical, they are likely to address the features of bipolar disorder comprehensively only when the client is willing to be transparent and is insightful about the self.

CONSEQUENCES OF MISDIAGNOSIS

Assessors who are called upon to address the question "Does this individual have a bipolar disorder?" may be challenged for not conducting a streamlined assessment. What must be recognized is that whenever the question of bipolar disorder is present, the stakes are high in that the consequences of misdiagnosis are great. If the individual is misdiagnosed as having a unipolar disorder, it is likely that the individual will be placed on an antidepressant. Such a medication regime increases the risk of a manic episode (Hirschfeld, 2014). In a naturalistic study, among individuals on the bipolar spectrum treated for unipolar disorder, 55% experienced a manic or hypomanic episode (Ghaemi et al., 2000).

Another consequence of the failure to diagnose bipolar disorder is that critical elements of treatment are likely to be withheld. Individuals with bipolar disorder are at greater risk than persons with other disorders—including those with unipolar depression—of having suicidal ideation, making suicide attempts, and completing such attempts (McIntyre et al., 2008). Moreover, delay in diagnosis appears to be associated with greater suicidality in this population (Undurraga et al., 2012). Once an accurate diagnosis of bipolar disorder, whether I or II, is made, the clinician is alerted to the need to assess for suicidality using specialized instruments for this population (e.g., the Concise Health Risk Tracking Self Report; Trivedi et al., 2011) as well as the likelihood that the management of suicidality will be an ongoing concern. Also, bipolar disorder is comorbid with a variety of psychological (e.g., drug abuse, anxiety) and physical (e.g., asthma disorders; Hossain et al., 2019) problems for which the clinician can look once an accurate bipolar diagnosis is made.

A bipolar diagnosis, when warranted, not only alerts the practitioner to safety concerns but also allows the assessor to recommend a treatment package containing elements that have been found to be crucial for competent treatment of this population. In addition to pointing to appropriate psychopharmacological interventions, an accurate bipolar diagnosis can reveal the importance of those psychosocial interventions associated with more favorable outcomes from this population. These include helping the individual to establish consistent social rhythms, alerting the client and family members to the importance of recognizing triggers and early warning signs of a manic episode, encouraging the avoidance of alcohol and other drugs, attending to comorbid medical conditions (Grande et al., 2016), and including the individual in all critical decision making to promote treatment adherence (Fountoulakis et al., 2017). Of course, the nature of the client's current mood state (depressed, manic, euthymic) and the phase of the episode (e.g., acute phase) must be considered in identifying an appropriate intervention strategy (Fountoulakis et al., 2017).

FINAL NOTE

Diagnosing individuals on the bipolar spectrum has proven to be a challenge for clinicians over many decades. This problem not only hinders individuals from obtaining the needed treatment but creates the potential for harm from inappropriate interventions producing unintended effects. One way in which psychological assessors can improve diagnostic accuracy is through the use of a multimethod approach. By tapping a multiplicity of methods, the clinician is aided in overcoming any one method's limitations, such as its vulnerability to the client's test-taking set and the clinician's bias, or its requirement that the client possess a certain level of insight about the self. Through the use of a multimethod approach, the assessor is likely to get information not only about symptomatology but also its personality underpinnings. Although this chapter has looked primarily at personality assessment, cognitive studies (e.g., Cotrena et al., 2020) show promise for identifying a distinctive pattern of weaknesses in individuals on the bipolar spectrum, such as difficulties with verbal memory, cognitive flexibility, inhibition, and planning, and for using the extent of the weaknesses to differentiate between bipolar I and II.

REFERENCES

Akinhanmi, M. O., Biernacka, J. M., Strakowski, S. M., McElroy, S. L., Balls Berry, J. E., Merikangas, K. R., Assari, S., McInnis, M. G., Schulze, T. G., LeBoyer, M., Tamminga, C., Patten, C., & Frye, M. A. (2018). Racial disparities in bipolar disorder treatment and research: A call to action. *Bipolar Disorders, 20*(6), 506–514. https://doi.org/10.1111/bdi.12638

American Psychiatric Association. (2022). *Diagnostic and statistical manual of mental disorders: DSM-5-TR* (5th ed., text rev.).

Andreasen, N. C. (1979). Thought, language, and communication disorders: I. Clinical assessment, definition of terms, and evaluation of their reliability. *Archives of General Psychiatry, 36*(12), 1315–1321. https://doi.org/10.1001/archpsyc.1979.01780120045006

Black, D. W., & Andreasen, N. C. (2021). *Introductory textbook of psychiatry* (7th ed.). American Psychiatric Association.

Blais, M. A., Hilsenroth, M. J., Castlebury, F., Fowler, J. C., & Baity, M. R. (2001). Predicting *DSM-IV* Cluster B personality disorder criteria from MMPI-2 and Rorschach data: A test of incremental validity. *Journal of Personality Assessment, 76*(1), 150–168. https://doi.org/10.1207/S15327752JPA7601_9

Bornstein, R. F., & Hopwood, C. J. (2014). Introduction to multimethod clinical assessment. In C. J. Hopwood & R. F. Bornstein (Eds.), *Multimethod clinical assessment* (pp. 1–18). Guilford Press.

Bowden, C. L. (2001). Strategies to reduce misdiagnosis of bipolar depression. *Psychiatric Services, 52*(1), 51–55. https://doi.org/10.1176/appi.ps.52.1.51

Boyette, L., & Noordhof, A. (2021). A commentary on "Developments in the Rorschach assessment of disordered thinking and communication" (Kleiger & Mihura, 2021). *Rorschachiana, 42*(2), 281–288. https://doi.org/10.1027/1192-5604/a000145

Bram, A. D., & Peebles, M. J. (2014). *Psychological testing that matters: Creating a road map for effective treatment.* American Psychological Association. https://doi.org/10.1037/14340-000

Bruchmüller, K., & Meyer, T. D. (2009). Diagnostically irrelevant information can affect the likelihood of a diagnosis of bipolar disorder. *Journal of Affective Disorders, 116*(1–2), 148–151. https://doi.org/10.1016/j.jad.2008.11.018

Butcher, J., Dahlstrom, W., Graham, J., Tellegen, A., & Kaemmer, B. (1989). *Manual for administering and scoring the MMPI-2.* University of Minnesota Press.

Cicero, D. C., Jonas, K. G., Chmielewski, M., Martin, E. A., Docherty, A. R., Berzon, J., Haltigan, J. D., Reininghaus, U., Caspi, A., Graziolplene, R. G., & Kotov, R. (2022). Development of the thought disorder measure for the hierarchical taxonomy of psychopathology. *Assessment, 29*(1), 46–61. https://doi.org/10.1177/10731911211015355

Cotrena, C., Damiani Branco, L., Ponsoni, A., Samamé, C., Milman Shansis, F., & Paz Fonseca, R. (2020). Executive functions and memory in bipolar disorders I and II: New insights from meta-analytic results. *Acta Psychiatrica Scandinavica, 141*(2), 110–130. https://doi.org/10.1111/acps.13121

Crisi, A., & Palm, J. A. (2018). *The Crisi Wartegg System (CWS): Manual for administration, scoring, and interpretation.* Routledge. https://doi.org/10.4324/9781315123929

Daniels, R. (2019). *Multimethod assessment of interpersonal dysfunction using the Rorschach and the MMPI-2-RF* [Unpublished doctoral dissertation]. Florida Institute of Technology.

First, M. B., Spitzer, R. L., Gibbon, M., & Williams, J. B. (1995). *Structured Clinical Interview for* DSM-IV *Axis I Disorders–Patient Edition (SCID-I/P, Version 2.0).* Biometrics Research Department, New York State Psychiatric Institute.

Fountoulakis, K. N., Grunze, H., Vieta, E., Young, A., Yatham, L., Blier, P., Kasper, S., & Moeller, H. J. (2017). The International College of Neuro-Psychopharmacology (CINP) treatment guidelines for bipolar disorder in adults (CINP-BD-2017), Part 3: The clinical guidelines. *International Journal of Neuropsychopharmacology, 20*(2), 180–195. https://doi.org/10.1093/ijnp/pyw109

Galione, J. N., & Oltmanns, T. F. (2013). Identifying personality pathology associated with major depressive episodes: Incremental validity of informant reports. *Journal of Personality Assessment, 95*(6), 625–632. https://doi.org/10.1080/00223891.2013.825624

Geddes, J. R., & Miklowitz, D. J. (2013). Treatment of bipolar disorder. *The Lancet, 381*(9878), 1672–1682. https://doi.org/10.1016/S0140-6736(13)60857-0

Ghaemi, S. N., Boiman, E. E., & Goodwin, F. K. (2000). Diagnosing bipolar disorder and the effect of antidepressants: A naturalistic study. *Journal of Clinical Psychiatry, 61*(10), 804–808. https://doi.org/10.4088/jcp.v61n1013

Ghaemi, S. N., Stoll, A. L., & Pope, H. G., Jr. (1995). Lack of insight in bipolar disorder. The acute manic episode. *Journal of Nervous and Mental Disease, 183*(7), 464–467. https://doi.org/10.1097/00005053-199507000-00007

Grande, I., Berk, M., Birmaher, B., & Vieta, E. (2016). Bipolar disorder. *The Lancet, 387*(10027), 1561–1572. https://doi.org/10.1016/S0140-6736(15)00241-X

Handler, L. (2014). Historical perspectives: Figure drawings. In L. Handler & A. D. Thomas (Eds.), *Drawings in assessment and psychotherapy: Research and application* (pp. 1–6). Routledge.

Hirschfeld, R. M., Williams, J. B. W., Spitzer, R. L., Calabrese, J. R., Flynn, L., Keck, P. E., Jr., Lewis, L., McElroy, S. L., Post, R. M., Rapport, D. J., Russell, J. M., Sachs, G. S., & Zajecka, J. (2000). Development and validation of a screening instrument for bipolar spectrum disorder: The mood disorder questionnaire. *The American Journal of Psychiatry, 157*(11), 1873–1875. https://doi.org/10.1176/appi.ajp.157.11.1873

Hirschfeld, R. M. A. (2014). Differential diagnosis of bipolar disorder and major depressive disorder. *Journal of Affective Disorders, 169*(Suppl. 1), S12–S16. https://doi.org/10.1016/S0165-0327(14)70004-7

Hirschfeld, R. M. A., Lewis, L., & Vornik, L. A. (2003). Perceptions and impact of bipolar disorder: How far have we really come? Results of the national depressive and manic-depressive association 2000 survey of individuals with bipolar disorder. *The Journal of Clinical Psychiatry, 64*(2), 161–174. https://doi.org/10.4088/JCP.v64n0209

Hirschfeld, R. M. A., & Vornik, L. A. (2004). Recognition and diagnosis of bipolar disorder. *The Journal of Clinical Psychiatry, 65*(Suppl. 15), 5–9.

Hopwood, C. J., & Waugh, M. H. (2020). Madeline G. and five assessment paradigms two decades on. In C. J. Hopwood & M. H. Waugh (Eds.), *Personality assessment paradigms and methods: A collaborative reassessment of Madeline G* (pp. 1–12). Routledge.

Hossain, S., Mainali, P., Bhimanadham, N. N., Imran, S., Ahmad, N., & Patel, R. S. (2019). Medical and psychiatric comorbidities in bipolar disorder: Insights from national inpatient population-based study. *Cureus, 11*(9), Article e5636. https://doi.org/10.7759/cureus.5636

Hunsley, J., & Meyer, G. J. (2003). The incremental validity of psychological testing and assessment: Conceptual, methodological, and statistical issues. *Psychological Assessment, 15*(4), 446–455. https://doi.org/10.1037/1040-3590.15.4.446

Kimura, H., Osaki, A., Kawashima, R., Inoue, T., Nakagawa, S., Suzuki, K., Asakura, S., Tanaka, T., Kitaichi, Y., Masui, T., Kitagawa, N., Kako, Y., Abekawa, T., Kusumi, I., Yamanaka, H., Denda, K., & Koyama, T. (2013). Differences between bipolar and unipolar depression on Rorschach testing. *Neuropsychiatric Disease and Treatment, 9*, 619–627. https://doi.org/10.2147/NDT.S42702

Kleiger, J., & Mihura, J. (2021). Developments in the assessment of disordered thinking and communication. *Rorschachiana, 42*(2), 265–280. https://doi.org/10.1027/1192-5604/a000132

Klopfer, B., Ainsworth, M. D., Klopfer, W. G., & Holt, R. R. (1954). *Developments in the Rorschach technique: Vol. 1. Technique and theory.* World Book.

Köllner, M. G., & Schultheiss, O. C. (2014). Meta-analytic evidence of low convergence between implicit and explicit measures of the needs for achievement, affiliation, and power. *Frontiers in Psychology, 5*, Article 826. https://doi.org/10.3389/fpsyg.2014.00826

Kotov, R., Krueger, R. F., Watson, D., Achenbach, T. M., Althoff, R. R., Bagby, R. M., Brown, T. A., Carpenter, W. T., Caspi, A., Clark, L. A., Eaton, N. R., Forbes, M. K., Forbush, K. T., Goldberg, D., Hasin, D., Hyman, S. E., Ivanova, M. Y., Lynam, D. R., Markon, K., . . . Zimmerman, M. (2017). The Hierarchical Taxonomy of Psychopathology (HiTOP): A dimensional alternative to traditional nosologies. *Journal of Abnormal Psychology, 126*(4), 454–477. https://doi.org/10.1037/abn0000258

Krishnamurthy, R., & Meyer, G. (2016). Psychopathology assessment. In J. C. Norcross, G. R. VandenBos, D. K. Freedheim, & R. Krishnamurthy (Eds.), *APA handbook of clinical psychology: Vol. 1. Applications and methods* (pp. 103–137). American Psychological Association. https://doi.org/10.1037/14861-006

Krueger, R. F., & Tackett, J. L. (2006). Introduction. In R. F. Krueger & J. L. Tackett (Eds.), *Personality and psychopathology* (pp. 1–6). Guilford Press.

MacCorquodale, K., & Meehl, P. E. (1948). On a distinction between hypothetical constructs and intervening variables. *Psychological Review, 55*(2), 95–107. https://doi.org/10.1037/h0056029

Martini, J., Leopold, K., Pfeiffer, S., Berndt, C., Boehme, A., Roessner, V., Fusar-Poli, P., Young, A. H., Correll, C. U., Bauer, M., & Pfennig, A. (2021). Early detection of bipolar disorders and treatment recommendations for help-seeking adolescents and young adults: Findings of the Early Detection and Intervention Center Dresden. *International Journal of Bipolar Disorders, 9*(1), Article 23. https://doi.org/10.1186/s40345-021-00227-3

McCrae, R. R., & Weiss, A. (2007). Observer ratings of personality. In R. Robins, R. C. Fraley, & R. F. Krueger (Eds.), *Handbook of research methods in personality psychology* (pp. 259–272). Guilford Press.

McIntyre, R. S., Muzina, D. J., Kemp, D. E., Blank, D., Woldeyohannes, H. O., Lofchy, J., Soczynska, J. K., Banik, S., & Konarski, J. Z. (2008). Bipolar disorder and suicide: Research synthesis and clinical translation. *Current Psychiatry Reports, 10*(1), 66–72. https://doi.org/10.1007/s11920-008-0012-7

Meyer, G. J. (2000). Incremental validity of the Rorschach Prognostic Rating Scale over the MMPI Ego Strength Scale and IQ. *Journal of Personality Assessment, 74*(3), 356–370. https://doi.org/10.1207/S15327752JPA7403_2

Meyer, G. J., Finn, S. E., Eyde, L. D., Kay, G. G., Moreland, K. L., Dies, R. R., Eisman, E. J., Kubiszyn, T. W., & Reed, G. M. (2001). Psychological testing and psychological assessment: A review of evidence and issues. *American Psychologist, 56*(2), 128–165. https://doi.org/10.1037/0003-066X.56.2.128

Mihura, J. L., & Graceffo, R. A. (2014). Multimethod assessment and treatment planning. In C. J. Hopwood & R. F. Bornstein (Eds.), *Multimethod clinical assessment* (pp. 285–318). Guilford Press.

Mihura, J. L., Roy, M., & Graceffo, R. A. (2017). Psychological assessment training in clinical psychology doctoral programs. *Journal of Personality Assessment, 99*(2), 153–164. https://doi.org/10.1080/00223891.2016.1201978

Miller, C. J., Johnson, S. L., & Eisner, L. (2009). Assessment tools for adult bipolar disorder. *Clinical Psychology: Science and Practice, 16*(2), 188–201. https://doi.org/10.1111/j.1468-2850.2009.01158.x

Momenian-Schneider, S. H., Brabender, V. M., & Nath, S. R. (2009). Psychophysiological reactions to the response phase of the Rorschach and 16PF. *Journal of Personality Assessment, 91*(5), 494–496. https://doi.org/10.1080/00223890903088727

Morcos, N., Bess, J. D., & Casher, M. I. (2020). The inpatient with mania. In M. I. Casher & J. S. Bess (Eds.), *Manual of inpatient psychiatry* (pp. 63–81). Cambridge University Press. https://doi.org/10.1017/9781108656672.005

Morgan, C. D., & Murray, H. H. (1935). A method for investigating fantasies: The Thematic Apperception Test. *Archives of Neurology and Psychiatry, 34*(2), 289–306. https://doi.org/10.1001/archneurpsyc.1935.02250200049005

Pagel, T., Baldessarini, R. J., Franklin, J., & Baethge, C. (2013). Characteristics of patients diagnosed with schizoaffective disorder compared with schizophrenia and bipolar disorder. *Bipolar Disorders, 15*(3), 229–239. https://doi.org/10.1111/bdi.12057

Paris, J. (2015). *A concise guide to personality disorders*. American Psychological Association. https://doi.org/10.1037/14642-000

Roche, E., Creed, L., MacMahon, D., Brennan, D., & Clarke, M. (2015). The epidemiology and associated phenomenology of formal thought disorder: A systematic review. *Schizophrenia Bulletin, 41*(4), 951–962. https://doi.org/10.1093/schbul/sbu129

Rorschach, H. (1942). *Psychodiagnostics* (5th ed.). Hans Huber. (Original work published 1921)

Sechrest, L. (1963). Incremental validity: A recommendation. *Educational and Psychological Measurement, 23*(1), 153–158. https://doi.org/10.1177/001316446302300113

Sellbom, M., Kremyar, A. J., & Wygant, D. B. (2021). Mapping MMPI-3 scales onto the hierarchical taxonomy of psychopathology. *Psychological Assessment, 33*(12), 1153–1168. https://doi.org/10.1037/pas0001049

Singer, H. K., & Brabender, V. (1993). The use of the Rorschach to differentiate unipolar and bipolar disorders. *Journal of Personality Assessment, 60*(2), 333–345. https://doi.org/10.1207/s15327752jpa6002_10

Smith, J. D., & Finn, S. E. (2014). Integration and therapeutic presentation of multimethod assessment results: An empirically supported framework and case example. In

C. J. Hopwood & R. F. Bornstein (Eds.), *Multimethod clinical assessment* (pp. 403–425). Guilford Press.

Stensland, M. D., Schultz, J. F., & Frytak, J. R. (2008). Diagnosis of unipolar depression following initial identification of bipolar disorder: A common and costly misdiagnosis. *The Journal of Clinical Psychiatry, 69*(5), 749–758. https://doi.org/10.4088/JCP. v69n0508

Trivedi, M. H., Wisniewski, S. R., Morris, D. W., Fava, M., Gollan, J. K., Warden, D., Nierenberg, A. A., Gaynes, B. N., Husain, M. M., Luther, J. F., Zisook, S., & Rush, A. J. (2011). Concise Health Risk Tracking scale: A brief self-report and clinician rating of suicidal risk. *The Journal of Clinical Psychiatry, 72*(6), 757–764. https://doi.org/10.4088/ JCP.11m06837

Undurraga, J., Baldessarini, R. J., Valenti, M., Pacchiarotti, I., & Vieta, E. (2012). Suicidal risk factors in bipolar I and II disorder patients. *The Journal of Clinical Psychiatry, 73*(6), 778–782. https://doi.org/10.4088/JCP.11m07041

Vazire, S. (2006). Informant reports: A cheap, fast, and easy method for personality assessment. *Journal of Research in Personality, 40*(5), 472–481. https://doi.org/10.1016/j. jrp.2005.03.003

Ventimiglia, G. (2020). A psychoanalytic interpretation of bipolar disorder. *International Forum of Psychoanalysis, 29*(2), 74–86. https://doi.org/10.1080/0803706X.2018. 1518595

Watson, C., Quilty, L. C., & Bagby, R. M. (2011). Differentiating bipolar disorder from major depressive disorder using the MMPI-2-RF: A receiver operating characteristics (ROC) analysis. *Journal of Psychopathology and Behavioral Assessment, 33*(3), 368–374. https://doi.org/10.1007/s10862-010-9212-7

Watson, D., Forbes, M. K., Levin-Aspenson, H. F., Ruggero, C. J., Kotelnikova, Y., Khoo, S., Bagby, R. M., Sunderland, M., Patalay, P., & Kotov, R. (2022). The development of preliminary HiTOP internalizing spectrum scales. *Assessment, 29*(1), 17–33. https:// doi.org/10.1177/10731911211003976

Waugh, M. H. (2019). Construct and paradigm in the AMPD 1. In C. J. Hopwood, A. L. Mulay, & M. H. Waugh (Eds.), *The DSM-5 alternative model for personality disorders* (pp. 1–47). Routledge. https://doi.org/10.4324/9781315205076-1

Weiner, I. B. (1997). *Psychodiagnosis in schizophrenia*. Lawrence Erlbaum.

Wolkenstein, L., Bruchmüller, K., Schmid, P., & Meyer, T. D. (2011). Misdiagnosing bipolar disorder—Do clinicians show heuristic biases? *Journal of Affective Disorders, 130*(3), 405–412. https://doi.org/10.1016/j.jad.2010.10.036

Yalincetin, B., Bora, E., Binbay, T., Ulas, H., Akdede, B. B., & Alptekin, K. (2017). Formal thought disorder in schizophrenia and bipolar disorder: A systematic review and meta-analysis. *Schizophrenia Research, 185*, 2–8. https://doi.org/10.1016/j.schres.2016.12.015

Zimmerman, M., Ruggero, C. J., Chelminski, I., & Young, D. (2008). Is bipolar disorder overdiagnosed? *The Journal of Clinical Psychiatry, 69*(6), 935–940. https://doi.org/10. 4088/JCP.v69n0608

II

INTERVIEW AND
SELF-REPORT METHODS

2

Clinical Interview Methods for Assessing Bipolar Spectrum Disorders

Ali Khadivi

The clinical interview is the most common and essential method for assessing bipolar spectrum disorders (BSDs; Goodwin & Jamison, 1990; Grande et al., 2016). It is often the first diagnostic procedure employed, and the clinician uses the interview to establish an assessment alliance, gather relevant clinical information, and prepare the patient for further assessment (Maruish, 2014).

This chapter focuses on applying traditional clinical interview methods for assessing BSDs that are commonly practiced in most settings (see Khadivi, 2021; Maruish, 2014; Shea, 2016). In this type of interview, the clinician uses a semistructured format to elicit and probe for symptoms, observe signs of a psychiatric disorder, obtain a clinically relevant history, and conduct a mental status examination to arrive at an initial diagnosis and treatment plan.

While the clinical interview is the primary diagnostic method in practice, establishing an accurate diagnosis of bipolar disorder remains a challenging task for three reasons: (a) A person with BSD can potentially present at different phases of the illness, requiring a retrospective assessment of bipolar symptoms; (b) there is considerable comorbidity in BSDs, resulting in overlapping clinical presentations; and (c) individuals with BSDs could have clinical presentations that might be similar to other psychiatric conditions (McIntyre et al., 2019; Singh & Rajport, 2006; see also Chapters 12–16 in this volume).

Although bipolar disorder was historically underdiagnosed in the United States (Andreasen & Grove, 1986), the current practice trend shows that BSD is both underdiagnosed and overdiagnosed (McIntyre et al., 2019). Research has

https://doi.org/10.1037/0000356-003
Psychological Assessment of Bipolar Spectrum Disorders, J. H. Kleiger and I. B. Weiner (Editors)

also shown a high rate of misdiagnosis (Singh & Rajport, 2006). Close to 70% of people with BSD are initially misdiagnosed, and more than one third of patients remain misdiagnosed for 10 years or more (Tracy, 2013). As described in this volume (see Chapters 12, 14, 15, and 16), BSD can be misdiagnosed as attention-deficit/hyperactivity disorder, schizophrenia, schizoaffective disorder, major depression, personality disorders, trauma spectrum, and anxiety disorders (Tracy, 2013). Chapter 13 in this volume also shows that underlying medical or drug-induced conditions may be misdiagnosed as BSD as well.

To improve the accuracy of bipolar diagnosis, the bipolar and related disorders *Diagnostic and Statistical Manual of Mental Disorders* (5th ed.; *DSM-5*; American Psychiatric Association, 2013) task committee made essential changes in the diagnostic criteria. They added that an increase in goal-directed actions and energy are core diagnostic criteria (see Black & Grant, 2014). This change was made because if the increase in activity and energy level is not assessed with mood symptoms, then mild manic or hypomanic episodes will go undetected in patients who present during depressed or eurythmic phases (Angst et al., 2012). Other changes included placing bipolar disorders in a separate diagnostic category and not under mood disorders and allowing bipolar II disorder to be diagnosed with mixed features, defined as having three manic and three depressive symptoms during a mood episode (Black & Grant, 2014; McIntyre et al., 2019). The following section discusses in more detail the assessment of manic and hypomanic episodes and core associated signs and symptoms.

MANIC AND HYPOMANIC EPISODES

In establishing a *DSM-5* diagnosis of BSDs, including bipolar I or bipolar II, it is essential to determine whether the person has had at least one manic (in the case of bipolar I) or one hypomanic episode (in bipolar II) in their lifetime. As such, the focus of the clinical interview is to establish the presence and the extent of current or past manic or hypomanic episodes. Given the new addition to the diagnostic criteria for bipolar disorder, the clinician must determine whether (a) the individual has had a lifetime history or is currently experiencing an elevated, expansive, or irritable mood concurrently with persistently increased activity and energy; (b) the mood symptoms and increase in energy are a significant deviation from the patient's baseline functioning; and (c) the patient is either currently, or has in the past, had other associated symptoms/signs of bipolar disorder (such as the diminished need for sleep, grandiosity, pressured speech, and racing thoughts) during the episode (American Psychiatric Association, 2013).

Because individuals in manic and hypomanic phases of BSD can have elevated or irritable moods, it is essential to inquire about them separately (First et al., 2016). It is best to ask about elevated mood plus an increase in energy and activity first and then inquire about irritable mood and an increase in the level of energy and movement.

The Structured Clinical Interview for *DSM-5* Disorders (SCID-5; First et al., 2016; see also Chapter 7 in this volume) offers one of the most comprehensive questions to assess all the above three diagnostic elements of manic/hypomanic episodes. The standard SCID-5 questions assess shifts in energy, activity level, and mood to help determine the existence of lifetime manic episodes.

1. *Energy and activity level*: "Have you ever had a period when you were feeling so good, high, excited, or on top of the world that other people thought you were not your usual self?" "Did you also feel like you were hyper or wired and had an unusual amount of energy?" "Were you much more active?"

2. *Mood*: "Have you ever had a period in your life that you felt so irritable, angry, or short-tempered for most of the day for at least several days that other people thought you were not your normal self?"

If the person's answers to these questions indicate that they have experienced any of the mood episodes with increased activity and energy, the clinician then has the person describe their experience ("What was the experience like?") and the duration of the episode ("How long did it last?" and "Was it most of day, nearly every day?"). This emphasis on the duration and the presence of symptoms nearly every day on the SCID-5 was made to help distinguish personality disordered and other individuals who have short-lived mood swings from those experiencing manic and hypomanic episodes (First et al., 2016). In assessing a current manic episode, the standard questions start with the phrase "In the past month or since one month ago, have you had a period that you felt so good, high, excited or on top of the world" (First et al., 2016, p. 17).

Also, First et al. (2016) recommended follow-up questions when substance abuse is involved. Specifically, if the person describes manic or hypomanic episodes in the context of substance use, ask whether there was ever another time when they were feeling this way when they did not use any drugs.

The same clinical interview questions are also used in assessing hypomania because the presentation is like mania except for the severity of impairment and duration of the episodes. First et al. (2016) argued that it is best to conceptualize hypomania as a change rather than an impairment in the level of functioning. It is more effective to inquire whether changes in energy and activity were uncharacteristic of the person and were observable to others. Moreover, during a hypomanic episode, many patients may experience mood symptoms as mild or may not recognize that elevated or irritable mood changes are a change from their unusual way of being (Skodol, 1989).

Lack of awareness of elevated mood is illustrated in the case of a 21-year-old male college student referred for diagnostic assessment by his parents for "mood changes." During the clinical interview, the patient insisted he has always been "upbeat and positive," and he was not able to describe changes in his mood; however, when asked about changes in his behavior, he reported increased goal-directed behavior focusing on multiple college projects, hypersexuality, sexting with numerous students, and diminished need for sleep. He and his family confirmed that his current behaviors were uncharacteristic and that they were a change from his baseline.

ASSESSMENT OF CORE ASSOCIATED SIGNS AND SYMPTOMS

During manic/hypomanic episodes in which sleep patterns, speech, thinking, and behavior are affected, the clinician must determine if and to what extent the other core signs and symptoms of BSD are present during the elevated or irritable mood state. According to the *Diagnostic and Statistical Manual of Mental Disorders* (5th ed., text rev.; *DSM-5-TR*), seven signs and symptoms need to be assessed. These include decreased need for sleep, being increasingly talkative or pressured to keep talking, flight of ideas or racing thoughts, inflated self-esteem, grandiosity, increased goal-directed or psychomotor activity, and excessive involvement in risky activities. Because some might find it difficult to remember these symptoms, mnemonics such as DIGFAST (see Table 2.1) may be helpful (Phelps, 2016).

After establishing that there has been an increase in energy or goal-directed actions combined with either elevated or irritable mood, the clinician should focus on assessing the other core manic signs and symptoms. However, to fully establish the presence of these core signs and symptoms, it is essential to understand them phenomenologically. An extensive literature (e.g., First et al., 2016; Skodol, 1989) describes the phenomenology of bipolar disorder, including the following core manic and hypomanic signs and symptoms that would need to be assessed.

Decreased Need for Sleep

Although insomnia is a nonspecific symptom in many psychiatric conditions, decreased need for sleep, as opposed to a decrease in sleep, is a unique phenomenon and a core symptom of manic and hypomanic episodes (Skodol, 1989). The best interviewing technique consists of asking open-ended questions about the patient's sleep and then following up with more specific

TABLE 2.1. DIGFAST Mnemonic for *DSM-5* Criterion B

Mnemonic	Symptoms and signs
D	Distractibility (unstable attention)
I	Impulsivity (excessive involvement in high-risk behaviors; e.g., spending, sexual activity, foolish investments)
G	Grandiosity (inflated self-esteem)
F	Flight of ideas (racing thoughts)
A	Activity increased (increased goal-directed activity)
S	Sleep decreased (decreased need for sleep)
T	Talkativeness (pressured speech)

Note. DSM-5 = Diagnostic and Statistical Manual of Mental Disorders, Fifth Edition. From *A Spectrum Approach to Mood Disorders: Not Fully Bipolar but Not Unipolar—Practical Management* (p. 11), by J. Phelps, 2016, W. W. Norton. Copyright 2016 by James Phelps. Used by permission of W. W. Norton & Company, Inc.

questions to differentiate between a decrease in sleep or a diminished need for sleep. It is especially helpful to inquire if the person felt rested without sleeping (First et al., 2016).

More Talkative Than Usual or Pressured to Keep Talking

During manic or hypomanic episodes, speech is accelerated and increased in quantity. Andreasen (1979) described the core characteristic of pressured speech as an increase in the rate and the amount of speech, which makes it challenging to interrupt the patient. Clinicians can retrospectively assess whether the patient has experienced pressured speech during a mood episode by asking, "Were you more talkative than usual, or did people ask you to slow down?" (First et al., 2016).

Flight of Ideas

Flight of ideas is a type of thought disorder observed during a clinical interview. It has been defined in different ways. Skodol (1989) stated that flight of ideas is more like a "rapid stream of speech, and it is not expressed simply by speech that shifts from one subject to another" (p. 260). However, Andreasen (1979) offered a more precise description based on her thought disorder research. She characterized flight of ideas as derailment (disorganized speech) with pressured speech. The *DSM-5* definition of flight of ideas, as evidenced in the SCID-5 manual (First et al., 2016), is more aligned with Andreasen's conceptualization. The best method of assessing the flight of ideas consists of asking open-ended questions that allow the person to speak uninterrupted for several minutes (Andreasen & Black, 2006).

An excellent example of pressured speech and flight of ideas can be found in a YouTube video from the University of Nottingham (2012).

Distractibility

Although distractibility can be seen in individuals with psychotic, depressive, and anxiety disorders, manic and hypomanic distractibility is characterized by an inability to filter out external stimuli. For example, a patient may become distracted by the examiner's clothes or sounds in the room. A related form of distractibility is distractible speech (Andreasen, 1979; Kleiger & Khadivi, 2015). The patient, while talking, becomes distracted by an external stimulus and suddenly shifts to a different topic and loses track of what they were saying. Here is an example: "Can you believe I left sunshine California for the Bronx? Who does that? Oh my god, are you wearing cufflinks? Have you ever had them in gold? It is my favorite color."

Grandiosity and Inflated Self-Esteem

In both mania and hypomania, patients experience inflated self-esteem. It is most useful to ask open-ended questions about how they experience themselves during episodes of mood disturbance and then follow up by asking them to give an example. A key differentiating feature of mania/hypomania inflated self-esteem is that it must be much more than a feeling of self-confidence (First et al., 2016).

Excessive Involvement in Activities That Have a High Potential for Painful Consequences

In both manic and hypomanic episodes, a person can engage in unrestrained spending, gambling, impulsive business investments, driving recklessly, and sexual disinhibitions. Since normal individuals, as well as persons with other psychological disorders, can engage in those behaviors, Skodol (1989) argued that to avoid misdiagnosis, it is essential to understand that these associated symptoms must occur with marked changes in mood and combine with an increase in energy or activity. Furthermore, one must consider the cultural and religious context in assessing these symptoms and tailor clinical questions accordingly (Kleiger & Khadivi, 2015; see also Chapter 18 in this volume). For example, patients in economically disadvantaged settings may not have the financial means to engage in unstrained shopping, or patients who live in religious communities may not have the opportunity to engage in any inter-personal sexual behavior.

INTERVIEWER REACTIONS

Clinicians' reactions and countertransference to patients as a source of diagnostic information have a long tradition in the psychiatric interview (Sullivan, 1954), psychodynamic-informed consultation (Racker, 1957), and personality assessment (Sugarman, 1981). Clinical experience has shown that patients in a manic phase of bipolar disorder could evoke unique reactions in clinicians, different from those elicited by patients presenting with psychosis and schizophrenia spectrum disorders (see Chapter 16 in this volume). The elevated mood of a manic patient can be contagious, causing the clinician to have a similar emotional response. Manic patients with pressured speech and flight of ideas can confuse and frustrate the clinician's ability to connect with the patient. Manic patients with irritable moods and increased energy can invoke anxiety in the interviewer and be challenging to engage in assessment.

DEPRESSIVE EPISODE

Depression is the prevalent mood state in BSDs, and the *DSM-5-TR*'s diagnostic criteria for major depressive disorder are identical to those for unipolar depression. Moreover, depression is often the first episode of a mood disturbance in bipolar disorder (Singh & Rajput, 2006). Two major survey studies conducted in 1999 and 2000 showed that almost 40% of BSD patients were initially misdiagnosed as having unipolar depression (Ghaemi et al., 1999, 2000). Therefore, it is essential to carefully assess bipolar disorder in any patient presenting with a depressive episode (Bowden, 2001).

Compared with unipolar depressed individuals, individuals with bipolar depression are more likely to have a functional impairment, be suicidal, have melancholic symptoms, and show psychomotor retardation (in bipolar I disorder) and atypical depressive symptoms such as hyper-insomnia and overeating (Hirschfeld et al., 2003). The National Institute of Mental Health Collaborative Prospective Depression study identified the severity of the depressive episode, acute onset, and presence of psychosis as predictors of bipolar disorder I (Coryell et al., 1989). In contrast, a depressive phase with substance abuse, early-onset disruption of psychosocial functioning, and a protracted course were the best predictors of bipolar disorder II (Winokur et al., 1994).

After determining whether a patient meets the criteria for a specific mood episode, it is imperative to assess for the presence of psychotic features, suicidal tendencies, violence risk, and substance abuse. Subsequent clinical interviews can focus on potential common comorbidities of bipolar disorder (McIntyre et al., 2019).

STRUCTURED CLINICAL INTERVIEWS IN ASSESSING BSDs

There are several structured and semistructured interview schedules that can be used to assess signs and symptoms of BSD in a standardized and systematic manner (see Chapter 7 in this volume). Given the high rate of misdiagnosis of bipolar disorders, these schedules can be especially useful as an adjunct to the clinical interview.

The clinician version of the SCID-5 (SCID-5-CV; First et al., 2016) is a semistructured interview schedule that has modules for assessing symptoms of bipolar disorder I and II, major depressive disorder, and other bipolar disorders. The bipolar disorder module is quite comprehensive and assesses both current (in the past month) as well as lifetime episodes. It also provides probes and questions to further elicit bipolar symptoms. The SCID-5-CV is focused on determining a diagnosis, and symptoms are scored as either present or absent, not for their severity.

A relatively new and shorter structured interview is the Quick Structured Clinical Interview for *DSM-5* Disorders (QuickSCID-5; First et al., 2016), a structured diagnostic instrument developed from the SCID-5. This briefer instrument has modules that assess bipolar I and II (lifetime and current episodes). It also assesses other specific bipolar disorders and current major depressive episodes. Unlike the questions on the SCID-5, the standard questions on the QuickSCID-5 are closed-ended and have no provision for follow-up questions.

Finally, the Mini-International Neuropsychiatric Interview (MINI; Sheehan et al., 1998) is a structured interview developed to rapidly assess major psychiatric disorders. The current version of this measure, named the MINI English Version 7.0.2 (MINI-7), is updated in accordance with the *DSM-5* diagnostic criteria. The MINI-7 (Sheehan, 2016) includes screening questions for the assessment of mania and hypomania that allow an examiner to determine whether a patient meets the core diagnostic criteria before proceeding with an inquiry. It assesses for the presence of manic and hypomanic episodes in two-time frames, both lifetime and in the past 2 weeks. Its questions are closed-ended and do not address the severity of symptoms.

CONCLUSION

Accurate assessment of BSDs is a challenging task. The clinical interview is an indispensable assessment method for these conditions. It offers considerable flexibility in exploring both past and current manic and hypomanic episodes. It allows the clinician to observe both overt and subtle signs of mood episodes and provides unlimited opportunity to pursue continuing inquiry. The availability of structured interview schedules enhances the systematic assessment of BSDs and increases the likelihood of an accurate diagnosis.

REFERENCES

American Psychiatric Association. (2013). *Diagnostic and statistical manual of mental disorders* (5th ed.).

American Psychiatric Association. (2022). *Diagnostic and statistical manual of mental disorders* (5th ed., text rev.). https://doi.org/10.1176/appi.books.9780890425787

Andreasen, N. C. (1979). Thought, language, and communication disorders. I. Clinical assessment, definition of terms, and evaluation of their reliability. *Archives of General Psychiatry, 36*(12), 1315–1321. https://doi.org/10.1001/archpsyc.1979.017801200 45006

Andreasen, N. C., & Black, D. W. (2006). *Introductory textbook of psychiatry* (4th ed.). American Psychiatric Association.

Andreasen, N. C., & Grove, W. M. (1986). Thought, language, and communication in schizophrenia: Diagnosis and prognosis. *Schizophrenia Bulletin, 12*(3), 348–359. https://doi.org/10.1093/schbul/12.3.348

Angst, J., Gamma, A., Bowden, C. L., Azorin, J. M., Perugi, G., Vieta, E., & Young, A. H. (2012). Diagnostic criteria for bipolarity based on an international sample of 5,635 patients with *DSM-IV* major depressive episodes. *European Archives of Psychiatry and Clinical Neuroscience, 262*(1), 3–11. https://doi.org/10.1007/s00406-011-0228-0

Black, D. W., & Grant, J. E. (2014). DSM-5 *guidebook: The essential companion to the diagnostic and statistical manual of mental disorders*. American Psychiatric Association.

Bowden, C. L. (2001). Strategies to reduce misdiagnosis of bipolar depression. *Psychiatric Services, 52*(1), 51–55. https://doi.org/10.1176/appi.ps.52.1.51

Coryell, W., Keller, M., Endicott, J., Andreasen, N., Clayton, P., Hirschfeld, R. (1989) Bipolar II illness: Course and outcome over a five-year period. *Psychological Medicine, 19*(1), 129–41. https://doi.org/10.1017/s0033291700011090

First, M. B., Williams, J. B. W., Karg, R. S., & Spitzer, R. L. (2016). *User's guide for the Structured Clinical Interview for* DSM-5 *Disorders, Clinician Version (SCID-5-CV)*. American Psychiatric Association.

Ghaemi, S. N., Boiman, E. E., & Goodwin, F. K. (2000). Diagnosing bipolar disorder and the effect of antidepressants: A naturalistic study. *The Journal of Clinical Psychiatry, 61*(10), 804–808. https://doi.org/10.4088/jcp.v61n1013

Ghaemi, S. N., Sachs, G. S., Chiou, A. M., Pandurangi, A. K., & Goodwin, K. (1999). Is bipolar disorder still underdiagnosed? Are antidepressants overutilized? *Journal of Affective Disorders, 52*(1–3), 135–144. https://doi.org/10.1016/s0165-0327(98)00076-7

Goodwin, F. K., & Jamison, K. R. (1990). *Manic-depressive illness.* Oxford University Press.

Grande, I., Berk, M., Birmaher, B., Vieta, E. (2016). Bipolar disorder. *The Lancet, 387*(10027), 1561–1572. https://doi.org/10.1016/S0140-6736(15)00241-X

Hirschfeld, R. M., Lewis, L., & Vornik, L. A. (2003). Perceptions and impact of bipolar disorder: How far have we really come? Results of the National Depressive and Manic-Depressive Association 2000 survey of individuals with bipolar disorder. *Journal of Clinical Psychiatry, 64*(2), 161–74. https://doi.org/10.4088/JCP.v64n0209

Khadivi, A. (2021). Clinical interview methods. In I. B. Weiner & J. H. Kleiger (Eds.), *Psychological assessment of disordered thinking and perception* (pp. 35–47). American Psychological Association.

Kleiger, J. H., & Khadivi, A. (2015). *Assessing psychosis: A clinician's guide.* Routledge.

Maruish, M. E. (2014). The clinical interview. In R. P. Archer & J. D. Smith (Eds.), *Personality assessment* (2nd ed., pp. 37–88). Routledge.

McIntyre, R. S., Zimmerman, M., Goldberg, J. F., & First, M. B. (2019). Differential diagnosis of major depressive disorder versus bipolar disorder: Current status and best clinical practices. *The Journal of Clinical Psychiatry, 80*(3), Article ot18043ah2. https://doi.org/10.4088/JCP.ot18043ah2

Phelps, J. (2016). *A spectrum approach to mood disorders. Not fully bipolar but not unipolar—Practical management.* W. W. Norton.

Racker, H. (1957). The meanings and uses of countertransference. *The Psychoanalytic Quarterly, 26*(3), 303–357. https://doi.org/10.1080/21674086.1957.11926061

Shea, S. C. (2016). *Psychiatric interviewing: The art of understanding, a practical guide for psychiatrists, psychologists, counselors, social workers, nurses and other mental health professionals* (3rd ed.). Elsevier.

Sheehan, D. (2016). *The mini international neuropsychiatric interview, English Version 7.0.2 for DSM-5.*

Sheehan, D. V., Lecrubier, Y., Sheehan, K. H., Amorim, P., Janavs, J., Weiller, E., Hergueta, T., Baker, R., & Dunbar, G. C. (1998). The Mini-International Neuropsychiatric Interview (M.I.N.I.): The development and validation of a structured diagnostic psychiatric interview for *DSM-IV* and *ICD-10. The Journal of Clinical Psychiatry, 59*(Suppl. 20), 22–33.

Singh, T., & Rajput, M. (2006). Misdiagnosis of bipolar disorder. *Psychiatry, 3*(10), 57–63.

Skodol, A. E. (1989). *Problems in differential diagnosis: From* DSM-III *to* DSM-III-R *in clinical practice.* American Psychiatric Association.

Sugarman, A. (1981). The diagnostic use of countertransference reactions in psychological testing. *Bulletin of the Menninger Clinic, 45*(6), 473–490.

Sullivan, H. S. (1954). *The psychiatric interview.* W. W. Norton.

Tracy, N. (2013). The danger of misdiagnosing bipolar disorder. *Healthy Place.* https://www.healthyplace.com/blogs/breakingbipolar/2013/12/dangers-misdiagnosing-bipolar-disorder

University of Nottingham. (2012, January 31). *Psychiatric interviews for teaching: Mania* [Video]. YouTube. https://www.youtube.com/watch?v=zA-fqvC02oM

Winokur, G., Coryell, W., Akiskal, H. S., Endicott, J., Keller, M., & Mueller, T. (1994). Manic-depressive (bipolar) disorder: The course in light of a prospective ten-year follow-up of 131 patients. *Acta Psychiatrica Scandinavica, 89*(2), 102–110. https://doi.org/10.1111/j.1600-0447.1994.tb01495.x

3

Minnesota Multiphasic Personality Inventory–3 (MMPI-3) Assessment of Bipolar Spectrum Disorders

Martin Sellbom and Megan R. Whitman

In this chapter, we describe how scores from the Minnesota Multiphasic Personality Inventory–3 (MMPI-3; Ben-Porath & Tellegen, 2020a) can be used to assess mood episodes associated with bipolar disorder, particularly from a spectrum perspective. We begin by briefly describing the development of the MMPI-3, its scale structure, and some psychometric considerations. Next, the majority of the chapter focuses on the MMPI-3 Validity and Substantive Scales that are particularly relevant to assessing response styles and psychological symptoms that are common to individuals presenting with bipolar spectrum disorders. We subsequently review the convergence between MMPI-3 scale scores with contemporary models of personality and psychopathology (with a focus on aspects relevant to mania and depression), and we describe research on its utility in the differential diagnosis of mood and thought disorders. Finally, we conclude by highlighting key practical takeaways and calling for research into the assessment of mania and depression symptoms using the MMPI-3.

OVERVIEW OF THE MMPI-3

The development of the MMPI began in the 1930s when Starke Hathaway and J. Charnley McKinley worked at the University of Minnesota Hospital and intended to create an inventory that could be used to efficiently assess common

https://doi.org/10.1037/0000356-004
Psychological Assessment of Bipolar Spectrum Disorders, J. H. Kleiger and I. B. Weiner (Editors)

presenting problems. Since then, the MMPI has evolved through several paradigm changes, with transitions from empirical keying scale construction to the interpretation of configural patterns, or code types, and from categorical code types to a dimensional, transdiagnostic structure and interpretive approach (see Ben-Porath & Tellegen, 2020b, for a detailed history). The evolution of the inventory has culminated in the MMPI-3, which was designed to build on the foundations of the MMPI-2–Restructured Form (MMPI-2-RF), including its efficiency, strong psychometric properties, and correspondence with contemporary models of personality and psychopathology (Sellbom, 2019).

The MMPI-3 development started with a series of preliminary studies to consider several possible changes, including item improvements and new item development for the purpose of increasing content coverage (see Ben-Porath & Tellegen, 2020b, for detail). Following preliminary studies and extensive consultation with MMPI experts, 95 new items were combined with the 338 MMPI-2-RF items to create the MMPI-2-RF–Expanded Form (MMPI-2-RF-EX; Ben-Porath & Tellegen, 2016), which was used to collect data from a large number of clinical and nonclinical settings. The MMPI-2-RF-EX was also translated into Spanish for similar data collections, including the collection of Spanish-language normative data. The data collected were used by the MMPI-3 authors to revise existing MMPI-2-RF scales and to develop new MMPI-3 scales. Because external criterion measures were also collected at many sites, a substantial amount of data were available for scale validation analyses. Further details are available in the *MMPI-3 Technical Manual* (Ben-Porath & Tellegen, 2020b).

The resulting MMPI-3 has 335 true/false items that aggregate onto 52 scales (see Ben-Porath & Tellegen, 2020a, for detailed descriptions of the scales). Ten Validity Scales measure response styles, which can invalidate an MMPI-3 protocol or indicate a need to qualify substantive scale interpretation. The 42 Substantive Scales are organized in a hierarchy that includes three Higher-Order (H-O) Scales on the first tier, reflecting general and pervasive dysfunction in their respective areas. Eight Restructured Clinical (RC) Scales are at the mid-tier level, and 26 Specific Problems (SP) Scales are at the bottom, comprising the most narrowband symptom and trait measures on the instrument. The SP Scales are organized into four thematic domains—somatic/cognitive, internalizing, externalizing, and interpersonal—which also reflect the general interpretive organization of the instrument. Last, the Personality Psychopathology Five Scales, which are dimensional measures of personality pathology, appear in parallel to this hierarchy. Ben-Porath and Tellegen (2020a) provided a detailed discussion of the underlying psychological constructs assessed by the MMPI-3 Substantive Scales, which is not repeated here.

The *MMPI-3 Technical Manual* (Ben-Porath & Tellegen, 2020b) also describes the MMPI-3 normative sample data collection in detail. In general, the normative sample ($n = 810$ men and 810 women) matches the 2020 U.S. census projections for age, race/ethnicity, and education, and it is geographically diverse, representing all U.S. regions. The U.S. Spanish translation of the MMPI-3 and its accompanying Spanish-language normative sample ($n = 275$ men and 275 women) are described in an MMPI-3 manual supplement (Ben-Porath et al., 2020). In both English and Spanish, the MMPI-3 utilizes nongendered uniform *T* scores for standardized score interpretation. Finally, the *MMPI-3 Technical Manual* provides extensive information about the psychometric properties of MMPI-3 scales, including reliability and construct validity data from multiple settings. These data include MMPI-2-RF and MMPI-3 scale correlations across various settings, which illustrate that, by and large, the scales that are meant to reflect the same underlying psychological constructs were very highly correlated across MMPI versions. Consequently, research supporting the construct validity of MMPI-2-RF scores, including over 500 peer-reviewed publications, can be applied to the use of the MMPI-3. The MMPI-2-RF research base informs much of our subsequent discussion, as MMPI-3-specific research is still in its infancy.

Relevance of the MMPI-3 Validity Scales to Assessment of Bipolar Spectrum Disorders

With respect to the assessment of bipolar spectrum disorders, we start with the discussion of a critical component of any psychological assessment: the consideration of the veracity of a test-taker's account of their psychological functioning (i.e., the protocol validity of an assessment). We also describe empirical support for the utility of MMPI-3 scales that measure threats to protocol validity, including three broad categories: content nonresponsiveness, overreporting, and underreporting (Burchett & Bagby, 2014). First, content nonresponsiveness includes nonresponding, inconsistent random responding, and inconsistent fixed responding (i.e., acquiescence or counter-acquiescence). These threats are assessed by MMPI-3 Cannot Say (CNS; a count of unscorable responses) and the Variable Response Inconsistency (VRIN) and True Response Inconsistency (TRIN) Scales, respectively. The Combined Response Inconsistency (CRIN) scale was added to the MMPI-3 to identify mixed content nonresponsiveness that may not elevate VRIN or TRIN.

Especially during manic or hypomanic episodes, cognitive problems can impair a test-taker's ability to read, comprehend, and respond appropriately to test items, resulting in some degree of content nonresponsiveness. Indeed, patients who present with current manic episodes are sometimes not referred for testing due to the relatively obvious clinical presentation and inability to cooperate with the testing process. Nevertheless, a large proportion of patients with manic symptoms can respond relevantly to the MMPI-3. For example, Sellbom and Bagby (2010) reported that 87% of hospitalized psychiatric inpatients with severe mental disorders produced valid MMPI-2-RF protocols. CNS, CRIN, VRIN, and TRIN scores can be used to assess content-inconsistent responding, and when these scales are excessively elevated, the remaining MMPI-3 Validity and Substantive Scales are invalid and should not be interpreted (Burchett et al., 2016).

Second, overreporting, or the exaggeration or fabrication of problems, can occur with respect to several domains of functioning. On the MMPI-3, Infrequent Responses (F), Infrequent Psychopathology Responses (Fp), and Infrequent

Somatic Responses (Fs) identify test-takers who provide an excessive number of responses that are infrequent among the normative sample, individuals in mental health treatment and medical patients, respectively. Like Fs, the Symptom Validity Scale (FBS) measures noncredible somatic complaints, and the Response Bias Scale (RBS) measures exaggerated memory complaints. MMPI-3 FBS and RBS are unchanged from their MMPI-2-RF counterparts.

Consideration of overreporting is especially important in contexts with potential for secondary gains, such as criminal and civil forensic evaluations (Rogers, 2008). The MMPI-3 F, Fp, Fs, FBS, and RBS Scales can identify potential attempts to overreport. Indeed, Ingram and Ternes (2016) conducted a meta-analysis on the utility of MMPI-2-RF Validity Scales for detecting overreported psychopathology. These authors concluded that the Validity Scales, particularly Fp-r, are effective at detecting general overreporting. Research has also supported the utility of MMPI-2-RF Validity Scales for identifying overreported depressive symptoms specifically. For example, Marion et al. (2011) demonstrated that participants instructed to overreport depression, including naïve simulators (undergraduate students) and sophisticated simulators (advanced mental health students and professionals), produced higher scores on MMPI-2-RF Validity Scales, particularly Fp-r, than patients with major depressive disorder who responded to the test items honestly. Recent research with the MMPI-3 Validity Scales has, by and large, replicated MMPI-2-RF findings (Morris et al., 2021; Reeves et al., 2022; Tylicki et al., 2022; Whitman, Tylicki, & Ben-Porath, 2021).

Finally, underreporting includes both the exaggeration of positive personal attributes and the minimization of genuine psychological problems. The MMPI-3 includes the Uncommon Virtues (L) and Adjustment Validity (K) Scales to assess these threats, respectively. Underreporting should also be considered when assessing individuals for bipolar spectrum disorders, particularly because test-takers may lack insight into their symptoms or be motivated to minimize their problems to avoid diagnosis, mood-stabilizing medications, or inpatient hospitalization. The utility of the MMPI-3 L and K Scales for detecting underreporting response styles has been demonstrated in simulation studies (e.g., Whitman, Tylicki, & Ben-Porath, 2021), among psychiatric patients (Sellbom & Bagby, 2008), and with other populations (e.g., Brown & Sellbom, 2020; Crighton et al., 2017). A test taker's scores on L and K can also provide information about their approach to extra-test components of the assessment process, which is especially useful when these measures do not include Validity Scales (Crighton et al., 2017; Forbey et al., 2013).

MMPI-3 SUBSTANTIVE SCALES IN THE ASSESSMENT OF MANIA AND DEPRESSION SYMPTOMS

In the development of the original MMPI, Hathaway and McKinley (1942; McKinley & Hathaway, 1944) recognized the necessity of assessing both mania/hypomania and depression via the Clinical Scales. Clinical Scales 2 (Depression) and 9 (Hypomania) reflected items that differentiated patients with depressive disorders and manic episodes, respectively, from a "normal" control group. These scales served as the foundation for three of the RC Scales that measure depressive (Demoralization [RCd] and Low Positive Emotions [RC2] from Scale 2) and manic symptoms (Hypomanic Activation [RC9] from Scale 9). In this section, we discuss a set of primary MMPI-3 markers of both depression and mania, as well as MMPI-3 scales that would have secondary relevance in symptom measurement. Tables 3.1 and 3.2 list our conceptual mapping of MMPI-3 scales and these disorder constructs, which has been informed by our knowledge of the construct validity of the MMPI-3 scale scores from the empirical literature. Indeed, in these tables, we provide example citations of relevant research that connects each scale with the mood episodes and/or individual symptoms listed.

MMPI-3 Scales for Assessing Mania

Bipolar spectrum disorders require the presence of at least one manic or hypomanic episode per the *Diagnostic and Statistical Manual of Mental Disorders* (5th ed., text rev.; *DSM-5-TR*; American Psychiatric Association, 2022) to differentiate them from unipolar mood disorders. As such, we start with a symptom assessment of mania/hypomania. It is important to make clear that it is difficult to explicitly differentiate mania and hypomania using self-report scales, as these are primarily differentiated based on the duration and severity of the mood episode (American Psychiatric Association, 2022). Nevertheless, the degree of scale elevation and the number of relevant scales with clinical elevations (discussed next) could assist with the latter severity determination.

As indicated in Table 3.1, there are two primary scales that assess a range of manic or hypomanic symptoms. RC9 is the broadest scale. Its item content reflects the key symptom of excitation and expansive mood as well as other symptoms, including decreased need for sleep, pressure to keep talking, subjective experience of racing thoughts, and excessive involvement in activities with high potential for negative consequences. As documented in a subsequent section, the RC9 scale correlates consistently with manic symptoms, bipolar disorder diagnosis, and a range of externalizing behaviors. Indeed, because the behavioral sequela of manic symptoms are so prominent, especially within this scale, RC9 is listed among the MMPI-3 externalizing scales.

The Activation (ACT) scale is a more specific version of RC9, which centers on the more classic manic symptoms. Its item content also reflects the key symptom of excitation and expansive mood, as well as decreased need for sleep, pressure to keep talking, and subjective experience of racing thoughts, but not externalizing behaviors. As discussed in the later section, ACT scores are the most robust predictor of manic symptomatology on the MMPI-2-RF/MMPI-3.[1] Although

---

[1] We note that the MMPI-2-RF and MMPI-3 versions of ACT are identical with respect to item content.

TABLE 3.1. MMPI-3 Scales Linked to *DSM-5-TR* and *ICD-11* Diagnostic Criteria for Manic Episodes

Scale	Diagnostic criteria	Key research
Primary		
RC9	Euphoria and expansive mood Reduced need for sleep Pressured speech Flight of ideas or racing thoughts Engagement in activities with high potential for consequences	C. Watson et al. (2011) Sellbom et al. (2012) Ben-Porath and Tellegen (2020b) Whitman, Tylicki, Mascioli, et al. (2021)
ACT[a]	Euphoria and expansive mood Reduced need for sleep Pressured speech Flight of ideas or racing thoughts	C. Watson et al. (2011) Sellbom et al. (2012) Ben-Porath and Tellegen (2020b) Whitman, Tylicki, Mascioli, et al. (2021)
Secondary		
ANP	Extreme irritability	Ben-Porath and Tellegen (2020b) Whitman, Tylicki, Mascioli, et al. (2021)
SFI	Increased self-esteem or grandiosity	Ben-Porath and Tellegen (2020b) Sellbom (2021) Whitman and Ben-Porath (2021) Whitman, Tylicki, Mascioli, et al. (2021)
COG	Distractibility	Ben-Porath and Tellegen (2020b) Gervais et al. (2009)
BXD	Engagement in activities with high potential for consequences	Ben-Porath and Tellegen (2020b) Whitman, Tylicki, Mascioli, et al. (2021)
RC4 & JCP	Engagement in activities with high potential for consequences	Ben-Porath and Tellegen (2020b) Whitman, Tylicki, Mascioli, et al. (2021)
SUB	Engagement in activities with high potential for consequences	Ben-Porath and Tellegen (2020b)
IMP	Engagement in activities with high potential for consequences	Ben-Porath and Tellegen (2020b) Whitman, Tylicki, Mascioli, et al. (2021)
DISC	Engagement in activities with high potential for consequences	Ben-Porath and Tellegen (2020b) Whitman, Tylicki, Mascioli, et al. (2021)

Note. MMPI-3 = Minnesota Multiphasic Personality Inventory–3; MMPI-2-RF = MMPI–2–Restructured Form; *DSM-5-TR* = *Diagnostic and Statistical Manual for Mental Disorders* (5th ed., text rev.); *ICD-11* = *International Statistical Classification of Diseases and Related Health Problems* (11th ed.); RC9 = Hypomanic Activation; ACT = Activation; ANP = Anger Proneness; SFI = Self-Importance; COG = Cognitive Complaints; BXD = Behavioral/Externalizing Dysfunction; RC4 = Antisocial Behavior; JCP = Juvenile Conduct Problems; SUB = Substance Abuse; IMP = Impulsivity; DISC = Disconstraint.
[a] MMPI-2-RF and MMPI-3 scale versions are identical with respect to item content.

listed as an externalizing MMPI-3 scale (as a facet of RC9), it is not surprising that multiple studies have shown that this scale tends to converge more prominently with thought dysfunction (Sellbom et al., 2021) and/or internalizing (McNulty & Overstreet, 2014), which is consistent with how other contemporary models of psychopathology treat mania (e.g., Kotov et al., 2017).

TABLE 3.2. MMPI-3 Scales Linked to *DSM-5-TR* and *ICD-11* Diagnostic Criteria for Major Depressive Episodes

Scale	Diagnostic criteria	Key research
	Primary	
EID	Depressed or dysphoric mood	Sellbom et al. (2012) Ben-Porath and Tellegen (2020b) Whitman, Tylicki, Mascioli, et al. (2021)
RCd	Depressed or dysphoric mood	Sellbom et al. (2012) Ben-Porath and Tellegen (2020b) Whitman, Tylicki, Mascioli, et al. (2021)
RC2	Depressed or dysphoric mood Reduced pleasure or interest in typically enjoyable activities Psychomotor retardation	Sellbom et al. (2012) Ben-Porath and Tellegen (2020b) Whitman, Tylicki, Mascioli, et al. (2021)
INTR	Reduced pleasure or interest in typically enjoyable activities Impaired social functioning or distress	Ben-Porath and Tellegen (2020b) Whitman, Tylicki, Mascioli, et al. (2021)
	Secondary	
HLP	Depressed or dysphoric mood	Ben-Porath and Tellegen (2020b) Whitman, Tylicki, Mascioli, et al. (2021)
MLS	Fatigue or reduced energy	Ben-Porath and Tellegen (2020b) Sellbom et al. (2012)
SFD	Sense of worthlessness or unjustified guilt	Ben-Porath and Tellegen (2020b) Sellbom et al. (2012) Whitman, Tylicki, Mascioli, et al. (2021)
SFI (−)	Sense of worthlessness	Sellbom et al. (2021) Whitman, Tylicki, Mascioli, et al. (2021)
COG & NFC	Subjective experience of difficulty concentrating and indecisiveness	Ben-Porath and Tellegen (2020b) Gervais et al. (2009) Whitman, Tylicki, Mascioli, et al. (2021)
SUI	Thoughts of death or suicide	Ben-Porath and Tellegen (2020b)
SHY[a] & SAV	Impaired social functioning or distress	Ben-Porath and Tellegen (2020b) Whitman, Tylicki, Mascioli, et al. (2021)

Note. MMPI-3 = Minnesota Multiphasic Personality Inventory–3; MMPI-2-RF = MMPI–2–Restructured Form; *DSM-5-TR* = *Diagnostic and Statistical Manual for Mental Disorders* (5th ed., text rev.); *ICD-11* = *International Statistical Classification of Diseases and Related Health Problems* (11th ed.); EID = Emotional/ Internalizing Dysfunction; RCd = Demoralization; RC2 = Low Positive Emotions; INTR = Introversion/Low Positive Emotionality; HLP = Helplessness/Hopelessness; MLS = Malaise; SFD = Self-Doubt; SFI = Self-Importance; COG = Cognitive Complaints; NFC = Inefficacy; SUI = Suicide/Death Ideation; SHY = Shyness; SAV = Social Avoidance.
[a] MMPI-2-RF and MMPI-3 scale versions are identical with respect to item content.

Table 3.1 also lists several MMPI-3 scales that are likely of secondary (but not trivial) relevance to the assessment of manic symptoms. The Anger Proneness (ANP) scale measures irritable mood, which is important in the context of expansive mood, particularly in hypomanic episodes (American Psychiatric Association, 2022). The Self-Importance (SFI) scale, which is new to the MMPI-3, consists of items that reflect grandiosity and inflated self-esteem (Sellbom, 2021; Whitman & Ben-Porath, 2021). The Cognitive Complaints (COG) is directly related to distractibility symptoms. Several externalizing MMPI-3 scales (Behavioral/Externalizing Dysfunction [BXD], Antisocial Behavior [RC4], Juvenile Conduct Problems [JCP], Substance Abuse [SUB], Impulsivity [IMP], and Disconstraint [DISC]) measure behaviors that might reflect excessive involvement in activities with a high potential for negative consequences. Of course, all these symptoms occur outside the context of mania as well, but they can nevertheless signal the presence of these symptoms when a manic or hypomanic episode is confirmed or suspected.

MMPI-3 Scales for Assessing Depression

Table 3.2 lists the primary and secondary MMPI-3 scales for the assessment of depressive episodes. As with mania, none of these scales are explicitly diagnostic of a major depressive episode (MDE), but they do measure symptoms associated with it. The Higher-Order scale Emotional/Internalizing Dysfunction (EID) is a broad measure of internalizing dysfunction and would be expected to be elevated in the context of an MDE. It is not specific to depression but is nevertheless highly correlated with depressed mood, general unhappiness, and dysphoria. RCd measures demoralization. Although this construct is meant to reflect nonspecific emotional distress, it is important to note that it primarily reflects the unhappiness and hopelessness associated with depressed mood, one of the two key criteria for an MDE. The second key criterion is loss of interest or pleasure in things typically enjoyed, also known as anhedonia, which separates depression from other internalizing disorders. RC2 and Introversion/Low Positive Emotionality (INTR) both measure anhedonia directly, though the latter scale also measures social disengagement/withdrawal, which is a key form of social impairment associated with an MDE. Moreover, RC2 is also linked to low energy and thus psychomotor retardation, which is another criterion for an MDE. Thus, in combination, RCd and RC2 would likely feature prominently in an individual with an MDE, with EID and INTR as somewhat broader scales quite likely being elevated as well.

Table 3.2 also lists several MMPI-3 SP scales that are relevant to the assessment of specific MDE symptoms. Helplessness/hopelessness (HLP) measures an explicit cognitive component of the MDE depressed mood criterion. Malaise (MLS) captures fatigue and loss of energy in the context of a somatization process. Self-Doubt (SFD) and low scores on SFI are both, in somewhat different ways (Whitman & Ben-Porath, 2021), associated with feelings of worthlessness. COG is directly related to the subjective experience of diminished ability to think or concentrate associated with MDEs, whereas inefficacy (NFC) measures indecisiveness. With respect to the suicidal ideation criterion of MDE, the Suicide/Death Ideation (SUI) scale measures this construct in a face-valid manner. Finally, the Shyness (SHY) and Social Avoidance (SAV) interpersonal scales are both relevant to social inhibition and withdrawal, which is a primary manifestation of social impairment for MDE. Again, none of these scales were designed to assess specific symptoms of MDE, but the constructs underlying these scales are highly relevant in the manner just described and, in constellation, could lead to strong hypotheses about the presence of MDE.

A Note on Psychotic Features

As the introductory chapter of this volume discusses, bipolar spectrum disorders, particularly in the more severe manifestations of the spectrum, often co-occur with thought disorder symptoms, such as poor reality testing, grandiose or paranoid delusions, thought disorganization, and hallucinations (see also Chapter 16 in this volume). The *DSM-5-TR*, for instance, suggests that in the case of bipolar spectrum disorders, the prevailing mood episode (mania/hypomania or MDE) manifests exclusively in mood-congruent psychotic symptoms (which are not present in the absence of disordered mood), to distinguish it from schizoaffective disorder, for which the prevailing condition is schizophrenia with mood episodes.

The MMPI-3 is unlikely to provide this degree of distinction in differential diagnosis, but its scales can signal the possible presence of psychotic symptoms concurrently with mood pathology. Specifically, elevations on some combination of the four scales of the MMPI-3 thought dysfunction spectrum, Thought Dysfunction (THD), Ideas of Persecution (RC6), Aberrant Experiences (RC8), and Psychoticism (PSYC), can indicate the presence of such symptoms, with RC6 and RC8 providing the most specific degree of abstraction.

CONVERGENCE BETWEEN THE MMPI-3 AND CONTEMPORARY PSYCHOPATHOLOGY MODELS

We believe that discussions of bipolar spectrum disorders assessment would be incomplete without considering contemporary developments in psychopathology science. These models focus on psychopathology constructs as dimensional entities that can be organized into a hierarchical framework. There is research that suggests that mania, for instance, is indeed multifactorial. Ruggero et al. (2014) reviewed 23 studies on the factor structure of manic symptoms, and all but one found mania to be multifactorial. The modal number of factors was three, with these subdimensions reflecting psychomotor activation/increased energy, excessive euphoria, and irritability-aggression. Ruggero et al. observed major methodological and statistical inconsistencies across the studies examined regarding how these dimensions were determined. These authors therefore conducted their own examination of a series of 24 distinct mania symptoms derived from the Interview for Mood and Anxiety Disorders (D. Watson et al., 2012) in multiple samples. They found support for a four-factor structure across samples, with subdimensions reflecting euphoric activation, hyperactive cognition, reckless overconfidence, and irritability. A detailed examination of the RC9 scale item content indicates that its items tap into each of these four domains. The ACT scale, being more specific, focuses on euphoric activation and hyperactive cognition, with more specific scales, like ANP and externalizing scales, tapping into the other domains.

More broadly, a recent model that has rapidly become influential is the Hierarchical Taxonomy of Psychopathology (HiTOP; Kotov et al., 2017).[2] The HiTOP model attempts to generate a hierarchical representation of psychopathology essentially based on research on covariance structures. HiTOP contains six broad psychopathology spectra: somatoform, internalizing, thought disorder, detachment, antagonistic-externalizing, and disinhibited-externalizing. Not surprisingly, there is considerable evidence that major depressive disorder, and its specific symptom dimensions, load on the internalizing spectrum. The evidence is more divided on bipolar spectrum disorders and mania, with the majority of evidence supporting a loading on the thought disorder spectrum, more so than internalizing (e.g., Kotov et al., 2020). Indeed, in a very comprehensive review, Kotov et al. (2020) articulated substantial etiological overlap between bipolar spectrum disorders and thought disorders, with thought disorders being distinct with respect to genetic liability from internalizing psychopathology.

Research with the MMPI-2-RF and MMPI-3 shows impressive consistency with this broader psychopathology literature (McNulty & Overstreet, 2014; Sellbom et al., 2021). MMPI-3 scales linked to depression as articulated earlier, by and large, tend to structurally load on a higher order internalizing factor, whereas ACT (in particular) consistently loads on a thought dysfunction factor along with THD, RC6, RC8, and PSYC across multiple samples.[3] These studies provide important evidence for construct validity and further emphasize the need to consider the assessment of bipolar spectrum disorders via the MMPI-3 in conjunction with these other scales.

EMPIRICAL RESEARCH ON THE MMPI-3 IN SYMPTOM MEASUREMENT AND DIFFERENTIAL DIAGNOSIS

In this section, we consider the empirical research literature on the assessment of manic and depressive symptomatology, particularly with the primary and secondary scales discussed earlier. We also review studies that have explicitly focused on differential diagnosis, particularly that distinguishing bipolar spectrum disorders from other mental disorders.

---

[2] At the time of this writing, the original HiTOP article, which had been published about 5 years earlier, has almost 1,600 citations according to Google Scholar.

[3] We note that the placement of the Specific Problem scale ACT on the MMPI-3 externalizing spectrum, for which there is no factor analytic evidence at all (see also Sellbom, 2016), is therefore not optimal, but a function of no thought dysfunction scales at this level of the MMPI-3 hierarchy.

First, research has demonstrated the validity of MMPI-3 scores for predicting bipolar spectrum disorder symptoms and diagnoses. For example, Arbisi et al. (2008) found that psychiatric inpatients with clinical elevations (≥65*T*) on MMPI-2-RF RC9 were about twice as likely to have racing thoughts and 1.5 times more likely to be prescribed lithium during hospitalization than individuals who scored <65*T*. More recently, Whitman, Tylicki, Mascioli, et al. (2021) found that in a sample of 197 neuropsychology examinees, ACT and RC9 scores yielded the strongest correlations with both mania and having a bipolar spectrum disorder diagnosis. Producing clinical elevations on these scales was associated with at least 2 times higher odds of having a prior manic episode and being diagnosed with a bipolar disorder relative to individuals without clinical elevations. With regard to relevant new scales on the MMPI-3, IMP scores yielded substantial associations with symptoms of mania and bipolar disorder diagnosis, and SFI scores yielded very small but meaningful correlations with these criteria. This latter finding likely reflects the more transient nature of grandiosity (relative to features such as activation) in bipolar spectrum disorders. Last, this study showed that the remaining scales we identified as having secondary relevance in mania assessments, including BXD, RC4, JCP, SUB, and DISC, were meaningfully associated with bipolar disorder diagnosis, but generally to a lesser degree than the primary scales.

A robust literature on the assessment of unipolar depressive symptoms using the MMPI-2-RF (e.g., Haber & Baum, 2014; Ingram et al., 2021) and MMPI-3 (Sellbom et al., 2021; Whitman, Tylicki, Mascioli, et al., 2021) has also accumulated. For example, Haber and Baum (2014) reported that EID, RCd, RC2, and SFD scores were most strongly correlated with depressive disorder diagnosis in a university-based psychological clinic setting. Ingram et al. (2021) reported moderate to very large associations between MMPI-2-RF scale scores (including EID, RCd, RC2, and INTR, as well as SUI, HLP, SFD, MLS, SAV, and SHY) and other measures of depression among veterans. Recent research using the MMPI-3 has demonstrated that key scales for assessing depressive symptoms were primary indicators of a distress factor in samples of mental health outpatients and male prison inmates (Sellbom et al., 2021). Additionally, Whitman, Tylicki, Mascioli, et al. (2021) found evidence that the MMPI-3 scales we identified as having primary relevance for assessing depressive symptoms, including EID, RC2, RCd, and INTR, yielded moderate to large associations with depressive disorder diagnosis, and several secondary scales, including HLP, MLS, SFD, SFI, COG, NFC, SHY, and SAV, yielded moderate to large correlations with this criterion.

In addition to specific symptom measurement, research indicates that the MMPI-2-RF and MMPI-3 can be used to aid in the differential diagnosis of bipolar spectrum disorders versus other mood and thought disorders (Menton, 2022; Sellbom et al., 2012; C. Watson et al., 2011). C. Watson et al. (2011) compared MMPI-2-RF substantive scale scores across Canadian psychiatric outpatients diagnosed with bipolar I, bipolar II, or major depressive disorder.

They found that ACT scores best differentiated patients with lifetime bipolar spectrum disorders and major depressive disorder, and that ACT scores were useful for differentiating between patients who met the criteria for a current depressive episode and who were diagnosed with either a bipolar spectrum disorder or major depressive disorder. Another study using partially overlapping data with C. Watson et al. (2011), Sellbom et al. (2012) reported that ACT was the most useful scale for differentiating between bipolar disorder and schizophrenia or major depression in a sample of mental health outpatients. These authors also reported that patients diagnosed with bipolar disorder scored higher than those with major depressive disorder on BXD, RC9, and ACT, whereas those with major depressive disorder scored higher on EID, RC1, RC2, MLS, and SAV.

Additionally, Menton (2022) used a combined sample of inpatients and outpatients who were tested at three mental health settings to construct a set of weighted indices for the MMPI-2-RF to guide the differential diagnosis of bipolar, schizophrenia, and major depressive disorder. He subsequently tested these indices in an independent subset of data and they outperformed scores on any single MMPI-2-RF scale for distinguishing groups. Menton also reported AUC values for MMPI-2-RF scales in differentiating between these three disorders. Of these, THD and RC6 scores best distinguished bipolar disorder from schizophrenia (with the schizophrenia group scoring higher on these scales), followed by ACT scores (with the bipolar disorder group scoring higher). Scores on EID, RCd, and RC2, as well as MLS, SFD, and SHY yielded some of the highest AUC estimates for distinguishing bipolar disorder from major depressive disorder. These findings are generally quite supportive of our conceptual mappings.

SUMMARY, CONCLUSION, AND FUTURE RECOMMENDATIONS

The MMPI instruments have been used to assess bipolar spectrum disorders since their inception. Over the past decades, research has culminated in the MMPI-3, and such measurement has been refined through scales that assess transdiagnostic psychological constructs rather than classic psychiatric syndromes. The MMPI-3 has several scales that, in conjunction, are conceptually and empirically linked to the assessment of both mania and depression symptom dimensions. There is considerable literature available on hierarchical structure, relevant empirical correlates, and differential diagnosis to support our general recommendations. We believe that RC9 and ACT are primary measures of the mania symptom dimension, with additional scales likely to reflect specific symptoms in the context of a manic or hypomanic episode (e.g., SFI for grandiosity). We also recommend that RCd and RC2 be used as primary markers of depression, again, alongside other specific scales (e.g., SUI for suicidal ideation). These recommendations notwithstanding, any MMPI-3 user needs to keep in mind that these scales can be elevated for several reasons and their interpretation should be in the context of extra-test information.

It will be important for future research to continue to empirically evaluate the conceptual MMPI-3 model put forth in this chapter. In addition to sampling from patients with bipolar spectrum disorder diagnoses, such research should also focus on empirically established symptom dimensions that cover the entire spectrum. It will be particularly important for such research to also align with movements in contemporary psychopathology science, including important symptom dimensions across psychopathology spectra (e.g., Kotov et al., 2017).

Key Practical Takeaways

- The MMPI-2-RF and MMPI-3 scales are intended to measure transdiagnostic, dimensional psychological constructs, such as activation and low positive emotionality, rather than syndromes, such as bipolar spectrum disorders.

- The MMPI-3 features well-validated measures of invalid response styles, including content-inconsistent responding, overreporting, and underreporting. Evaluating all three threats to protocol validity is critical in the assessment of individuals presenting with bipolar disorder symptomatology.

- The MMPI-3 RC9 and ACT scales are most directly relevant to the assessment of mania and hypomania, and several additional scales can be used to assess additional features of bipolar disorder.

- Similarly, MMPI-3 EID and INTR at the broadest level, and RCd and RC2 at the mid-tier level, are particularly relevant to the assessment of depressive symptoms. Additional scales can be used to assess other features of major depressive episodes.

- A large and growing empirical literature can be used to guide the interpretation of MMPI-3 scores in the assessment of bipolar spectrum disorders. This research provides impressive support for the construct validity and clinical utility of MMPI-3 scores and links the MMPI-3 to contemporary psychopathology models.

REFERENCES

American Psychiatric Association. (2022). *Diagnostic and statistical manual of mental disorders* (5th ed., text rev.).

Arbisi, P. A., Sellbom, M., & Ben-Porath, Y. S. (2008). Empirical correlates of the MMPI-2 Restructured Clinical (RC) scales in psychiatric inpatients. *Journal of Personality Assessment, 90*(2), 122–128. https://doi.org/10.1080/00223890701845146

Ben-Porath, Y. S., & Tellegen, A. (2016). *The MMPI-2-RF expanded form.* University of Minnesota Press.

Ben-Porath, Y. S., & Tellegen, A. (2020a). *MMPI-3 manual for administration, scoring, and interpretation.* University of Minnesota Press.

Ben-Porath, Y. S., & Tellegen, A. (2020b). *MMPI-3 technical manual.* University of Minnesota Press.

Ben-Porath, Y. S., Tellegen, A., & Puente, A. E. (2020). *Minnesota Multiphasic Personality Inventory–3 (MMPI-3): Manual supplement for the U.S. Spanish translation.* University of Minnesota Press.

Brown, T. A., & Sellbom, M. (2020). The utility of the MMPI-2-RF validity scales in detecting underreporting. *Journal of Personality Assessment, 102*(1), 66–74. https://doi.org/10.1080/00223891.2018.1539003

Burchett, D., & Bagby, R. M. (2014). Multimethod assessment of distortion: Integrating data from interviews, collateral records, and standardized assessment tools. In C. J. Hopwood & R. F. Bornstein (Eds.), *Multimethod clinical assessment* (pp. 345–378). Guilford Press.

Burchett, D., Dragon, W. R., Smith Holbert, A. M., Tarescavage, A. M., Mattson, C. A., Handel, R. W., & Ben-Porath, Y. S. (2016). "False feigners": Examining the impact of non-content-based invalid responding on the Minnesota Multiphasic Personality Inventory–2 Restructured Form content-based invalid responding indicators. *Psychological Assessment, 28*(5), 458–470. https://doi.org/10.1037/pas0000205

Crighton, A. H., Tarescavage, A. M., Gervais, R. O., & Ben-Porath, Y. S. (2017). The generalizability of overreporting across a battery of self-report measures: An investigation with the Minnesota Multiphasic Personality Inventory–2–Restructured Form and the Personality Assessment Inventory in a civil disability sample. *Assessment, 24*(5), 555–574. https://doi.org/10.1177/1073191115621791

Forbey, J. D., Lee, T. T. C., Ben-Porath, Y. S., Arbisi, P. A., & Gartland, D. (2013). Associations between MMPI-2-RF validity scale scores and extra-test measures of personality and psychopathology. *Assessment, 20*(4), 448–461. https://doi.org/10.1177/1073191113478154

Gervais, R. O., Ben-Porath, Y. S., & Wygant, D. B. (2009). Empirical correlates and interpretation of the MMPI-2-RF Cognitive Complaints (COG) scale. *The Clinical Neuropsychologist, 23*(6), 996–1015. https://doi.org/10.1080/13854040902748249

Haber, J. C., & Baum, L. J. (2014). Minnesota Multiphasic Personality Inventory–2–Restructured Form (MMPI-2-RF) scales as predictors of psychiatric diagnoses. *South African Journal of Psychology/Suid-Afrikaanse Tydskrif vir Sielkunde, 44*(4), 439–453. https://doi.org/10.1177/0081246314532788

Hathaway, S. R., & McKinley, J. C. (1942). A multiphasic personality schedule (Minnesota): III. The measurement of symptomatic depression. *The Journal of Psychology, 14*(1), 73–84. https://doi.org/10.1080/00223980.1942.9917111

Ingram, P. B., Tarescavage, A. M., Ben-Porath, Y. S., Oehlert, M. E., & Bergquist, B. K. (2021). External correlates of the MMPI–2–Restrcutured Form across a national sample of veterans. *Journal of Personality Assessment, 103*(1), 19–26. https://doi.org/10.1080/00223891.2020.1732995

Ingram, P. B., & Ternes, M. S. (2016). The detection of content-based invalid responding: A meta-analysis of the MMPI–2–Restructured Form's (MMPI-2-RF) over-reporting validity scales. *The Clinical Neuropsychologist, 30*(4), 473–496. https://doi.org/10.1080/13854046.2016.1187769

Kotov, R., Jonas, K. G., Carpenter, W. T., Dretsch, M. N., Eaton, N. R., Forbes, M. K., Forbush, K. T., Hobbs, K., Reininghaus, U., Slade, T., South, S. C., Sunderland, M., Waszczuk, M. A., Widiger, T. A., Wright, A. G. C., Zald, D. H., Krueger, R. F., Watson, D., & the HiTOP Utility Workgroup. (2020). Validity and utility of Hierarchical Taxonomy of Psychopathology (HiTOP): I. Psychosis superspectrum. *World Psychiatry, 19*(2), 151–172. https://doi.org/10.1002/wps.20730

Kotov, R., Krueger, R. F., Watson, D., Achenbach, T. M., Althoff, R. R., Bagby, R. M., Brown, T. A., Carpenter, W. T., Caspi, A., Clark, L. A., Eaton, N. R., Forbes, M. K., Forbush, K. T., Goldberg, D., Hasin, D., Hyman, S. E., Ivanova, M. Y., Lynam, D. R., Markon, K., . . . Zimmerman, M. (2017). The Hierarchical Taxonomy of Psychopathology (HiTOP): A dimensional alternative to traditional nosologies. *Journal of Abnormal Psychology, 126*(4), 454–477. https://doi.org/10.1037/abn0000258

Marion, B. E., Sellbom, M., & Bagby, R. M. (2011). The detection of feigned psychiatric disorders using the MMPI-2-RF overreporting validity scales: An analog investigation. *Psychological Injury and Law, 4*(1), 1–12. https://doi.org/10.1007/s12207-011-9097-0

McKinley, J. C., & Hathaway, S. R. (1944). The Minnesota Multiphasic Personality Inventory. V. Hysteria, hypomania and psychopathic deviate. *Journal of Applied Psychology, 28*(2), 153–174. https://doi.org/10.1037/h0059245

McNulty, J. L., & Overstreet, S. R. (2014). Viewing the MMPI-2-RF structure through the Personality Psychopathology Five (PSY-5) lens. *Journal of Personality Assessment, 96*(2), 151–157. https://doi.org/10.1080/00223891.2013.840305

Menton, W. H. (2022). Development and initial validation of differential diagnostic indices for the MMPI-2-RF. *Assessment, 29*(3), 410–424. https://doi.org/10.1177/1073191120978797

Morris, N. M., Mattera, J., Golden, B., Moses, S., & Ingram, P. B. (2021). Evaluating the performance of the MMPI-3 over-reporting scales: Sophisticated simulators and the effects of comorbid conditions. *The Clinical Neuropsychologist*. Advance online publication. https://doi.org/10.1080/13854046.2021.1968037

Reeves, C. K., Brown, T. A., & Sellbom, M. (2022). An examination of the MMPI-3 validity scales in detecting overreporting of psychological problems. *Psychological Assessment, 34*(6), 517–527. https://doi.org/10.1037/pas0001112

Rogers, R. (Ed.). (2008). *Clinical assessment of malingering and deception* (3rd ed.). Guilford Press.

Ruggero, C. J., Kotov, R., Watson, D., Kilmer, J. N., Perlman, G., & Liu, K. (2014). Beyond a single index of mania symptoms: Structure and validity of subdimensions. *Journal of Affective Disorders, 161*, 8–15. https://doi.org/10.1016/j.jad.2014.02.044

Sellbom, M. (2016). Elucidating the validity of the externalizing spectrum of psychopathology in correctional, forensic, and community samples. *Journal of Abnormal Psychology, 125*(8), 1027–1038. https://doi.org/10.1037/abn0000171

Sellbom, M. (2019). The MMPI–2–Restructured Form (MMPI-2-RF): Assessment of personality and psychopathology in the twenty-first century. *Annual Review of Clinical Psychology, 15*(1), 149–177. https://doi.org/10.1146/annurev-clinpsy-050718-095701

Sellbom, M. (2021). Examining the criterion and incremental validity of the MMPI-3 Self-Importance scale. *Psychological Assessment, 33*(4), 363–368. https://doi.org/10.1037/pas0000975

Sellbom, M., & Bagby, R. M. (2008). Validity of the MMPI–2–RF (restructured form) L-r and K-r scales in detecting underreporting in clinical and nonclinical samples. *Psychological Assessment, 20*(4), 370–376. https://doi.org/10.1037/a0012952

Sellbom, M., & Bagby, R. M. (2010). Detection of overreported psychopathology with the MMPI-2-RF [corrected] validity scales. *Psychological Assessment, 22*(4), 757–767. https://doi.org/10.1037/a0020825

Sellbom, M., Bagby, R. M., Kushner, S., Quilty, L. C., & Ayearst, L. E. (2012). Diagnostic construct validity of MMPI–2–Restructured Form (MMPI-2-RF) scale scores. *Assessment, 19*(2), 176–186. https://doi.org/10.1177/1073191111428763

Sellbom, M., Kremyar, A. J., & Wygant, D. B. (2021). Mapping MMPI-3 scales onto the hierarchical taxonomy of psychopathology. *Psychological Assessment, 33*(12), 1153–1168. https://doi.org/10.1037/pas0001049

Tylicki, J. L., Gervais, R. O., & Ben-Porath, Y. S. (2022). Examination of the MMPI-3 over-reporting scales in a forensic disability sample. *The Clinical Neuropsychologist, 36*(7), 1878–1901. https://doi.org/10.1080/13854046.2020.1856414

Watson, C., Quilty, L. C., & Bagby, R. M. (2011). Differentiating bipolar disorder from major depressive disorder using the MMPI-2-RF: A receiver operating characteristics (ROC) analysis. *Journal of Psychopathology and Behavioral Assessment, 33*(3), 368–374. https://doi.org/10.1007/s10862-010-9212-7

Watson, D., O'Hara, M. W., Naragon-Gainey, K., Koffel, E., Chmielewski, M., Kotov, R., Stasik, S. M., & Ruggero, C. J. (2012). Development and validation of new anxiety and bipolar symptom scales for an expanded version of the IDAS (the IDAS-II). *Assessment, 19*(4), 399–420. https://doi.org/10.1177/1073191112449857

Whitman, M. R., & Ben-Porath, Y. S. (2021). Distinctiveness of the MMPI-3 Self-Importance and Self-Doubt Scales. *Journal of Personality Assessment, 103*(5), 613–620. https://doi.org/10.1080/00223891.2021.1883628

Whitman, M. R., Tylicki, J. L., & Ben-Porath, Y. S. (2021). Utility of the MMPI-3 validity scales for detecting overreporting and underreporting and their effects on substantive scale validity: A simulation study. *Psychological Assessment, 33*(5), 411–426. https://doi.org/10.1037/pas0000988

Whitman, M. R., Tylicki, J. L., Mascioli, R., Pickle, J., & Ben-Porath, Y. S. (2021). Psychometric properties of the Minnesota Multiphasic Personality Inventory–3 (MMPI-3) in a clinical neuropsychology setting. *Psychological Assessment, 33*(2), 142–155. https://doi.org/10.1037/pas0000969

4

Personality Assessment Inventory (PAI) Assessment of Bipolar Spectrum Disorders

Morgan N. McCredie, Christopher J. Hopwood, and Leslie C. Morey

The Personality Assessment Inventory (PAI; Morey, 1991) is a multiscale, self-report questionnaire developed to offer a comprehensive assessment of client personality and psychopathology. The measure comprises 344 items with a 4-point response scale, including *false, not at all true* (F), *slightly true* (ST), *mainly true* (MT), and *very true* (VT). These items form 22 distinct scales of four different types: four validity scales, 11 clinical scales, five treatment scales, and two interpersonal scales. Ten of the full scales are further broken down into subscales that offer a breadth of coverage within clinical constructs, and several supplemental indicators have been developed following the test's initial publication to aid in more extensive interpretation. The PAI is currently employed in a variety of clinical, research, and training settings (Archer et al., 2006; Stedman et al., 2018) and has practical applications across many specialty assessment areas, including health, forensics, and personnel selection. This chapter offers a brief overview of the PAI, describes and provides interpretive guidelines for the PAI scales and indices most relevant to the assessment of bipolar spectrum disorders, and summarizes noteworthy research in this area. A more thorough description of the theory, development, administration, and scoring protocol of the PAI is provided in Chapter 5 of *Psychological Assessment of Disordered Thinking and Perception* (McCredie et al., 2021). Primary resources

https://doi.org/10.1037/0000356-005
Psychological Assessment of Bipolar Spectrum Disorders, J. H. Kleiger and I. B. Weiner (Editors)

should be consulted for a more comprehensive discussion of specific features and applications of the PAI beyond the scope of these chapters (Blais et al., 2010; Morey, 1996, 2003, 2007b; Morey & Hopwood, 2007).

OVERVIEW OF THE PERSONALITY ASSESSMENT INVENTORY

Theory and Development

The PAI was developed using a construct validation framework that simultaneously took a theoretically informed approach to item development and selection while also empirically evaluating the psychometric properties of those items. Importance was placed on both the *breadth* and *depth* of content coverage, striving to provide a balanced sampling of the core aspects of each psychological construct assessed. Content *breadth* refers to the extent of the representation of the diversity of clinical features encompassed by a psychological domain. For example, in order to measure the construct of mania, it is important to assess both the behavioral expression (e.g., heightened activity level) as well as the cognitive and affective manifestations (e.g., grandiosity, irritability). The *depth* of content coverage refers to the assessment of a clinical construct across varying degrees of severity. PAI scales were developed to include items that represent the mildest to most severe manifestations of a given clinical phenomenon; for instance, depressive cognitions can range from mild cynicism to extreme hopelessness and despair. Thus, the PAI includes items that represent a diverse range of symptoms and features at varying degrees of severity in order to adequately capture the full range of possible clinical presentations within a given construct.

PAI Scales

The PAI contains four types of scales: validity, clinical, treatment consideration, and interpersonal. The four validity scales were designed to identify response patterns that suggest deviation from accurate and honest responding, including random response tendencies (Inconsistency [ICN], Infrequency [INF]) and systematic negative (Negative Impression Management [NIM]) and positive (Positive Impression Management [PIM]) responding. The 11 clinical scales of the PAI were designed to assess for a range of diagnostically important phenomena. There are four neurotic spectrum scales, Somatic Complaints (SOM), Anxiety (ANX), Anxiety-Related Disorders (ARD), and Depression (DEP), and three psychotic spectrum scales, Paranoia (PAR), Schizophrenia (SCZ), and Mania (MAN). The other four clinical scales assess syndromes with distinguishing externalizing features: two scales for the assessment of personality pathology, Borderline Features (BOR) and Antisocial Features (ANT), and two scales for the assessment of substance use and related consequences, Alcohol Problems (ALC) and Drug Problems (DRG).

The five treatment consideration scales were designed to offer clinically relevant information for individual treatment planning, such as the degree to which a client may pose a risk of harm to themselves or others (the Suicidal Ideation [SUI] scale and the Aggression [AGG] scale), the situational or environmental factors that may be exacerbating psychological difficulties (Stress [STR] scale and Nonsupport [NON] scale), and their degree of treatment motivation and readiness (Treatment Rejection [RXR] scale). Last, the PAI includes two interpersonal scales, Dominance (DOM) and Warmth (WRM), corresponding to the relatively normally distributed axes (Ansell et al., 2011) of interpersonal style: (a) dominant control versus meek submission and (b) warm affiliation versus cold rejection.

In addition to the 22 basic PAI scales, a host of supplemental indicators have been developed to help address issues of profile validity and clinical decision making. Some of these have been extensively cross-validated (Morey, 2007b), while others have received limited research attention (McCredie & Morey, 2018). Many of these indicators can be scored using scoring software, as described in the next section (Morey, 2020).

Administration and Scoring

The PAI was developed and standardized to be used as a clinical assessment instrument with adults 18 years of age and older; a parallel version, the PAI–Adolescent (PAI-A; Morey, 2007a), is available for use with individuals aged 12 to 18. Raw PAI scale and subscale scores are linearly transformed to *T* scores (mean of 50, standard deviation of 10) to allow for interpretation relative to a census-matched standardization sample of 1,000 community-dwelling adults. Several procedures were employed throughout the process of item selection to identify and eliminate any items at risk of being biased by demographic characteristics. With very few exceptions, differences in item responses as a function of demographic features were minimal in the community standardization sample. In order to facilitate the interpretation of scale elevations relative to other clinical respondents, the PAI profile form also indicates *T* scores that correspond to marked elevations when referenced against a representative clinical sample of 1,246 clients selected from a variety of clinical settings. Thus, PAI profiles can be interpreted with respect to both community and clinical norms as deemed appropriate for the testing context.

Computerization

A few different computer software packages are available to enhance the use of the PAI in clinical (Morey, 2020), correctional (i.e., inmate assessment; Edens & Ruiz, 2005), and public safety personnel selection (Roberts et al., 2000) assessment contexts. The PAI Software Portfolio (Morey, 2020) can be used for online administration and scoring of the test and provides a narrative report of results, diagnostic hypotheses, and critical items relevant to clinical assessment.

ASSESSMENT OF BIPOLAR SPECTRUM DISORDERS

Given the complex and fluctuating nature of their symptoms, bipolar spectrum disorders are particularly challenging from a measurement standpoint. The PAI contains two scales of particular relevance to the assessment of bipolar spectrum disorders, DEP and MAN, which assess depressive and manic/hypomanic symptomatology, respectively. The interpretive guidelines for these scales are described in greater detail in the following sections. Several additional scales and subscales that are informative with respect to bipolar spectrum disorder differential diagnosis and treatment planning are also discussed. It should be noted that in mood disorders of a cyclical nature, the pattern of elevations is likely to vary somewhat depending on whether the individual is currently experiencing a depressed, euthymic, or manic/hypomanic mood state, and the PAI is primarily a marker of current mental status. Thus, a variety of sources of information, reflecting both historic and current presentation, should be considered in the evaluation of bipolar spectrum disorders.

Bipolar Spectrum Disorder Diagnostic Considerations

DEP Scale

The DEP scale (standard error of measurement [SEm] = 3.6T) assesses the affective, cognitive, and physiological elements of depression across a spectrum of clinical severity, ranging from mild symptoms to very severe. Average scores (below 60T) on DEP are reflective of an individual who is generally feeling optimistic and self-confident and experiencing minimal unhappiness and distress. Scores in the mildly elevated range (60–70T) suggest some degree of unhappiness, pessimism, or self-doubt, at least part of the time. An individual with a bipolar spectrum disorder currently experiencing a manic or hypomanic episode may demonstrate mild elevations on DEP due to the reporting of historic depressive symptoms, despite not appearing to be depressed at the time of testing. Moderately elevated scores (70–80T) indicate a clinical presentation in which unhappiness and dysphoria are prominent, likely marked by feelings of guilt, moodiness, and withdrawal from previously pleasurable activities. Very high scores on DEP (above 80T) increase the likelihood of a diagnosis of a major depressive episode, with marked elevations (above 95T) strongly supporting such a diagnosis. Individuals scoring in this range likely are experiencing feelings of worthlessness and view their circumstances as hopeless. Their very low energy levels and motivation make it difficult to accomplish even basic everyday tasks, and they are socially withdrawn. Suicidal ideation is common among scorers in this range, thus warranting careful consideration of co-occurring elevations on SUI and the Suicide Potential Index (SPI; discussed later).

DEP comprises three subscales representing the Cognitive (DEP-C; SEm = 4.8T), Affective (DEP-A; SEm = 3.9T), and Physiological (DEP-P; SEm = 5.0T) elements of depression. DEP-C assesses the degree to which one's beliefs and expectancies reflect feelings of worthlessness, hopelessness, and personal failure, as well as difficulties with concentration and decisiveness. Elevated scores on DEP-C are suggestive of an individual with low self-worth and poor self-efficacy, who is feeling helpless and pessimistic about their capacity to bring about positive changes in their life. Conversely, low scores on DEP-C (e.g., below 40*T*) may reflect unwarranted optimism regarding the limits of one's capabilities. Thus, very low scores on DEP-C may be present if an individual is experiencing a current manic or hypomanic episode. DEP-A assesses the affective component of depression, such as feeling unhappy, sad, distressed, "down," or "blue." Elevations on DEP-A are often accompanied by feelings of subjective sadness, loss of interest in daily activities, and a loss of pleasure in previously enjoyed activities. As such, DEP-A represents the purest indicator of overall life satisfaction on the PAI. Finally, DEP-P assesses aspects of physical functioning which are relevant to depressive disorders, such as low activity levels, poor sleep, and changes in appetite. Elevated scores on DEP-P are suggestive of an individual who is fatigued, lacks energy and drive, and has experienced recent changes in eating, sleeping, and/or sexual interest.

The DEP subscale configuration is informative with respect to the diagnostic implications of an elevated DEP score. When all three DEP subscales are elevated beyond 70*T*, it is quite likely that the respondent meets the criteria for a current major depressive episode. Elevations on DEP-C and DEP-A, but not DEP-P, are more likely to represent a milder form of depression, such as persistent depressive disorder (formerly dysthymic disorder). However, elevations on DEP may not be specific to a depressive disorder but may instead reflect subjective distress associated with another psychiatric condition, particularly when DEP is elevated in the context of other PAI scale elevations. As noted, an individual who is currently experiencing a manic episode of a cyclical mood disorder may demonstrate only modest elevations on DEP, due to the reporting of historical symptoms, whereas elevations on DEP are likely to be much more pronounced when testing occurs during a depressive episode.

MAN Scale

The MAN scale (*SE*m = 4.1*T*) measures aspects of the clinical presentation pertinent to mania or hypomania, including externalizing, internalizing, and psychotic elements. These elements encompass a diverse array of symptoms, including elevated mood, grandiosity, heightened activity level, irritability, and poor frustration tolerance. Elevations on MAN tend to be relatively rare in clinical settings as compared with elevations on the other PAI clinical scales, in part because relatively few individuals presenting for evaluation of emotional problems experience features such as heightened activity levels and self-esteem. Furthermore, those that might present with such symptoms, such as an individual in an acute, severe manic episode, are often unable or unwilling to complete a relatively lengthy self-report questionnaire such as the 344-item PAI. Thus, the critical thresholds for identifying MAN scores as a prominent clinical issue tend to be lower than the thresholds used for other clinical scales, given that average scores on MAN are nearly identical in the community and clinical standardization samples. Notably, the clinical issues represented by MAN are fairly heterogenous, and thus an elevated score on MAN (particularly one driven by a single subscale) is not necessarily specific to a bipolar diagnosis. Elevations on the MAN scale and subscales can occur across a variety of psychological disorders, necessitating interpretation of a MAN elevation within the context of the broader PAI profile.

Average MAN scores, roughly 54T or below, are indicative of an individual with few if any features of mania or hypomania. However, it should be noted that although individuals experiencing a depressive episode typically do not demonstrate heightened activity levels or grandiosity, depression is often associated with irritability. Thus, a depressive episode will not necessarily be associated with a low MAN score. Respondents with scores ranging from 55T to 64T may appear active, outgoing, self-confident, and ambitious, although individuals at the higher end of this range may also present as impatient, quick-tempered, or somewhat hostile. Scores in the 64T to 74T range suggest an individual who presents as restless and impulsive with noticeably high energy levels; others may perceive such individuals as confrontational or lacking sensitivity. Markedly elevated MAN scores (above 75T) are typically associated with the presence of mania, hypomania, or cyclothymia. Such individuals are typically attempting to engage in a number of activities disproportionate to their capability to do so effectively or in an organized manner, and they may respond with anger to those who suggest they slow down or reduce their overinvolvement. They are often impulsive, particularly in self-destructive areas, and they likely have impaired judgment impacting role functioning. Interpersonal relationships may be strained due to others' perceptions of the individual as narcissistic, hostile, or unsympathetic.

MAN comprises three subscales, including Activity Level (MAN-A; *SE*m = 5.7T), Grandiosity (MAN-G; *SE*m = 4.4T), and Irritability (MAN-I; *SE*m = 4.6T). MAN-A assesses the extent to which the respondent's ideas (e.g., flight of ideas) and behaviors (e.g., motor activity) are accelerated in both speed and intensity. It is important to note that while the *quantity* of activity increases with elevations on MAN-A, the quality of activity decreases as the ideation and overt behaviors become increasingly pressured and disorganized. Scores in the lowest range (below 30T) are indicative of very low activity levels and marked apathy and indifference, typically seen in a severe depressive episode. Mild elevations (55–65T) indicate a somewhat higher than normal activity level; individuals high in this range may be involved in a variety of activities, but this level of involvement may remain functional and not necessarily disorganized. Elevations in this range have also been associated with attention-deficit/hyperactivity disorder (e.g., Watson & Liljequist, 2018). Moderate elevations (65–75T) indicate a level of overinvolvement in a variety of activities that is noticeable to a casual observer and increases the likelihood of disorganized involvement and impaired performance, for at least some of those activities. Individuals scoring in this range may also be experiencing accelerated thought processes (e.g., flight of ideas). At markedly high levels (exceeding 75T), the individual appears confused and is difficult for others to understand due to the accelerated thought processes; scores in this range are rare on the PAI given the focused attention needed to respond to a lengthy self-report questionnaire.

MAN-G is reflective of the extent to which an individual demonstrates an exaggerated self-concept, marked by inflated self-esteem, expansiveness, and grandiosity. At very low scores, MAN-G can indicate internalized low self-worth, such that the respondent feels inadequate and is unable or unwilling to acknowledge positive aspects of themselves, which may occur in the context of a depressive episode. Moderately elevated scores on MAN-G (60–70*T*) indicate an optimistic and confident self-perception, with the possibility of inflated self-esteem increasing at the upper end of this range. Such individuals may appear to be driven and focused on strategies for success and achievement. High scores (above 70*T*) are quite rare in clinical settings and reflect the possibility of psychotic or narcissistic grandiosity. Such individuals report that they possess many unique talents and abilities, and they may endorse borderline delusional beliefs regarding the likelihood of those special talents leading to fame or fortune. Others are likely to view such individuals as self-centered or narcissistic.

MAN-I assesses the extent to which a respondent demonstrates irritability associated with others' inability or unwillingness to keep up with their plans, demands, and potentially unrealistic ideas. Although mania is often associated with elevated mood, manic affect more commonly manifests as volatility, particularly in response to frustration. Items on MAN-I are thus reflective of a combination of ambition (albeit often disorganized in its manifestation) and poor frustration tolerance. Low scores (40*T* and below) indicate someone who portrays themself as exceptionally patient and relatively immune to frustrations. Mild elevations (60–70*T*) indicate some impatience and poor frustration tolerance. Respondents scoring in this range are likely to become frustrated with others who they view as uncooperative with their plans and unable to keep up with their activities; others are likely to view these respondents as demanding. At higher elevations (70*T* or above), the respondent's relationships with others are likely strained due to the demanding presentation of the respondent. Respondents scoring in this range are likely to accuse others of attempting to thwart their potentially unrealistic plans for success and achievement and to externalize blame onto others for failures. Marked elevations (above 80*T*) indicate marked volatility in response to frustration. Individuals scoring in this range are likely to experience rapid fluctuations in mood state and will be prone to lashing out at others whom they view as sources of their frustrations.

Given the heterogeneity of MAN, the diagnostic implications of a MAN elevation will vary depending upon the subscale configuration. When all three subscales are elevated, a manic episode within a bipolar spectrum disorder should be a central diagnostic consideration. However, in cases in which one subscale is primarily driving the full-scale elevation, other diagnostic hypotheses should be considered. In cases in which MAN-G is the predominant elevation, the individual may be demonstrating prominent narcissistic personality pathology, such as in the case of narcissistic or antisocial personality disorder. Conversely, very low scores on MAN-G may be associated with low self-esteem and feelings of worthlessness characteristic of a depressive episode. When MAN-I is the predominant elevation, the respondent is likely having difficulties with frustration tolerance, impulse control, and anger management. Although some level of impatience or poor frustration tolerance is common among depressed individuals, co-occurring marked elevations on the AGG scale may indicate a diagnosis such as intermittent explosive disorder.

Differential Diagnosis and Treatment Planning Considerations

Affective Instability Scale

The Affective Instability (BOR-A) scale assesses the propensity for an individual to experience rapid mood fluctuations, typically within the realm of negative affectivity (e.g., shifts between anger, irritability, anxiety, and depression in rapid succession). This type of rapid mood fluctuation typically reflects extreme emotional responsivity (e.g., triggered by an interpersonal interaction) such as that associated with borderline personality disorder, as opposed to cyclical changes in mood as in the case of bipolar spectrum disorders (see also Chapter 14 in this volume). Nevertheless, a BOR-A elevation independent of the other BOR subscales may be indicative of a bipolar spectrum disorder diagnosis, particularly if there also happens to be a personality component. The highest range scores on the subscale (above 80T) are indicative of an individual experiencing mood shifts representing the full range of negative affect, including poorly controlled anger. Moderately elevated scores (70–80T) may indicate a propensity toward experiencing a particular variant of negative affect, and examination of elevations on other scales may help to determine whether depression (DEP-A), anxiety (ANX-A or ARD-P), or anger (AGG-A) is the most typical emotional response.

Self-Harm/Impulsivity Scale

The Self-Harm/Impulsivity (BOR-S) scale assesses the tendency for an individual to act impulsively, often in a self-damaging manner, without significant regard for the consequences of those actions. BOR-S is not a direct indicator of suicidal behavior or nonsuicidal self-injury, although individuals high on BOR-S may be more at risk of such behaviors. Although impulsivity is generally associated with manic/hypomanic episodes of bipolar spectrum disorders, research has suggested that heightened impulsivity may be a core feature of bipolar disorder across the various mood phases of the disorder, including euthymia (Najt et al., 2007). Thus, BOR-S may offer a useful indicator of an individual's level of trait-like impulsivity in the assessment of bipolar spectrum disorders.

Antisocial Scale

The ANT scale assesses both the personological (Egocentricity [ANT-E] and Stimulus-Seeking [ANT-S]) and behavioral (Antisocial Behaviors [ANT-A]) features associated with antisocial personality disorder. Although markedly elevated scores on ANT (above 82*T*) are suggestive of antisocial personality pathology, moderate elevations (approximately 70–80*T*), particularly when driven by ANT-S, may also reflect the lack of inhibition associated with a manic episode and thus are not uncommon with bipolar spectrum disorders.

Aggression Scale and Violence Potential Index

AGG provides an assessment of the attitudinal (Aggressive Attitudes [AGG-A]) and behavioral (Verbal Aggression [AGG-V] and Physical Aggression [AGG-P]) features of aggression, anger, and hostility, independent of psychiatric diagnosis. Although its clinical presentation is heterogenous, bipolar disorder has been associated with an increased risk of aggression, particularly during acute episodes (e.g., Ballester et al., 2012, 2014). As such, an individual's aggressive tendencies and capacity to act out aggressively should be considered in the assessment of bipolar spectrum disorders. Scores above 70*T* on AGG are suggestive of an individual who experiences chronic anger issues and is likely to express their anger; examination of the relative elevations on AGG-V and AGG-P may help elucidate the nature by which their anger is typically expressed. Very high scores (above 82*T*) indicate the presence of a considerable degree of anger and the potential for aggressive behavior. The Violence Potential Index (VPI; Morey, 1996) includes 20 configural features of the PAI profile related to violence risk and can be consulted in conjunction with AGG to determine one's risk of violent behavior. Scores above nine (1 *SD* above the clinical standardization mean) and 17 (2 *SD*s above the clinical standardization mean) are associated with moderate and marked risk of violence, respectively.

Suicidal Ideation Scale and Suicide Potential Index

SUI assesses the extent to which an individual is experiencing suicidal ideation across a spectrum of severity, ranging from vague thoughts about death to active, serious consideration of suicide. Bipolar disorder is associated with one of the highest rates of suicide of all psychiatric conditions, with a prevalence that is 20 to 30 times larger than that of the general population (Miller & Black, 2020). As such, evaluation of suicidal ideation and risk is essential to bipolar spectrum disorder assessment. Clinical respondents generally score in the moderate range (approximately 60–69*T*) on SUI, indicating at least periodic thoughts of self-harm. Scores in the moderately elevated range (approximately 70–84*T*) suggest recurrent thoughts of suicide and self-harm and should be considered a significant warning sign for suicide potential, particularly in the context of other risk factors. The intensity of the suicidal ideation increases as scores exceed 85*T*, with many individuals scoring in this range requiring suicide precautions.

Although some degree of suicidal ideation is common among clinical respondents (as well as, to a lesser extent, community respondents), any elevation on SUI warrants follow-up discussion with the client regarding the details of suicidal thoughts and the potential for suicidal behavior. However, it should be noted that the SUI scale assesses suicidal ideation, not suicide potential. The SPI (Morey, 1996) includes 20 configural features of the PAI profile related to suicide risk and can be consulted in conjunction with SUI to determine one's risk of suicidal behavior. Scores above 13 (1 *SD* above the clinical standardization mean) suggest that an individual is endorsing a number of risk factors for suicidality, thus warranting a thorough suicide risk assessment and careful monitoring.

Structural Summary Configuration for Bipolar Spectrum Disorders

Several of the scales described in the previous sections are included in the PAI structural summary approach (Morey & Hopwood, 2007), which was designed to aid in the diagnosis of a variety of common psychiatric disorders, including bipolar disorder. Simultaneous elevations on both MAN and DEP exceeding 60*T* are generally rare in clinical samples and thus warrant careful consideration of a bipolar spectrum disorder diagnosis, particularly when BOR-A is also elevated. Typically, such a pattern of scores is reflective of a combination of current and historical reporting, although mixed-mood episodes are possible. A manic episode is typically associated with elevations on all three MAN subscales and may also be accompanied by elevations on BOR-S and ANT-S, indicating impulsivity, disinhibition, and poor judgment, as well as a suppressed score on DEP-C, indicating an unwarranted degree of optimism. Interpersonally, an individual experiencing manic symptoms may demonstrate an elevation on DOM, indicating a (likely unrealistic) belief in themselves as a highly effective leader, as well as an average or above average score on WRM, reflective of their largely uninhibited interactions with others. The persecution (PAR-P) subscale may also be elevated, as a reflection of their belief that others are attempting to interfere with their important plans and ideas; however, these persecutory beliefs are generally not associated with feelings of bitterness and resentment (PAR-R) as seen in more pure paranoia. Finally, RXR may be at or above 50*T*, suggesting a lack of insight into the severity of presenting problems.

NOTEWORTHY RESEARCH FINDINGS

It should be noted that the empirical literature base regarding the use of the PAI in the diagnosis of bipolar spectrum disorders remains limited relative to other diagnostic categories. This is particularly the case for research examining the PAI profiles of individuals experiencing a current manic episode, given previously noted challenges associated with the administration of a relatively lengthy self-report questionnaire to an individual in an acute manic state. The following subsections provide a summary of the empirical evidence regarding the use of the PAI with respect to the diagnosis of bipolar spectrum disorders, as well as the literature examining relationships between PAI scales and a variety of correlates associated with bipolar spectrum disorders.

Relationships With Bipolar Spectrum Disorder Symptomatology

A small number of studies have examined the PAI's capacity for differential diagnosis between bipolar disorder and a range of other disorders with overlapping symptomatology. For instance, Rogers et al. (1995) reported a modest correlation between the MAN scale and bipolar disorder diagnosis (correlation $r = .24$) among correctional inmates, as assessed by the Schedule of Affective Disorders and Schizophrenia–Change Version (Spitzer & Endicott, 1978b), whereas relationships between MAN and Schizophrenia ($r = .12$) and Depression ($r = .10$) diagnoses were smaller in magnitude. Similarly, Mullen-Magbalon (2008) evaluated the PAI's capacity to discriminate between bipolar disorder, borderline personality disorder (BPD), and posttraumatic stress disorder (PTSD) at a university counseling center. MAN-A, but not MAN-G or MAN-I, significantly predicted the diagnostic category and was found to be significantly higher on average in those with a bipolar diagnosis ($64T$) as compared with those with a BPD ($56T$) or PTSD ($55T$) diagnosis. Among South Korean respondents, Lee et al. (2016) found that individuals diagnosed with bipolar disorder demonstrated significantly higher scores on MAN (Cohen's $d = .52$) and AGG ($d = .69$) than individuals with unipolar depression; at the subscale level, MAN-G ($d = .48$), BOR-N ($d = .61$), ANT-S ($d = .62$), AGG-A ($d = .80$), and AGG-P ($d = .51$) were found to be higher among the bipolar patients. Notably, however, scores on these scales for the bipolar diagnosis group were only in the normal to moderate range ($48–64T$), with DEP and SUI being the only full scales to reach clinical significance (i.e., $T > 70$) for both groups. Although the unipolar depression group demonstrated slightly higher scores on both DEP ($d = .41$) and SUI ($d = .14$), these differences were not statistically significant.

Several studies have additionally examined the MAN and DEP scales as indicators of manic and depressive symptomatology, respectively, in diverse samples. For instance, Rogers et al. (1998) reported a modest correlation among correctional inmates between the MAN scale and manic symptomatology ($r = .31$) as assessed by the SADS (Spitzer & Endicott, 1978a). However, a stronger relationship was observed between the DEP scale and SADS depressive symptom constellation ($r = .67$). Blais et al. (2021) examined relationships between the PAI and SPECTRA: Indices of Psychopathology (SPECTRA; Blais & Sinclair, 2018), a relatively novel instrument designed to align with contemporary hierarchical-dimensional models of psychopathology, among psychiatric inpatients. Consistent with expectations, MAN-A was found to correlate significantly with the Manic Activation scale of the SPECTRA ($r = .39$), while MAN-G correlated significantly with the Grandiose Ideation scale ($r = .48$). Also as expected, DEP correlated significantly with the Depression domain ($r = .76$). Also among psychiatric inpatients, Ban et al. (1993) reported convergent relationships between the MAN scale and the Grandiosity ($r = .48$), Conceptual Disorganization ($r = .40$), and Unusual Thought Content ($r = .42$) scales of the Brief Psychiatric Rating Scale (Overall & Gorham, 1962). Similarly, Briere and Runtz (2002) reported moderate-sized correlations between MAN and the Affect Dysregulation ($r = .46$), Susceptibility to Influence ($r = .42$), and

Idealization-Disillusionment ($r = .44$) scales of their self-developed Inventory of Altered Self-Capacities in a small sample of clinical participants. Among veteran clients, Rielage (2005) found significant correlations between the MAN scale and the Bipolar: Manic ($r = .58$) scale of the Millon Clinical Multiaxial Inventory–II (MCMI-II; Millon, 1994). In addition, the DEP scale demonstrated robust correlations with the MCMI-II scales for Dysthymia ($r = .75$) and Major Depression ($r = .74$). Finally, MAN has been shown to correlate significantly with the Mania scale of the Emotional Assessment System (Choca et al., 2001) in both community ($r = .56$; Dunkel, 2005) and clinical ($r = .60$; Francis, 2019) samples.

Correlates Relevant to Bipolar Spectrum Disorders

In addition to bipolar spectrum disorder diagnosis, relationships between MAN and DEP and a variety of psychological constructs relevant to bipolar spectrum disorder have also been examined.

Aggression

Some studies have noted relationships between MAN and indicators of aggressive behavior, in line with the previously noted relationship between bipolar disorder and increased risk of aggression. Helfritz and Stanford (2006) reported significantly higher scores on MAN among college students identified as impulsive aggressors ($65.7T$) as compared with nonaggressive control students ($48.6T$). However, impulsive aggressors were also found to be higher on DEP ($63.4T$) than nonaggressive students ($43.2T$), suggesting a global elevation in psychopathology not necessarily specific to severe manic symptoms. Likewise, Blais et al. (2021) reported that the SPECTRA Severe Aggression scale correlated significantly with MAN ($r = .36$), and to a lesser extent also DEP ($r = .26$). Diamond and Magaletta (2006) similarly reported significant correlations between the MAN scale and the Physical ($r = .29$) and Verbal Aggression ($r = .35$) scales of the Short-Form Buss–Perry Aggression Questionnaire. In a related area of research, Sinclair et al. (2012) noted that individuals with a history of mania demonstrated significantly higher scores on the PAI VPI ($64.5T$) than individuals without a history of mania ($54.2T$; $d = .66$).

Impulsivity

Several studies have examined the relationships between MAN and various indicators of impulsivity. For instance, significant, medium effect size relationships have been reported between the MAN-A subscale and the Barrett Impulsiveness Scale–11 (BIS-11; Patton et al., 1995) total score across studies ($r = .37$: Fields et al., 2015; $r = .37$: Ruiz et al., 2010). Fields et al. (2015) also noted a significant correlation between the MAN scale and BIS-11 total score ($r = .19$). Likewise, Hopwood et al. (2013) reported a significant correlation between MAN-A and the Impulsivity facet ($r = .40$) of the Personality Inventory for *Diagnostic and Statistical Manual of Mental Disorders* (5th ed.; PID-5;

Krueger et al., 2012), while the relationship between MAN-A and Risk Taking (r = .19) was more modest.

Suicidality

Bipolar spectrum disorders are associated with a heightened risk of suicide relative to other psychiatric disorders (Miller & Black, 2020). As such, some studies have examined relationships between bipolar symptomatology and a history of suicide attempts and psychological hospitalization. Sinclair et al. (2012) found that individuals with a history of mania demonstrated significantly higher scores on the SPI (70.9T) than individuals without a history of mania (63.2T; d = .52). A history of depression was also associated with higher scores on the SPI (68.6T) relative to those with no history of depression (49.5T; d = 1.28). Notably, however, Slavin-Mulford et al. (2012) found that neither MAN nor DEP significantly predicted suicide attempt history, and only DEP was a significant predictor of past psychiatric hospitalizations (r = .26). These findings highlight the importance of considering multiple indicators in the evaluation of suicide risk associated with bipolar spectrum disorders.

CONCLUSION AND FUTURE DIRECTIONS

The PAI offers clinically useful information pertinent to diagnostic and treatment planning considerations in the assessment of bipolar spectrum disorders. The PAI contains two scales, MAN and DEP, that assess the diverse range of clinical features associated with manic/hypomanic and depressive symptomatology, respectively, at varying degrees of severity. Furthermore, several additional scales are informative with respect to the differential diagnosis and treatment of bipolar spectrum disorders, such as scales and indices assessing impulsivity (BOR-S), affective lability (BOR-A), aggression (AGG, VPI), and suicidality (SUI, SPI). Furthermore, existing research has offered support for the validity of the PAI in the assessment of bipolar spectrum disorders and related clinical phenomena.

Future research examining the PAI in the context of bipolar spectrum disorders may be particularly informative given the PAI's capacity to assess similar constructs as those represented on contemporary dimensional models of psychopathology, such as the hierarchical taxonomy of psychopathology (HiTOP) model (Kotov et al., 2017). Research regarding the internal structure of the PAI has revealed a similar hierarchical structure with overarching internalizing and externalizing dimensions (e.g., Hopwood & Moser, 2011; Ruiz & Edens, 2008), as well as specific scales aligning conceptually with other elements of the model relevant to bipolar disorder, such as thought problems (SCZ-T), emotional lability (BOR-A), euphoric activation and hyperactive cognition (MAN-A), reckless overconfidence (MAN-G; ANT-S), and irritability (MAN-I). There has been some debate regarding the positioning of Mania on the internalizing or thought disorder spectrum of the HiTOP model

(Watson et al., 2022), and future research examining bipolar spectrum disorders with the PAI may offer further clarity on this issue. Additionally, future research involving multimethod, longitudinal assessment of bipolar spectrum disorders using the PAI may also help to elucidate the ways in which the PAI score pattern may vary as a function of the current mood phase of the disorder.

REFERENCES

Ansell, E. B., Kurtz, J. E., DeMoor, R. M., & Markey, P. M. (2011). Validity of the PAI interpersonal scales for measuring the dimensions of the interpersonal circumplex. *Journal of Personality Assessment, 93*(1), 33–39. https://doi.org/10.1080/00223891.2011.529013

Archer, R. P., Buffington-Vollum, J. K., Stredny, R. V., & Handel, R. W. (2006). A survey of psychological test use patterns among forensic psychologists. *Journal of Personality Assessment, 87*(1), 84–94. https://doi.org/10.1207/s15327752jpa8701_07

Ballester, J., Goldstein, B., Goldstein, T. R., Yu, H., Axelson, D., Monk, K., Hickey, M. B., Diler, R. S., Sakolsky, D. J., Sparks, G., Iyengar, S., Kupfer, D. J., Brent, D. A., & Birmaher, B. (2014). Prospective longitudinal course of aggression among adults with bipolar disorder. *Bipolar Disorders, 16*(3), 262–269. https://doi.org/10.1111/bdi.12168

Ballester, J., Goldstein, T., Goldstein, B., Obreja, M., Axelson, D., Monk, K., Hickey, M., Iyengar, S., Farchione, T., Kupfer, D. J., Brent, D., & Birmaher, B. (2012). Is bipolar disorder specifically associated with aggression? *Bipolar Disorders, 14*(3), 283–290. https://doi.org/10.1111/j.1399-5618.2012.01006.x

Ban, T. A., Fjetland, O. K., Kutcher, M., & Morey, L. C. (1993). CODE-DD: Development of a diagnostic scale for depressive disorders. In I. Hindmarch & P. Stonier (Eds.), *Human psychopharmacology: Measures and methods* (Vol. 4, pp. 73–86). Wiley.

Blais, M. A., Baity, M. R., & Hopwood, C. J. (2010). *Clinical applications of the Personality Assessment Inventory*. Routledge.

Blais, M., & Sinclair, S. (2018). *SPECTRA: Indices of psychopathology: Professional manual*. Psychological Assessment Resources.

Blais, M. A., Sinclair, S. J., Richardson, L. A., Massey, C., & Stein, M. B. (2021). External correlates of the SPECTRA: Indices of psychopathology (SPECTRA) in a clinical sample. *Clinical Psychology & Psychotherapy, 28*(4), 929–938. https://doi.org/10.1002/cpp.2546

Briere, J., & Runtz, M. (2002). The Inventory of Altered Self-Capacities (IASC): A standardized measure of identity, affect regulation, and relationship disturbance. *Assessment, 9*(3), 230–239. https://doi.org/10.1177/1073191102009003002

Choca, J., Laatsch, L., O'Keefe, G., Strack, S., Greenblatt, R., Szucko, J., Craig, R., & Rossini, E. (2001). *The emotional assessment system manual*. Roosevelt University.

Diamond, P. M., & Magaletta, P. R. (2006). The short-form Buss–Perry Aggression Questionnaire (BPAQ-SF): A validation study with federal offenders. *Assessment, 13*(3), 227–240. https://doi.org/10.1177/1073191106287666

Dunkel, T. M. (2005). *Concurrent validation of the Emotional Assessment System and the Personality Assessment Inventory* [Doctoral dissertation, Roosevelt University]. ProQuest.

Edens, J. F., & Ruiz, M. A. (2005). *PAI interpretive report for correctional settings (PAI-CS)*. Psychological Assessment Resources.

Fields, S., Edens, J. F., Smith, S. T., Rulseh, A., Donnellan, M. B., Ruiz, M. A., McDermott, B. E., & Douglas, K. S. (2015). Examining the psychometric properties of the Barratt Impulsiveness Scale–Brief Form in justice-involved samples. *Psychological Assessment, 27*(4), 1211–1218. https://doi.org/10.1037/a0039109

Francis, C. (2019). *Testing the emotional assessment system and the Personality Assessment Inventory in clinical practice* [Doctoral dissertation, Roosevelt University]. ProQuest.

Helfritz, L. E., & Stanford, M. S. (2006). Personality and psychopathology in an impulsive aggressive college sample. *Aggressive Behavior: Official Journal of the International Society for Research on Aggression, 32*(1), 28–37. https://doi.org/10.1002/ab.20103

Hopwood, C. J., & Moser, J. S. (2011). Personality Assessment Inventory internalizing and externalizing structure in college students: Invariance across sex and ethnicity. *Personality and Individual Differences, 50*(1), 116–119. https://doi.org/10.1016/j.paid.2010.08.013

Hopwood, C. J., Wright, A. G., Krueger, R. F., Schade, N., Markon, K. E., & Morey, L. C. (2013). *DSM-5* pathological personality traits and the Personality Assessment Inventory. *Assessment, 20*(3), 269–285. https://doi.org/10.1177/1073191113486286

Kotov, R., Krueger, R. F., Watson, D., Achenbach, T. M., Althoff, R. R., Bagby, R. M., Brown, T. A., Carpenter, W. T., Caspi, A., Clark, L. A., Eaton, N. R., Forbes, M. K., Forbush, K. T., Goldberg, D., Hasin, D., Hyman, S. E., Ivanova, M. Y., Lynam, D. R., Markon, K., . . . Zimmerman, M. (2017). The Hierarchical Taxonomy of Psychopathology (HiTOP): A dimensional alternative to traditional nosologies. *Journal of Abnormal Psychology, 126*(4), 454–477. https://doi.org/10.1037/abn0000258

Krueger, R. F., Derringer, J., Markon, K. E., Watson, D., & Skodol, A. E. (2012). Initial construction of a maladaptive personality trait model and inventory for *DSM-5. Psychological Medicine, 42*(9), 1879–1890. https://doi.org/10.1017/S0033291711002674

Lee, J. S., Lee, S. Y., Lee, K. H., & Paik, Y. S. (2016). Comparison of psychometric properties between bipolar and unipolar depression. *Mood and Emotion, 14*(3), 131–136. http://www.moodandemotion.org/journal/view.html?uid=58&vmd=Full

McCredie, M. N., Hopwood, C. J., & Morey, L. C. (2021). Personality Assessment Inventory (PAI) for assessing disordered thought and perception. In I. B. Weiner & J. H. Kleiger (Eds.), *Psychological assessment of disordered thinking and perception* (pp. 79–98). American Psychological Association. https://doi.org/10.1037/0000245-006

McCredie, M. N., & Morey, L. C. (2018). Evaluating new supplemental indicators for the Personality Assessment Inventory: Standardization and cross-validation. *Psychological Assessment, 30*(10), 1292–1299. https://doi.org/10.1037/pas0000574

Miller, J. N., & Black, D. W. (2020). Bipolar disorder and suicide: A review. *Current Psychiatry Reports, 22*(2), Article 6. https://doi.org/10.1007/s11920-020-1130-0

Millon, T. (1994). *Manual for the MCMI-III.* National Computer Systems.

Morey, L. C. (1991). *Personality Assessment Inventory professional manual.* Psychological Assessment Resources.

Morey, L. C. (1996). *An interpretive guide to the Personality Assessment Inventory.* Psychological Assessment Resources.

Morey, L. C. (2003). *Essentials of PAI assessment.* Wiley.

Morey, L. C. (2007a). *Personality Assessment Inventory–Adolescent (PAI-A).* Psychological Assessment Resources.

Morey, L. C. (2007b). *Personality Assessment Inventory professional manual* (2nd ed.). Psychological Assessment Resources.

Morey, L. C. (2020). *PAI Software Portfolio manual.* Psychological Assessment Resources.

Morey, L. C., & Hopwood, C. J. (2007). *Casebook for the Personality Assessment Inventory: A structural summary approach.* Psychological Assessment Resources.

Mullen-Magbalon, S. D. (2008). *Using the Personality Assessment Inventory to discriminate among borderline personality disorder, bipolar disorder, and post-traumatic stress disorder* [Doctoral dissertation, University of Tennessee, Knoxville]. Tennessee Research and Creative Exchange.

Najt, P., Perez, J., Sanches, M., Peluso, M. A. M., Glahn, D., & Soares, J. C. (2007). Impulsivity and bipolar disorder. *European Neuropsychopharmacology, 17*(5), 313–320. https://doi.org/10.1016/j.euroneuro.2006.10.002

Overall, J. E., & Gorham, D. R. (1962). The Brief Psychiatric Rating Scale. *Psychological Reports, 10*(3), 799–812. https://doi.org/10.2466/pr0.1962.10.3.799

Patton, J. H., Stanford, M. S., & Barratt, E. S. (1995). Factor structure of the Barratt Impulsiveness Scale. *Journal of Clinical Psychology, 51*(6), 768–774. https://doi.org/10.1002/1097-4679(199511)51:6<768::AID-JCLP2270510607>3.0.CO;2-1

Rielage, J. K. (2005). *Assessing the association between veterans' personality traits, suicidal ideation, and suicide risk with the PAI and MCMI-II* [Doctoral dissertation, Southern Illinois University, Carbondale]. ProQuest.

Roberts, M. D., Thompson, J. A., & Johnson, M. (2000). *PAI law enforcement, corrections, and public safety selection report module*. Psychological Assessment Resources.

Rogers, R., Sewell, K. W., Ustad, K., Reinhardt, V., & Edwards, W. (1995). The Referral Decision Scale with mentally disordered inmates. *Law and Human Behavior, 19*(5), 481–492. https://doi.org/10.1007/BF01499339

Rogers, R., Ustad, K. L., & Salekin, R. T. (1998). Convergent validity of the Personality Assessment Inventory: A study of emergency referrals in a correctional setting. *Assessment, 5*(1), 3–12. https://doi.org/10.1177/107319119800500102

Ruiz, M. A., & Edens, J. F. (2008). Recovery and replication of internalizing and externalizing dimensions within the Personality Assessment Inventory. *Journal of Personality Assessment, 90*(6), 585–592. https://doi.org/10.1080/00223890802388574

Ruiz, M. A., Skeem, J. L., Poythress, N. G., Douglas, K. S., & Lilienfeld, S. O. (2010). Structure and correlates of the Barratt Impulsiveness Scale (BIS-11) in offenders: Implications for psychopathy and externalizing pathology. *International Journal of Forensic Mental Health, 9*(3), 237–244. https://doi.org/10.1080/14999013.2010.517258

Sinclair, S. J., Bello, I., Nyer, M., Slavin-Mulford, J., Stein, M. B., Renna, M., Antonius, D., & Blais, M. A. (2012). The Suicide (SPI) and Violence Potential Indices (VPI) from the Personality Assessment Inventory: A preliminary exploration of validity in an outpatient psychiatric sample. *Journal of Psychopathology and Behavioral Assessment, 34*, 423–431. https://doi.org/10.1007/s10862-012-9277-6

Slavin-Mulford, J., Sinclair, S. J., Stein, M., Malone, J., Bello, I., & Blais, M. A. (2012). External validity of the Personality Assessment Inventory (PAI) in a clinical sample. *Journal of Personality Assessment, 94*(6), 593–600. https://doi.org/10.1080/00223891.2012.681817

Spitzer, R. L., & Endicott, J. (1978a). *Schedule for affective disorders and schizophrenia (SADS)*. Biometrics Research.

Spitzer, R. L., & Endicott, J. (1978b). *Schedule for affective disorders and schizophrenia–Change version (SADS-C)*. Biometrics Research.

Stedman, J. M., McGeary, C. A., & Essery, J. (2018). Current patterns of training in personality assessment during internship. *Journal of Clinical Psychology, 74*(3), 398–406. https://doi.org/10.1002/jclp.22496

Watson, D., Levin-Aspenson, H. F., Waszczuk, M. A., Conway, C. C., Dalgleish, T., Dretsch, M. N., Eaton, N. R., Forbes, M. K., Forbush, K. T., Hobbs, K. A., Michelini, G., Nelson, B. D., Sellbom, M., Slade, T., South, S. C., Sunderland, M., Waldman, I., Witthöft, M., Wright, A. G. C., . . . the HiTOP Utility Workgroup. (2022). Validity and utility of Hierarchical Taxonomy of Psychopathology (HiTOP): III. Emotional dysfunction superspectrum. *World Psychiatry, 21*(1), 26–54. https://doi.org/10.1002/wps.20943

Watson, J., & Liljequist, L. (2018). Using the Personality Assessment Inventory to identify ADHD-like symptoms. *Journal of Attention Disorders, 22*(11), 1049–1055. https://doi.org/10.1177/1087054714567133

5

Millon Clinical Multiaxial Inventory–IV (MCMI–IV) Assessment of Bipolar Spectrum Disorders

James P. Choca

While I was working at a hospital, we took turns carrying the emergency room pager. My turn was Wednesday afternoons. One such Wednesday, I headed down to the first-floor emergency room from my office on the 15th floor after the pager went off. I was shown into a small medical examining room where a man and a woman were seated. The 26-year-old man needed a shave. He wore a loud Hawaiian shirt, black pants, and loafers. The woman was more conservatively dressed in a white blouse and green skirt. The man responded to my question of how I could help by telling me that there was nothing wrong with him, but that his girlfriend insisted on his being "checked." He was hoping I would convince his girlfriend that he was OK so they could both go home. Laughing, he volunteered that he had no idea why his girlfriend thought he needed to be "checked." I did not respond and waited in silence until the girlfriend spoke.

The girlfriend explained that her boyfriend wanted to quit his job because he believed he knew more about the warehouse vehicle tires business than anyone else in the world. "The other workers in the office are morons," he interjected. According to the girlfriend, the man I will call "Don" had no savings and needed to keep working in order to eat and pay his part of their rent. He interrupted her to say that he planned to sell his car. The girlfriend continued by noting that Don wanted to start his own company but did not have any of the resources needed.

https://doi.org/10.1037/0000356-006
Psychological Assessment of Bipolar Spectrum Disorders, J. H. Kleiger and I. B. Weiner (Editors)

Visibly irritated, he told her in a loud voice that "all" he needed was to find a partner with funding, and that it would be easy money for his partner!

The girlfriend worried because Don had been sleeping only 3 or 4 hours a night and had been getting up in the early morning hours to do the laundry, clean the apartment, and even wash his car on the street. He claimed he did not need more sleep. Facing him, she pointed out that he had been getting to work late, had already been reprimanded, and could possibly be fired if he kept this up. He dismissed the idea that his job could be in jeopardy, claiming he was a most important part of the office. Looking a little embarrassed, the girlfriend told me that Don had been wanting to have sex all of the time, wanting sex so often that it had been physically painful for her. He shouted, "Aw, come on! You love it!" At home, she said, he had trouble watching TV or relaxing. Don claimed the TV was "boring! Boring! Too boring!" Turning toward him, she told him that she had trouble having a conversation with him because he wouldn't stop talking and would not listen to anything she says. Right now, she pointed out, he was not taking into account anything she was saying. She felt that he could not be doing a good job at work because he was too "hyper."

After we admitted the patient into the psychiatric ward, in what appeared to be a manic state, we learned that he had had a similar episode in the military and had received a medical discharge. Initial assessment included the Millon Clinical Multiaxial Inventory (MCMI-III; Millon, 1983). Table 5.1 shows the results of Don's MCMI-III.

FEATURES OF BIPOLARITY IN DON'S MCMI-III

In considering the issue of a bipolar spectrum disorders (BSDs), we first examine the Modifier Indexes of the MCMI-III to decide how revealing or useful the rest of the record may be. Consistent with Don's presentation, we discover a significant elevation of the Desirability Scale (Scale Y). This scale is made up of socially positive items, and the finding suggested that he was making an attempt to look his best. This finding was consistent with Don's superficial claim that there was nothing wrong with him. I am calling this claim "superficial" because, despite his assertions, he had no trouble signing himself into the hospital as a voluntary patient, suggesting that somehow he knew there was something wrong. Next, we look at the Clinical Symptom scales, where we find no elevations; it was noteworthy that there were many low raw scores indicating, once more, that Don was not endorsing any symptomatology. In my own work, I group the personality "B" scales with the Severe Personality scales because I see them as inherently more pathological than Millon's original eight types. The pattern seen with the Clinical Symptom scales was replicated in the Severe Personality section, which showed no elevations and low raw scores. Finally, we examine the Personality Style section to discover a very pronounced elevation of the Histrionic Scale (Scale 4), and a significant elevation of the Narcissistic Scale (Scale 5), both of which may reflect personality characteristics

TABLE 5.1. Don's Millon Clinical Multiaxial Inventory-III

MCMI scale	Raw score	Base rate	Elevation
1—Schizoid	0	5	
2A—Avoidant	0	5	
3—Dependent	1	12	
4—Dramatic	22	101	Very high
5—Narcissistic	15	81	High
6A—Antisocial	3	41	
7—Compulsive	14	69	
8A—Explosive	2	18	
2B—Depressive	0	5	
6B—Sadistic	2	29	
8B—Masochistic	0	5	
S—Schizotypal	0	3	
C—Borderline	1	11	
P—Paraphrenic	0	3	
A— Generalized Anxiety	0	3	
H—Somatic Symptom	0	3	
N—Bipolar Spectrum	3	39	
D—Persistent Depression	2	16	
B—Alcohol Use	1	28	
T—Drug Use	2	63	
R—Posttraumatic Stress	1	13	
SS—Schizophrenic Spectrum	2	20	
CC—Major Depression	1	11	
PP—Delusional	2	63	
X—Disclosure	54	26	
Y—Desirability	17	80	High
Z—Debasement	2	38	
V—Validity	0		

Note. MCMI = Millon Clinical Multiaxial Inventory.

associated with BSDs. An example of how I may describe this 4–5-personality pattern follows:

> Individuals with high histrionic-narcissistic scores on the MCMI have a need for attention and conspicuousness. They typically feel they are a very "special" kind of person and view themselves as intelligent, outgoing, charming, and sophisticated. Often they discuss their own abilities in an exaggerated manner, constructing rationalizations to inflate their own worth, and belittling others who refuse to enhance the image they try to project. They make good first impressions, since they are able to express their feelings, have a flair for the dramatic, and have a natural ability to draw attention to themselves. They are also colorful and may have a good sense of humor. Don is probably seen as a friendly and helpful person; he may be actively solicitous of praise and may be entertaining and somewhat seductive. However, Don is probably easily bored, and his search for approval leaves him with a somewhat undefined identity when apart from others.

In this description we see many elements related to a manic state that were obvious during the initial meeting: namely, Don's thinking he was very gifted, his high aspirations, his attempts to be charming and engaging, his emotiveness, his tendency toward easy boredom, and his annoyance when his girlfriend contradicted him.

Don had taken the MCMI-III. A scale of the new MCMI-IV (Millon et al., 2015), the Turbulent Scale (4B), did not exist at the time. This scale has eight items with adjectives such as "exciting," "energetic," "animated," "optimistic," "enthusiastic," and "vigorous." The correlation between the Turbulent Scale and the Histrionic Scale (Scale 4A) is .72 (Millon et al., 2015). Since Don had a very high elevation on the Histrionic Scale of the MCMI-III and would have been expected to endorse the descriptors noted for the Turbulent Scale, I would expect that the Turbulent Scale would be elevated if Don were to take the newer version. On previous versions of the MCMI, bipolar manic patients were found to be more histrionic, narcissistic, antisocial, and compulsive than euthymic patients (Alexander et al., 1987; Alnaes & Torgersen, 1991; Turley et al., 1992; Wetzler & Marlowe, 1993). Thus, the pattern of scores Don obtained was very similar to what the literature indicates is the typical manic profile.

BSDs AND THE MCMI-IV

The MCMI-IV consists of 195 true–false self-report items (Millon et al., 2015). Of these, I (Choca, 2021) found that 122, or 70% of the items, were taken from its predecessor, the MCMI-III (Millon, 1983). Outside of what appears in the MCMI-IV Manual, there was little published data on the newer version at the time of this writing. Because so many of the items were taken from the previous version, I have included research done with that version in this chapter.

The scale designed to test for bipolar disorders is now called the Bipolar Spectrum Scale and has 13 items. All five of the prototypal items of the MCMI-III's Bipolar Manic Scale remained in the MCMI-IV, and an item added for the Turbulent Scale has become an additional prototypal Bipolar Spectrum item. Of the eight nonprototypal bipolar items of the MCMI-III, only two remained on the MCMI-IV; the five nonprototypal items that made up the new Bipolar Spectrum Scale already existed in the MCMI-III but were assigned to other scales. The fact that these items could be so easily changed from one scale to another pointed to one of the problems with the MCMI: It has high interscale correlations, with too few items for the number of scales it offers. More specifically, counting the Grossman Facet scales, the MCMI-IV has 71 scales, leading to an uncomfortably low 2.75 items per scale. In any event, the correlation between the MCMI-IV's Bipolar Spectrum Scale and the MCMI-III's Bipolar Manic Scale is .89, a figure that is actually higher than the test–retest correlation of the MCMI-IV scale (.78; Millon et al., 2015). These data argue for the contention that the new scale is the same as its predecessor.

Millon developed the MCMI after proposing a theory of personality (Millon, 1969). I was very much taken by his original theory, which included eight personality profiles mapped out in a simple and elegant manner (see Figure 5.1).

FIGURE 5.1. Original Rendition of Millon's Personality Theory

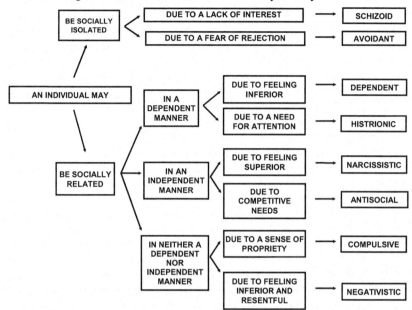

Note. Adapted from *Interpretive Guide to the Millon Clinical Multiaxial Inventory* (3rd ed., p. 59), by J. P. Choca, 2004, American Psychological Association. Copyright 2004 by the American Psychological Association.

Although there may be an infinite number of possible personality prototypes, the eight types Millon chose were profiles that were very familiar to the clinical community. His descriptions were thorough and readable. His theory included the idea that a milder and less pathological description of these personality profiles could be applied to individuals in everyday life and often represented, in fact, good coping mechanisms for the individual. For instance, the healthy correlates of histrionic, narcissistic, and compulsive styles have been repeatedly shown (e.g., Boyle & Le Déan, 2000).

After Millon became an influential member of the personality task force for the third edition of the *Diagnostic and Statistical Manual of Mental Disorders* (*DSM-III*; American Psychiatric Association, 1980), this classification system adopted much of what he had proposed. The result was that the original MCMI and the personality section of the *DSM-III* had much in common. Unfortunately, Millon became interested in adding increasing complexity to his theory in a way that made it much more intricate and pulled it away from the personality entities of our current classification system (*DSM-5*; American Psychiatric Association, 2013). Interested in explaining personality using concepts from the theory of evolution, Millon's new theory relied on the use of three domains (Replication Strategy, Survival Aim, and Adaptive Mode), in addition to eight functional and structural domains. He also added four personality styles (as described later) that are not in the *DSM-5*.

Human beings are very complex, and a good clinical theory is one that simplifies that complexity. I find it is easier to think of the dependent personality style, for instance, in terms of traits (a social person with feelings of inadequacy who tends to relate in a subordinate manner with others) than in terms of Millon's domains (an individual with *another* replication strategy and a *passive* adaptive mode and who is neutral in the Survival Aim domain, where the reader would have to understand what Millon means by each of these domains). Millon argued for the usefulness of his concepts in treatment planning, but I believe good treatment planning can be accomplished better with the simpler trait conceptualization that even our clients will be able to follow easily.

You do not have to understand Millon's theory in order to use the MCMI productively. In fact, there are indications that the MCMI does not measure Millon's theory well. For example, Piersma and his colleagues used the polarity scales that Millon created for the Millon Index of Personality Styles (MIPS; Millon et al., 1994) and correlated those values with the results of the MCMI-III administered to the same individuals. They found that approximately 60% of the time the MCMI-III did not correlate with the polarity scales of the MIPS, and that 11% of the time the correlation was actually in the opposite direction of what Millon would have predicted (Piersma et al., 2002). However, if you, my reader, have more appreciation for complexity than I do, there are excellent renditions of Millon's theory that should be pleasing to you (e.g., Grossman, 2020; Millon, 2011; Millon et al., 2015).

The greatest advantage the MCMI has over other broad-range inventories is the personality scales (Wise et al., 2010). The MCMI is the only broad-range commercially available instrument with scales that resemble the personality profiles of the *DSM-5*. (I have a computerized *DSM-5* questionnaire with both personality and clinical syndrome scales that my readers are welcome to download from https://www.choca-assessments.com/.) In the case of bipolar affective disorders, as was seen with Don, the personality scales were extremely helpful. As previously noted, the typical manic MCMI profile relies heavily on personality findings. Our experience was that once the acute problems the patient presented were more or less resolved, the person was left to cope with personality issues, personality issues that had often been associated with those problems. As Kleiger and Weiner note in the introductory chapter of this book, there is much support for the spectrum model for bipolar disorders. That model proposes that personality traits are the subclinical foundations of the clinical syndrome. The competing pathoplasty model proposes that both the personality traits and the clinical syndrome result from a common underlying substrate (Farmer & Nelson-Gray, 1990; Klein et al., 1993). Whichever turns out to be more obvious with a particular individual, the fact remains that attention should be paid to the personality of the individual.

OVERVIEW OF THE MCMI

To start with, I discuss the basic facts of the MCMI by focusing on the controversies. I should note first that the MCMI has been the instrument I have preferred using all of my professional life, and I have used it to great benefit. At Lakeside VA Hospital I gave the test, whenever possible, to every patient we took in. Being the shortest broadband self-report inventory, it did not take much time for the patient to complete, and I made every effort to have the results in the patient's chart as soon as possible. I trained the staff to look at the score table, like the one shown in Table 5.1, and abstract useful information about the patient. It is a good screening instrument that, in contrast to other tools, will almost always provide scale elevations to consider.

During the acute phase of a newly admitted individual, the usual recommendation is to be "supportive" in order to lower the amount of stress the patient is experiencing. But what does that mean? The parental-like interactions that would seem supportive to a dependent individual would be taken as abrasively condescending by a person with a narcissistic make-up; the emotional displays of acceptance that would be welcomed by the histrionic would be threatening to a person with schizoid tendencies and would appear unprofessional to the compulsive. Having a sense of the individual's personality makeup provides a handle on the approach that may be most helpful. These were relatively easy concepts to learn and use.

CONTROVERSIES SURROUNDING THE MCMI

I have already mentioned the issues I have with the increased complexity of Millon's theory. As part of the increased complexity, Millon kept adding personality prototypes (depressive, sadistic, masochistic, and turbulent). The first three of these prototypes had actually been considered and rejected by the clinical community. Another issue, that of the high interscale correlations, has also been noted.

Every scale the MCMI-IV has items that are considered "prototypical" for that scale, and items that are nonprototypical. A prototypical item is one theoretically deemed to represent the core concept of that scale. A prototypical item for the Dependent Scale of the MCMI-IV, for instance, is "I could never handle the world on my own"; the Narcissistic Scale has "I am very confident" as a prototypical item. The idea of having prototypical and nonprototypical items for each scale seems theoretically sound. What is controversial is that the test assigns 2 raw score points to the prototypical items and 1 point to the non-prototypical. Retzlaff and colleagues argued that the weighted score added complexity to the scoring system without improving the performance of the test. They showed that the correlation between the weighted raw score and an unweighted raw score was .97 (Retzlaff et al., 1990). Streiner and Miller (1989) demonstrated mathematically that the weighting could not have a significant effect.

Once the raw scores are obtained for all scales, they are transformed into base rate (BR) scores. Millon noted that the *T* score commonly used by other instruments did not take into account the prevalence of the disorder. If the

T score is set at 65 or 1.5 standard deviations above the mean, as is commonly done, it will statistically flag 8% of the population. That figure is on target for a common disorder such as depression (8.4% in the United States according to the National Institute of Mental Health [NIMH], 2022b) but will be too high for a less prevalent condition such as bipolar disorder (2.8%; NIMH, 2022a). Although the BR score idea makes sense, it presents the problem of determining the prevalence of the entity being measured. In some cases, such as those noted above, national figures may be available, even though there are no indications that Millon used such figures. Moreover, for the great majority of the MCMI scales, the national prevalence is unknown (e.g., what is the prevalence of the turbulent personality?). If the prevalence was determined using data from the normative sample, as I presume it was, then the BR scores are going to be inaccurate for any sample that is significantly different from the normative sample.

The MCMI-IV makes two adjustments to the BR scores of most of the scales by taking into account high or low scores of the Disclosure Scale (Scale X) and elevations of the Anxiety and Major Depression scales. Even if those adjustments make theoretical sense, it is not clear how the amount of the adjustment was determined. Moreover, adjustments of that kind seldom take care of the problem (a denial of psychopathology in Don's case) and cloud the findings by introducing a filter that need not be there. For myself, I would prefer if our instruments would give us the data unaltered; none of our tools can take the place of a good insightful clinician.

THE MCMI-IV AND ITS SCALES

I extracted the information that follows from the test manual (Millon et al., 2015). The MCMI-IV was normed with 1,547 psychiatric participants. In contrast to the sample used for earlier MCMIs, the normative sample for the MCMI-IV happily approximated the U. S. census data. With the exception of the Compulsive Scale (Scale 7), all of the MCMI-IV scales have an acceptable internal consistency level (a Cronbach's α above .7). Test–retest reliability was invariably high. Concurrent validation data against the Brief Symptom Inventory (BSI; Derogatis, 1993) were as high as .77 for the Persistent Depression Scale (Scale D) of the MCMI-IV and the DEP of the BSI, and as low as −.26 for the corresponding compulsive scales. In most cases, even when the correlation was high with the corresponding scales, similarly high correlations were found between the BSI scale and other MCMI-IV scales. The DEP scale of the BSI, for instance, also had a high correlation with the Melancholic (Scale 2B; .73), Borderline (Scale C; .70), Major Depression (Scale CC; .75), Masochistic (Scale 8B; .65), and Avoidant (Scale 2A; .60) scales. There was also concurrent validity against the Minnesota Multiphasic Personality Inventory–2–Restructured Form (MMPI-2-RF; Ben-Porath & Tellegen, 2008/2011). Those values went as high as .68 for the Melancholic (Scale 2B) and Low Positive

Emotions (RC2) of the MMPI-2-RF, and as low as .01 for the Persistent Depression (Scale CC) and Hypomanic Activation (RC9) scale of the MMPI-2-RF.

Once more, as was the case with the BSI, correlations of similar values were shown between the MMPI-2-RF scales and multiple MCMI-IV scales. I would remind you that concurrent validation data simply tell us whether the two scales are measuring a similar construct and do not indicate which of the two scales is doing a better job. It is obvious, for instance, that the two compulsive scales of the MCMI-IV and the BSI are very different, but the data do not tell us which one is better. In this case, the difference between these two compulsive scales may be due to the MCMI-IV scale measuring compulsive personality traits while the BSI scale may be measuring the pathological symptoms of an obsessive–compulsive disorder. The concurrent validity data do suggest that the MCMI-IV scales are not very discriminating; they are not "pure" in that their elevation may be indicating a number of different attributes or disorders. The MCMI-IV may be seen as sensitive in that it easily elevates with psychopathology, but as lacking specificity in that an elevation of one scale may not be very indicative of a particular syndrome.

As opposed to other instruments of its kind, the MCMI-IV offers diagnostic validity statistics. Offering such statistics is a very laudable effort because it tells us how well the instrument actually measures what it was designed to measure, and it is a risky effort that other instruments have not been willing to make. I should note, however, that the way it was done for the MCMI-IV was not "blind" and, consequently, the results have to be taken with much caution. The way it was done was by clinicians rating to what extent the MCMI-IV scores agreed with the *DSM* diagnosis or—in the absence of a corresponding *DSM* diagnosis—to what extent the MCMI-IV scores reflected a dysfunction.

To review what is meant by diagnostic statistics, the *sensitivity* of a scale is the true-positive value or the chance that the scale is elevated when the attribute is present. The lowest sensitivity value of the MCMI-IV given in the Manual (Millon et al., 2015) was obtained with the Masochistic Scale (Scale 8B; value: .22), and the most sensitive sale was Major Depression (Scale CC; value: .83). The Bipolar Spectrum Scale (Scale N) had acceptable sensitivity, elevating 58% of the time when the disorder was present. *Specificity* is the true-negative value, the percentage of the time the scale was not elevated when the attribute was not present. The most specific of the MCMI-IV scales was the Schizophrenic Spectrum Scale (Scale SS; .95) and the least was Generalized Anxiety (Scale A; .48). The Bipolar Spectrum Scale (Scale N) was not elevated 79% of the time when the bipolar disorder was not present.

We can compare those values from the manual to those reported by Mohammadi and his group (Mohammadi et al., 2022) in Iran. The study examined the personality clusters and clinical syndromes obtained through a structured clinical interview and the scales of the MCMI-IV with recently diagnosed psychiatric patients. The Kappa agreement ranged from .23 to .39. Sensitivity ranged from 23.08 on the Somatic Symptom Scale (Scale H) to 66.7

in Alcohol Use (Scale B). Specificity ranged from 72.52 in Generalized Anxiety (Scale A) to 95.61 for Schizophrenic Spectrum (Scale SS). The authors concluded that the overall validity indexes had improved from previous versions of the test but that the validity of some clinical scales was not yet acceptable.

The MCMI-IV includes the eight original personality scales (Schizoid [Scale 1], Avoidant [Scale 2A], Dependent [Scale 3], Histrionic [Scale 4A], Narcissistic [Scale 5], Antisocial [Scale 6A], Compulsive [Scale 7], and Negativistic [Scale 8A]). These scales were designed to measure personality patterns, and almost everyone taking the MCMI will elevate at least one of these basic personality scales (perhaps indicating they have a personality). A mistake that has been made with the MCMI in the past is to see an elevation of one or more of the personality scales as indicative of a personality disorder. The determination that the person suffers from a personality disorder must be made by the clinician by taking into account the level of functioning of the individual when the person is not acutely disturbed. An individual with a schizoid personality may have traits that do not interfere with their daily functioning. But if that same individual was struggling in their career and with their adjustment to the environment, they might have a personality disorder that is impairing their daily functioning. Acute symptomatology often exacerbates personality traits: A depressed individual may appear more schizoid, or dependent, than they were premorbidly; a manic person will seem more histrionic or narcissistic. The determination of how functional the individual's personality is can be made during the acute phase by taking a careful history and talking to relatives or close friends (see Choca, 2004, for more information about this issue).

As noted, with the further developments of his theory, Millon added four personality prototypes (Melancholic [Scale 2B], Turbulent [Scale 4B], Sadistic [Scale 6B], and Masochistic [Scale 8B]). The MCMI-IV has three scales to measure severe personality disturbances (Schizotypal [Scale S], Borderline [Scale C], and Paranoid [Scale P]). There are seven clinical syndrome scales (Generalized Anxiety [Scale A], Somatic Symptom [Scale H], Bipolar Spectrum [Scale N], Persistent Depression [Scale D], Alcohol Use [Scale B], Drug Use [Scale T], and Post-Traumatic Stress [Scale R]) and three severe clinical syndrome scales (Schizophrenic Spectrum [Scale SS], Major Depression [Scale CC], and Delusional [Scale PP]).

The test has five Modifier Indices or validity scales. The Debasement Scale (Scale Z) is the other side of the coin from the Desirability Scale (Scale Y), a scale that was elevated in Don's profile as he was seen to be endorsing more socially desirable items than the average person. To elevate the Debasement Scale an individual would have to endorse more socially undesirable items. The Invalidity Scale (Scale V) is made up of three items that are very unlikely to be true, such as claiming to have flown across the Atlantic 30 times during the last year. The Inconsistency Scale (Scale W) has 25 item pairs that are so highly correlated that they are expected to be answered in the same manner; this scale is mostly used to identify random responses. The Disclosure Scale (Scale X) is the sum of endorsements in 121 items of the personality scales. A low Disclosure Index suggests underreporting while a high Disclosure Index may indicate a tendency to exaggerate attributes or symptomatology. A note of caution: Working in a psychiatric ward, I sometimes obtained results with elevated Debasement and Disclosure scales that would ordinarily be indicative of exaggeration but that were valid indications of a very disturbed individual.

As already noted, individuals in the manic phase of a bipolar disorder typically elevate personality scales on the MCMI. At least in theory, such persons would also elevate the Bipolar Spectrum Scale. In practice, that scale may not elevate because the individual is in denial of the symptomatology, as was the case with Don, or because the person may not be aware of the symptoms. The goal of the therapy should be, in part, to increase awareness and responsiveness, so that the person comes in for treatment as soon as the symptoms start.

A self-report questionnaire such as the MCMI is likely to be more sensitive during the depressive phase of the disorder than the manic phase. During the depressive phase, the individual is more likely to be aware of the symptoms and to endorse the appropriate items in the inventory. In the case of the MCMI-IV, the scales that measure depressive symptoms and that may be elevated include the Melancholic (Scale 2B), Masochistic (Scale 8B), Persistent Depression (Scale D), and Major Depression (Scale CC) scales. Given the nature of a depressive episode, there may be personality scales that may be temporarily elevated during the depressive phase of a bipolar disorder, as was the case with the manic phase. Those scales may include Schizoid (Scale 1) due to the isolationism, Avoidant (Scale 2A) due to the tension and anxiety, and Dependent (Scale 3) due to feelings of inadequacy. As was mentioned with regard to the manic phase, the clinician will have to assess whether any of the personality attributes shown by the inventory were present prior to the onset of the bipolar disorder, and constituted a premorbid exacerbating factor.

Forty-five Grossman Facet scales were developed to help the clinician understand what may be contributing to the elevation of personality scales. There are three Facet scales for each personality scale that, in theory, highlight the aspects that contributed to the elevation of the personality scale. For instance, the Grossman Facet scales for the Schizoid Personality are Interpersonally Unengaged, Meager Content, and Temperamentally Apathetic. One problem with these scales is that, in order to have enough items, Grossman added items that were not in the parent scale. For instance, of the nine items of the Meager Content Facet Scale, only two are items of the Schizoid Personality Scale. At the very least, what that means is that there are many other personality styles or emotional disorders that are marked by meagerness of content. And, since the facets supposedly came from Millon's definitions of the different styles, the fact that Grossman had to repeatedly go beyond the items of the parent scale actually questions the usefulness of Millon's description. I personally do not pay attention to the Facet scales but some clinicians have found them useful (e.g., Loinaz et al., 2012).

CONCLUDING REMARKS

Different clinical sites have different populations, needs, and requirements. During the years I worked at a Veterans Administration medical center, the MCMI served me well as a brief measure of psychopathology. After I left the VA, doing full case diagnostic work in my private practice, most of the patients I saw were interested in the test results and were very willing to spend time completing questionnaires. So, if I spaced the questionnaires out so that they did not become cumbersome, I could use more than one broad-range instrument.

Each of the broad-range instruments has its own characteristics, and having the results from more than one can be useful. At times the results supported each other. When two bipolar scales are both elevated, the finding increased my confidence in the diagnosis; when only one was elevated, I had to consider the difference between the two scales in order to interpret the findings accurately. Finally, the results of the broad-range instruments can be supplemented by the results of questionnaires designed to measure only one type of pathology (e.g., depression, anxiety, eating disorder, post-traumatic stress) that can add substantially to what is known about the individual.

As Don was treated and the manic behavior receded, the narcissistic elements shown as part of his original presentation receded, and what was left was a clearly histrionic personality style. His presentation then was typically dramatic, emotional, and attention seeking. In his case, his personality was not only functional but was actually one of his biggest assets. It was this engaging, sociable, and affable personality that allowed him to be as effective as he was in the business of selling warehouse vehicle tires. Happily, that allowed for the therapy to emphasize the detection of hypomanic behaviors or depressive feelings that represented the beginning of another episode.

Additionally, we were able to examine the presumed psychodynamics of a bipolar disorder during his treatment. Although the exact neuropathology is still to be found, current thinking highlights the role that neurochemicals play in bipolar mood fluctuations. Without contradicting the validity of that position, it is possible to also consider the psychological aspects of the disorder. Traditional psychodynamics proposed that the individual had grown up to believe in having an outstanding destiny. From this point of view, the manic behavior represents the individual's attempt to reach that goal; the depressive feelings arise from a realization that the outstanding goals may not be reachable. Don was able to discuss the expectations that his parents had of their only child and their disappointment when his achievements turned out to be more modest than expected.

To conclude, I hope I have been able to show the many advantages that the MCMI-IV may have as a screening tool or as part of a full evaluation of an individual.

REFERENCES

Alexander, G. E., Choca, J. P., DeWolfe, A. S., Bresolin, L. B., Johnson, J. E., & Ostrow, D. G. (1987, August). *Interaction between personality and mood in unipolar and bipolar patients* [Paper presentation]. 95th Annual Convention of the American Psychological Association, New York, NY, United States.

Alnaes, R., & Torgersen, S. (1991). Personality and personality disorders among patients with various affective disorders. *Journal of Personality Disorders, 5*(2), 107–121. https://doi.org/10.1521/pedi.1991.5.2.107

American Psychiatric Association. (1980). *Diagnostic and statistical manual of mental disorders* (3rd ed.).

American Psychiatric Association. (2013). *Diagnostic and statistical manual of mental disorders* (5th ed.).

Ben-Porath, Y. S., & Tellegen, A. (2011). *MMPI-2-RF: Manual for administration, scoring and interpretation.* University of Minnesota Press. (Original work published 2008)

Boyle, G. J., & Le Déan, L. (2000). Discriminant validity of the illness behavior questionnaire and Millon Clinical Multiaxial Inventory–III in a heterogeneous sample of psychiatric outpatients. *Journal of Clinical Psychology, 56*(6), 779–791. https://doi.org/10.1002/(SICI)1097-4679(200006)56:6<779::AID-JCLP7>3.0.CO;2-7

Choca, J. P. (2004). *Interpretive guide to the Millon Clinical Multiaxial Inventory* (3rd ed.). American Psychological Association.

Choca, J. P. (2021). Millon Clinical Multiaxial Inventory (MCMI-IV) for assessing disordered thought and perception. In I. B. Weiner & J. H. Kleiger (Eds.), *Psychological assessment of disordered thinking and perception* (pp. 99–113). American Psychological Association. https://doi.org/10.1037/0000245-007

Derogatis, L. R. (1993). *BSI Brief Symptom Inventory: Administration, scoring, and procedure manual* (4th ed.). National Computer Systems.

Farmer, R., & Nelson-Gray, R. (1990). Personality disorders and depression: Hypothetical relations, empirical findings, and methodological considerations. *Clinical Psychology Review, 10*(4), 453–476. https://doi.org/10.1016/0272-7358(90)90048-F

Grossman, S. (2020). The Millon Clinical Multiaxial Inventory–IV. In M. Sellborn & J. A. Suhr (Eds.), *The Cambridge handbook of clinical assessment* (pp. 249–262). Cambridge University Press.

Klein, M. H., Wonderlich, S., & Shea, M. T. (1993). Models of relationships between personality and depression: Toward a framework for theory and research. In M. H. Klein, D. J. Kupfer, & M. T. Shea (Eds.), *Personality and depression* (pp. 1–54). Guilford Press.

Loinaz, I., Ortiz-Tallo, M., & Ferragut, M. (2012). MCMI-III Grossman personality facets among partner-violent men in prison. *International Journal of Clinical and Health Psychology, 12*(3), 389–404.

Millon, T. (1969). *Modern psychopathology: A biosocial approach to maladaptive learning and functioning.* W. B. Saunders.

Millon, T. (1983). *Millon Clinical Multiaxial Inventory manual* (3rd ed.). National Computer Systems.

Millon, T. (2011). *Disorders of the personality: Introducing a DSM/ICD spectrum from normal to abnormal.* Wiley. https://doi.org/10.1002/9781118099254

Millon, T., Grossman, S., & Millon, C. (2015). *MCMI-IV manual.* NCS Pearson.

Millon, T., Weiss, L., Millon, C., & Davis, R. D. (1994). *MIPS: Millon index of personality styles.* Psychological Corporation.

Mohammadi, M. R., Hooshyari, Z., Delavar, A., Amanat, M., Mohammadi, A., Abasi, I., & Salehi, M. (2022). Diagnostic validity of Millon Clinical Multiaxial Inventory–IV (MCMI-IV). *Current Psychology,* 249–262. https://doi.org/10.1007/s12144-022-02972-9

National Institute of Mental Health. (2022a). *Prevalence of bipolar disorder.* https://www.nimh.nih.gov/health/statistics/bipolar-disorder

National Institute of Mental Health. (2022b). *Prevalence of major depression.* https://www. nimh.nih.gov/health/statistics/major-depression

Piersma, H. L., Ohnishi, H., Lee, D. J., & Metcalfe, W. E. (2002). An empirical evaluation of Millon's dimensional polarities. *Journal of Psychopathology and Behavioral Assessment, 24*(3), 151–158. https://doi.org/10.1023/A:1016006616346

Retzlaff, P. D., Sheehan, E. P., & Lorr, M. (1990). MCMI-II scoring: Weighted and unweighted algorithms. *Journal of Personality Assessment, 55*(1–2), 219–223. https:// doi.org/10.1080/00223891.1990.9674061

Streiner, D. L., & Miller, H. R. (1989). The MCMI-II: How much better than the MCMI? *Journal of Personality Assessment, 53*(1), 81–84. https://doi.org/10.1207/s15327752 jpa5301_9

Turley, B., Bates, G. W., Edwards, J., & Jackson, H. J. (1992). MCMI-II personality disorders in recent-onset bipolar disorders. *Journal of Clinical Psychology, 48*(3), 320–329. https://doi.org/10.1002/1097-4679(199205)48:3<320::AID-JCLP2270480309>3.0. CO;2-F

Wetzler, S., & Marlowe, D. B. (1993). The diagnosis and assessment of depression, mania, and psychosis by self-report. *Journal of Personality Assessment, 60*(1), 1–31. https:// doi.org/10.1207/s15327752jpa6001_1

Wise, E. A., Streiner, D. L., & Walfish, S. (2010). A review and comparison of the reliabilities of the MMPI-2, MCMI-III, and PAI presented in their respective test manuals. *Measurement and Evaluation in Counseling and Development, 42*(4), 246–254. https://doi.org/10.1177/0748175609354594

6

SPECTRA Assessment of Bipolar Spectrum Disorders

Mark A. Blais and Samuel Justin Sinclair

Our conceptualization of psychopathology is evolving. While the fifth edition of the American Psychiatric Association's (2022) *Diagnostic and Statistical Manual of Mental Disorders* (5th ed., text rev.; *DSM-5-TR*) categorical depiction of mental disorders as distinct, bounded entities dominates clinical practice, contemporary research has produced an appealing alternative model. Whether measured as discrete disorders or continuous dimensions, psychopathology demonstrates substantial covariation and comorbidity. Emerging research over the last several decades has shown that the observed comorbidity reflects a few broad, higherorder spectra that give rise to a wide range of mental health conditions. The most widely replicated of these contemporary models organizes psychopathology into three broad spectra, or dimensions: Internalizing, Externalizing, and Reality Impairing (Kotov et al., 2011; Krueger, 1999; Krueger & Markon, 2006; Wright et al., 2013). The tridimensional model offers an empirically based framework for conceptualizing and assessing a wide range of mental disorders that is both compelling and parsimonious. SPECTRA: Indices of Psychopathology (SPECTRA; Blais & Sinclair, 2018) is a broadband assessment inventory based on the tridimensional hierarchical model of psychopathology. SPECTRA data offer assessment psychologists valuable and unique information to supplement and complement data from existing instruments.

An exciting although somewhat controversial finding from this research is the presence of an overarching general psychopathology factor called the P-factor (Smith et al., 2020). The P-factor appears to capture an individual's vulnerability to developing any and all forms of psychopathology (Caspi et al., 2014; Lahey et al., 2012). The P-factor has been widely replicated in studies using diverse

https://doi.org/10.1037/0000356-007
Psychological Assessment of Bipolar Spectrum Disorders, J. H. Kleiger and I. B. Weiner (Editors)

samples and measurement methods (e. g., *DSM* diagnoses, psychological tests, and symptoms/items; Smith et al., 2020), and it has been shown to be stable over time (Snyder et al., 2017). Conceptually, the P-factor is similar to Spearman's G-factor of global intelligence (Spearman, 1904). As the G-factor reflects a more global marker of cognitive ability, the P-factor similarly seems to represent an overall susceptibility (or vulnerability) to any form of psychopathology. Individuals with a high P-factor suffer more severe and persistent life impairment, greater comorbidity and relapse rates, have greater neurocognitive impairment, and are prone to experiencing a suboptimal or atypical response to standard treatments (Caspi et al., 2014; Lahey et al., 2012).

While there is solid empirical support for the presence of the P-factor (for a review, see Smith et al., 2020), there is still considerable debate as to the substantive meaning of P (Fried et al., 2021). This debate notwithstanding, Smith et al. (2020) argued that psychological assessment would benefit from instruments that assess the P-factor. While some instruments, including the Minnesota Multiphasic Personality Inventory–2–Restructured Form (MMPI-2-RF; Ben-Porath & Tellegen, 2008) and Minnesota Multiphasic Personality Inventory–3 (MMPI-3; Ben-Porath & Tellegen, 2020), have scales measuring the higher order dimensions of Internalizing, Externalizing, and Thought Dysfunction, only SPECTRA has a dedicated P-factor measure.

SPECTRA is a 96-item broadband psychological inventory that was designed to assess psychopathology at multiple levels of the tridimensional model hierarchy. At the narrowest level, 12 SPECTRA clinical scales measure the symptomatic expression of Depression (DEP), Anxiety (ANX), Social Anxiety (SOC), Post-Traumatic Stress (PTS), Alcohol Problems (ALC), Drug Problems (DRG), Severe Aggression (AGG), Antisocial Behavior (ANTI), Psychosis (PSY), Paranoid Ideation (PAR), Manic Activity (MAN), and Grandiosity (GRA). At the Spectra level, the clinical scales organize into three Higher-Order domains: Internalizing (DEP, ANX, SOC, and PTS), Externalizing (DRG, ALC, ANTI, and AGG) and Reality Impairing (PSY, PAR, MAN, and GRA). The Spectra-level scales are formed by adding up the raw scores of the four associated clinical scales. For example, the Internalizing Spectra scale (INT-Spectra) is the sum of the raw scores of items making up the four internalizing clinical scales (DEP, ANX, SOC, and PTS), converted to a *T* score based on the normative sample. At the broadest level of assessment, the three Spectra Scales (Internalizing, Externalizing, and Reality Impairing) combine to form the General Psychopathology Index (GPI), a global measure of psycho-pathological burden. The hierarchical dimensional structure of SPECTRA's clinical scales can be found in the professional manual (Blais & Sinclair, 2018; see also Blais, Stein, et al. 2021).

SPECTRA also contains three Supplemental scales measuring cognitive complaints (COG), psychosocial functioning (PF), and suicidal ideation (SUI). The COG scale measures subjective cognitive difficulties impacting daily func-tioning. The PF scale measures well-being, self-efficacy, social support, and access to basic needs (see Ro & Clark, 2009). The SUI scale assesses suicidal ideation, an important component of any clinical evaluation. Finally, SPECTRA has two profile validity indicators, the Infrequency scale (INF) and the Profile Classification Index (PCI). The INF scale assesses idiosyncratic responding and is useful in identifying careless, random, or confused response styles. In turn, the PCI provides information on symptom overreporting.

The professional manual (Blais & Sinclair, 2018) presents substantial evidence of construct validity for all SPECTRA scales. For example, the 12 SPECTRA clinical scales had an average correlation of 0.67 with matched Personality Assessment Inventory (PAI; Morey, 1991) Full Scales (range of correlation r 0.33–0.87; median r = 0.67) and 0.68 for matched PAI Sub-Scales (range of r 0.43–0.88; median r = 0.70). Further, a recent study (Blais, Stein et al., 2021) showed that the SPECTRA clinical and higher order scales had significant and meaningful correlations, with a wide range of external (nontest) criteria. Finally, construct validity and sensitivity to change were also recently supported in an inpatient psychiatric sample (Sinclair et al., 2022).

SPECTRA INTERPRETATION

SPECTRA profile analysis takes a somewhat different approach from most multiscale inventories. We recommend that SPECTRA findings be interpreted moving down the assessment hierarchy from broad to narrow. Figure 6.1 illustrates SPECTRA's hierarchical approach to assessment and measurement.

FIGURE 6.1. *SPECTRA*'s Hierarchical Assessment of Psychopathology

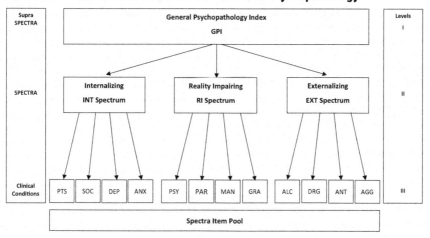

Note. GPI = general psychopathology index; INT = internalizing; RI = reality impairing; EXT = externalizing; PTS = post traumatic stress; SOC = social anxiety; DEP = depression; ANX = anxiety; PSY = psychosis; PAR = paranoid ideation; MAN = manic activity; ALC = alcohol problems; DRG = drug problems; ANTI = antisocial behavior; AGG = severe aggression; GRA = grandiose ideation. Adapted from *SPECTRA: Indices of Psychopathology: Professional Manual* (p. 2), by M. A. Blais and S. J. Sinclair, 2018, Psychological Assessment Resources. Copyright 2018 by Psychological Assessment Resources, Inc. Adapted with permission.

After inspecting the validity indicators (INF and PCI), clinicians should consider the GPI, as this reveals the patient's overall burden of psychiatric illness. The GPI has important implications for treatment and prognosis. Consistent with its conceptual model, the GPI and Spectra scales should be interpreted dimensionally, much like an IQ score, without concern for arbitrary cut scores (T score > 69). For example, GPI or Spectra scale T scores of 45 or below are considered Low, 46–56 are Normal, 57–63 are Mild, 64–69 are Moderate, 70–89 are Severe, and 90 or above are Extreme. This recommendation is especially relevant to the assessment of bipolar spectrum disorders, as identifying milder (subclinical) presentations increases the likelihood that patients will receive appropriate treatment in a timely manner (Angst, 2007).

Next, the Spectra level Internalizing (INT), Externalizing (EXT), and Reality Impairing (RI) scales should be reviewed. The patient's standing on these scales (dimensions of psychopathology) identifies their primary area of psychiatric difficulty. Like the GPI, Spectra scores should also be interpreted as fully dimensional. When a single Spectra is prominent in a profile, it indicates a broad liability for symptoms, syndromes, and conditions associated with that dimension. For example, a single prominent elevation of the EXT scale would suggest the presence of a wide range of signs and symptoms associated with behavioral dysregulation, impaired self-control, and hostility.

When multiple Spectra scales are elevated, it indicates a more complicated clinical presentation, with symptoms spanning multiple dimensions of psychopathology. Such complex clinical presentations often require an intensive multimodal approach to treatment. Focusing clinical interpretation (and assessment) at the Spectra level transforms troublesome comorbidity and disorder heterogeneity into valuable clinical information. Comorbidity is most common among disorders within the same spectra, such as anxiety and depression (Krueger & Markon, 2006), so most comorbid conditions will contribute to the same Spectra level score. The impact of intradisorder heterogeneity (i.e., disorders like depression which can be composed of different combinations of *DSM* symptoms) is also minimized, as all configurations of the disorder, regardless of their symptom composition, are integrated into the Internalizing Spectra scale. Likewise, subclinical conditions (i.e., conditions with symptom counts falling below the *DSM* diagnostic threshold but which are associated with meaningful impairment) also contribute to Spectra-level scores, rather than being overlooked or discounted (Hyman, 2011) as unimportant. These features combine to make Spectra-level scores important for assessing the complexity and primary nature (cognitive, affective, or behavioral) of psychopathology and potential treatment options.

Last, reviewing the 12 clinical scales using a dimensional perspective provides a more comprehensive representation of the patient's current symptomatic presentation at the level of each clinical syndrome. The clinical scales provide important information regarding immediate primary treatment targets and are the most direct reflection of the patient's current experience of their psychiatric condition. This information is often easier to present to patients, treating clinicians, or family members when feedback is requested. While not intended to specifically measure *DSM-5* disorders, many of the concurrent validity scales used in SPECTRA's development were selected from Section III, Emerging Measures and Models, of the *DSM-5* (American Psychiatric Association, 2013). Those validity correlations presented in the professional manual (p. 53) show that the SPECTRA clinical scales are meaningfully associated with their corresponding *DSM-5* disorders, thus allowing clinicians to infer potential *DSM* diagnoses if desired.

The SPECTRA profile analysis concludes with a review of the three Supplemental scales: Cognitive Complaints (COG), PF, and Suicidal Ideation (SUI). SPECTRA's COG and PF scales provide valuable information regarding the patient's perceived functional capacity, quality of life, and suicide risk. In addition to informing care, the COG and PF scales can also serve as non-symptom-based measures for monitoring treatment progress and considering other potential clinical referrals (e.g., neuropsychological testing).

BIPOLAR DISORDER AND PSYCHIATRIC NOSOLOGY

Since Kraepelin (1886/1921) first described manic-depressive illness as a condition with alternating periods of euphoria, dysphoria, irritability, mental and physical acceleration, and impaired thought quality, psychiatry has struggled to successfully classify it within a categorical diagnostic system. Debate continues over whether it is best classified as a mood disorder or as a schizophrenia spectrum disorder. The identification of "soft" bipolar presentations (i.e., other specified bipolar disorder, cyclothymia, bipolar II disorder) brought more confusion by raising the possibility of a spectrum of bipolar conditions, all having the same underlying pathophysiology, but differing in severity (Hafeman et al., 2016; see also the Introduction in this volume). Likewise, given that bipolar disorders involve dysregulation of mood, cognition, and behavior, situating it within contemporary dimensional models of psychopathology has also proven challenging (see Forbes et al., 2021). However, despite its phenotypic complexity, advances in genomics, neuroimaging, cognitive science, and epidemiology have identified strong associations between bipolar illness and other schizophrenic spectrum (reality impairing) conditions (Cuthbert & Morris, 2021; see also Chapter 16 in this volume). Regardless, a condition as complex and variable as bipolar illness presents significant challenges for clinical assessment.

THE SPECTRA ASSESSMENT OF BIPOLAR SPECTRUM DISORDERS

The development of SPECTRA was guided by two primary goals: accurately capturing the tridimensional hierarchical structure of psychopathology and maintaining clinical utility. Toward these ends, SPECTRA includes two scales reflecting the Reality Impairing aspects of bipolar disorders—Manic Activation

(MAN) and Grandiose Ideation (GRA). Factor analytic findings show that these scales consistently load with the Psychosis (PSY) and Paranoid Ideation (PAR) scales to form SPECTRA's Reality Impairing Spectra scale (Blais & Sinclair, 2018; Blais, Stein, et al., 2021). The MAN scale taps the mental and physical acceleration associated with manic episodes (e.g., "Recently I've had so much energy, I get hyper or irritable"), while GRA taps the expansive and grandiose quality of manic thinking (e.g., "I am destined to accomplish amazing things"). A study of SPECTRA's external correlates showed the MAN scale to be significantly correlated with a history of psychotic experiences, paranoid ideation, manic episodes, and suicide attempts, while both MAN and GRA scales were associated with a history of taking mood-stabilizing medication, nonsuicidal self-injury, and a history of arrest (Blais, Sinclair, et al., 2021).

As is true for most broadband assessment inventories, SPECTRA's clinical utility comes mostly from profile analysis rather than from a review of isolated scales. Profile analysis is especially important when assessing patients for bipolar spectrum disorders as they can experience concurrent dysregulation of mood, behavior, and cognition. For example, it is not uncommon for patients with bipolar disorders to experience symptoms of both depression and mania simulations, as in a mixed state, or report significant residual symptoms of depression and anxiety between full-blown episodes (Perlis, 2010). Likewise, the grandiose ideation, distractibility, and impulsive behavior common in bipolar spectrum conditions can result in a host of life-complicating outcomes, such as substance abuse, legal difficulties, and aggressive behavior. Given its evaluated lifetime risk for suicide, suicide assessment is crucial in evaluating bipolar patients. Clearly, patients with bipolar spectrum disorders are likely to generate complex assessment profiles featuring a wide range of diverse symptoms.

Group Differences

The Psychological Evaluation and Research Laboratory (PEaRL) at Massachusetts General Hospital maintains an institutional review board (IRB)–approved de-identified database that currently has SPECTRA data from over 200 clinical assessments. Using these data, we compared SPECTRA profiles for 25 patients with a well-established preassessment diagnosis of bipolar disorders and 151 patients without bipolar disorders (patients with provisional diagnoses were not included). Table 6.1 presents the mean SPECTRA profiles (in T scores) for both groups.

As Table 6.1 illustrates, patients with a bipolar diagnosis scored significantly higher on three of the four higher order Spectra scales (GPI, EXT, and RI), with effect sizes in the small-to-medium range. Starting at the broadest assessment level, the group with bipolar disorder reported a higher overall burden of psychopathology than the group without bipolar disorder, GPI (T scores 63 and 58, respectively, Cohen's $d = 0.48$). This finding captures the severity, chronicity, heightened morbidity, and all-cause mortality associated with the condition (Angst, 2007). The group with bipolar disorder also scored significantly

TABLE 6.1. Mean SPECTRA Clinical and Spectra Scale Scores for Bipolar and Nonbipolar Patients Evaluated at the PEaRL

Scale	BPI	Non-BPI	Sig.*	d**
GPI	63	58	Sig.	.48
INT	66	66	NS	—
EXT	63	55	Sig.	.66
RI	55	50	Sig.	.46
DEP	65	68	NS	—
ANX	69	65	NS	—
SOC	59	63	NS	—
PTS	63	60	NS	—
ALC	58	52	Sig.	.43
DRG	61	50	Sig.	.81
AGG	55	54	NS	—
ANTI	63	55	Sig.	.60
PSY	54	51	NS	—
PAR	52	51	NS	—
MAN	60	49	Sig.	.93
GRA	50	47	NS	—
COG	70	72	NS	—
PF	38	41	NS	—
SUI	56	57	NS	—

Note. BPI = bipolar Dx (n = 25); Non-BPI = other Dx (n = 151); PEaRL = Psychological Evaluation and Research Laboratory; GPI = General Psychopathology Index; NS = nonsignificant; INT = Internalizing; EXT = Externalizing; RI = Reality Impairing; DEP = Depression; ANX = Anxiety; SOC = Social Anxiety; PTS = Post Traumatic Stress; ALC = Alcohol Problems; DRG = Drug Problems; AGG = Severe Aggression; ANTI = Antisocial Behavior; PSY = Psychosis; PAR = Paranoid Ideation; MAN = Manic Activity; GRA = Grandiosity; COG = Cognitive; PF = Psychosocial Functioning; SUI = Suicidal Ideation.
*Sig = significantly different mean scores (p < .05).   **Cohen's *d* effect size.

higher on the RI and EXT Spectra scales with effect sizes of 0.46 and 0.66, respectively. The group's highest Spectra score was on the INT scale (*T* score of 66). While not significantly different from patients without bipolar disorder, this points to the prominent role of depressive and anxiety-related symptoms in the bipolar presentation. These Spectra-level findings reflect the wide range of dysregulation associated with bipolar spectrum disorders (affective, cognitive, and behavioral). And while affective (internalizing) symptoms are very prominent, what seems to distinguish bipolar patients from others is their degree of behavioral and cognitive dysregulation.

At the narrowest assessment level, four of the 12 clinical scales were also found to be significantly different between the two groups: MAN (d = 0.93), DRG (d = 0.81), ANTI (d = 0.60), and ALC (d = 0.43). Both the MAN and DRG scales achieved effect sizes within the large range, suggesting these are the most distinctive SPECTRA features of the bipolar group. It is informative that three of these four clinical scales (ALC, DRG, and ANTI) capture externalizing psychopathology. This finding highlights the diagnostic importance (and life-disrupting impact) of the impulsive/disinhibited behavior so common to bipolar spectrum patients (Alloy et al., 2012). However, as with the Spectra-level findings, the bipolar group's highest elevations came on the Internalizing clinical scales DEP ($T = 65$) and ANX ($T = 69$). While anxiety is not part of the *DSM-5* bipolar diagnostic criteria, some have argued it is a core feature of bipolarity (see Phelps, 2016; see also the Introduction in this volume). Clinicians focusing exclusively on high point-scale elevations at both the Spectra and clinical scale levels might miss the distinguishing features of bipolar spectrum disorders.

The Supplemental scales show that the group with bipolar disorder reported considerable cognitive difficulties (COG $T = 70$) and weak PF ($T = 38$). While not differing from those of the group without bipolar disorder, these Supplemental scale findings document the broad range of impairment associated with a bipolar diagnosis. Reviewing these scales allows the clinician to assess functional impairment apart from symptom severity, providing a more complete picture of the patient's current life situation. The final Supplemental scales SUI ($T = 56$) was not especially elevated in this sample, but as should be obvious, assessing suicide risk is an important component of all clinical evaluations.

Case Example

Michael is a 24-year-old college student who took medical leave during his sophomore year due to emerging mental health problems. Initially diagnosed with depression, he was treated with medication only. Despite some improvement, two attempts to return to school were unsuccessful. Each time, he became withdrawn, missed classes, and engaged in binge drinking. A psychologist, new to his care, referred him to our clinic for diagnostic clarity and treatment recommendations. SPECTRA was given as part of a comprehensive psychological and neurocognitive test battery.[1]

Figure 6.2 presents Michael's SPECTRA Hierarchical Interpretation Worksheet. We recommend clinicians use the worksheet, which can be reproduced from Appendix E in the professional manual (Blais & Sinclair, 2018, p. 88), as they learn SPECTRA to help maintain fidelity with the measurement model. A review of Michael's Validity Indices shows that both INF and PCI were "Acceptable" indicating that clinical interpretation can proceed. SPECTRA profile interpretation begins with the GPI, the broadest level of assessment. The GPI captures global psychiatric severity, chronicity, and burden of illness. This information helps inform treatment recommendations (e.g., level of care, intensity, and duration) and prognosis. Michael's GPI score fell within the moderate range ($T = 68$), his GPI score surpassed that of 81% of patients evaluated at the PEaRL. A score within this range is associated with significant psychiatric burden, chronicity, and functional impairment. Moderate-range GPI scores also suggest an increased risk for relapse and the potential for a suboptimal or atypical response to standard treatments. Furthermore, a GPI score at the upper end of the moderate range suggests that the patient may initially require

---

[1] The clinical example, Michael, combines actual deidentified SPECTRA data from our IRB-approved database with fictionalized background and demographic information. The identity of this individual has been carefully disguised to protect their privacy.

FIGURE 6.2. SPECTRA Hierarchical Interpretation Worksheet

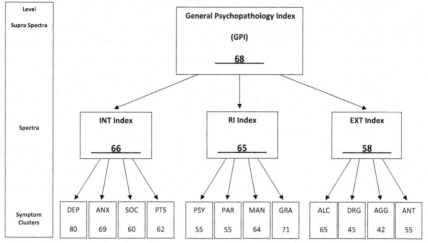

Note. Supplemental Scales: COG = 59, PF = 52, and SUI = 60. Protocol classification: INF (5) Acceptable and PCI (0) Acceptable. GPI = General Psychopathology Index; INT = Internalizing; RI = Reality Impairing; EXT = Externalizing; DEP = Depression; ANX = Anxiety; SOC = Social Anxiety; PTS = Post Traumatic Stress; PSY = Psychosis; PAR = Paranoid Ideation; MAN = Manic Activity; GRA = Grandiosity; ALC = Alcohol Problems; AGG = Severe Aggression; ANTI = Antisocial Behavior; DRG = Drug Problems. Adapted from *SPECTRA: Indices of Psychopathology: Professional Manual* (p. 88), by M. A. Blais and S. J. Sinclair, 2018, Psychological Assessment Resources. Copyright 2018 by Psychological Assessment Resources, Inc. Adapted with permission.

intensive outpatient care, multiple sessions weekly, or a partial hospital program to achieve stabilization followed by ongoing multimodal treatment (psychotherapy and pharmacotherapy). After stabilization, they are likely to require long-term mental health treatment and make uneven progress with improvement intermixed with relapses and setbacks.

Next, the interpretation moves to the Spectra level. The Spectra scales provide information about the complexity of the clinical presentation and potential treatments. At the Spectra level, there were elevations on all three scales: INT ($T = 66$, moderate), RI ($T = 65$, moderate), and EXT ($T = 58$, mild). Multiple Spectra elevations suggest a high degree of symptom complexity and the likelihood of cross-spectra comorbidity. In such cases, treaters should be on alert for disorders or symptom clusters that do not commonly co-occur. In addition, treating clinicians may have difficulty identifying a primary treatment target as divergent symptom clusters are likely to become problematic at different times. This type of changing clinical presentation often requires periods of polypharmacy and shifts in psychotherapeutic techniques.

The Clinical scales offer the narrowest, most specific assessment of psychopathology. Information from this level of assessment is key for understanding the patient's current symptom expression. At the Clinical-scale level, Michael's results showed meaningful elevations on scales from all three Spectra of psychopathology. On the Internalizing Clinical scales, there was an extreme elevation of DEP ($T = 80$), along with moderate elevations of ANX ($T = 69$), SOC ($T = 60$), and PTS ($T = 62$). Consistent with SPECTRA's hierarchical dimensional measurement model, clinical scales with elevations in the low 60s are interpreted as they contribute to the parent Spectra scale. In addition, symptoms associated with mild scale elevations may become prominent in the future as the expression of the higher order (Spectra-level) psychopathology can fluctuate.

The RI clinical scales show strong evidence of current bipolar symptoms for Michael (GRA $T = 71$ and MAN $T = 64$). Last, the profile also reveals a moderate degree of problematic alcohol use (ALC $T = 65$). While symptoms of depression and anxiety (or mixed negative affect) may dominate Michael's clinical presentation, signs of expansive, divergent thinking, grandiose self-appraisal, and physical or mental acceleration will also be present, if explored. Without the benefit of multiscale assessment data, a clinician might risk prematurely "closing" the diagnostic process and assigning a diagnosis consistent with the prominent Internalizing symptoms. Such premature closure would have overlooked the symptoms related to mania and needlessly delayed effective treatment.

The Supplemental scales are also informative in this case, as they reveal only mild subjective cognitive difficulty (COG $T = 59$) and average range PF ($T = 52$). So, despite experiencing significant life setbacks and ongoing struggles, Michael sees himself as functioning as well as the average person. This implies a lack of insight and raises the possibility of limited treatment motivation as he does not fully recognize his functional difficulties. Michael's level of suicidal ideation falls at the lower bound of the moderate range (SUI $T = 60$) and while not immediately concerning, should be closely monitored.

Differential Diagnosis

Before settling on a "suggested" *DSM* diagnosis, it is important to rule out (R/O) other potential conditions. With Michael's case, the three most likely R/Os would be unipolar major depression, schizoaffective disorder, and borderline personality disorder (BPD). Differentiating unipolar depression from bipolar disorder is critical, as approximately 37% of bipolar patients are initially diagnosed with major depression and treated with antidepressants only, which is less effective for bipolar depression and can often increase the risk of rapid cycling (Ghaemi et al., 2003). While there is strong evidence of clinical depression (DEP $T = 80$), unipolar depression would seem contraindicated given elevations on the MAN and GRA scales. This is particularly so for the GRA scale, as an excessively positive self-image is rarely present in severe unipolar depression. The lack of significant subjective cognitive difficulties (COG $T = 59$) would also argue against unipolar depression. Schizoaffective disorder should also be considered as it has features of mood and thought dysregulation. In this case, the absence of frank psychotic experiences (e.g., hallucinations, paranoia, and prominent delusions [PSY $T = 55$ and PAR $T = 55$]) seems to make this condition less likely. BPD is an important R/O as there is an ongoing debate about its relationship to the bipolar spectrum (Bayes et al., 2019). This R/O is a little more challenging, as SPECTRA does not assess abnormal personality traits. However, other dimensional models that include personality traits (hierarchical taxonomy of psychopathology [HiTOP]; see Forbes et al., 2021) represent BPD as a combination of Internalizing (Distress) and Externalizing (Antagonism) psychopathology (Ringwald et al., 2021). The lack of elevations on either the AGG or ANTI externalizing clinical scales would not support the presence of antagonistic personality traits, and the mild elevation on SUI ($T = 60$) is inconsistent with the prominent suicidal ideation (and threats) seen in BPD patients. Taken together, these data seem to make BPD less likely for Michael.

Although, in our view, psychological assessment does not provide direct correspondence with discrete psychiatric diagnoses, the present SPECTRA findings would seem most consistent with a *DSM-5* diagnosis of bipolar disorder, mixed-state, or what is often referred to clinically as an agitated bipolar depression. Support for this diagnosis is taken from the elevated Internalizing and Reality Impairing Spectra scales and the prominent symptoms associated with DEP, GRA, ANX, and MAN at the Clinical-scale level. Following the *DSM-5*, Michael's condition would likely be classified as bipolar II, given the lack of a clear, well-documented manic episode.

CONCLUSION

Beyond yielding a *DSM* diagnosis, the utility of a comprehensive psychological assessment resides in the clinical insights and guidance it provides, especially when evaluating challenging conditions like bipolar spectrum disorders. In fact, bipolar spectrum disorders with their broad multidomain dysregulation (e.g., mood, behavior, cognition) and varying severity provide an excellent illustration of SPECTRA's integrated hierarchical dimensional measurement approach. Each assessment level provides important clinical information that is specific to different assessment concerns, and together they offer a more differentiated picture of the individual's functioning. Information from the broadest Supra-Spectra level informs illness severity (impairment and chronicity), prognosis (treatment response and relapse), and the level of initial care (routine outpatient, intensive outpatient, or partial hospital inpatient). Mid-range Spectra-level assessment clarifies clinical complexity both within and across domains, identifying the primary areas of psychopathology vulnerability (Mood, Cognition, or Behavioral dysregulation), which broadly inform treatment selection. Assessment at the narrowest Clinical-scale level provides fine-grained, experience near information about the patient's current symptom profile. This information reveals the nature of the patient's current distress, helps refine initial treatment targets, and provides a language for feedback and discussion between patient and treaters. Information from the SPECTRA Supplemental scales further enriches the clinical picture by assessing the patient's perception of their functioning (cognitive and psychosocial) and suicide risk. Perceived functioning provides an important complement to the assessment of severity obtained from the psychopathology scales and helps evaluate insight, self-awareness, and treatment motivation.

REFERENCES

Alloy, L. B., Urošević, S., Abramson, L. Y., Jager-Hyman, S., Nusslock, R., Whitehouse, W. G., & Hogan, M. (2012). Progression along the bipolar spectrum: A longitudinal study of predictors of conversion from bipolar spectrum conditions to bipolar I and II disorders. *Journal of Abnormal Psychology, 121*(1), 16–27. https://doi.org/10.1037/a0023973

American Psychiatric Association. (2013). *Diagnostic and statistical manual of mental disorders: DSM-5* (5th ed.).

American Psychiatric Association. (2022). *Diagnostic and statistical manual of mental disorders: DSM-5-TR* (5th ed., text rev.).

Angst, J. (2007). The bipolar spectrum. *The British Journal of Psychiatry, 190*(3), 189–191. https://doi.org/10.1192/bjp.bp.106.030957

Bayes, A., Parker, G., & Paris, J. (2019). Differential diagnosis of bipolar II disorder and borderline personality disorder. *Current Psychiatry Reports, 21*, 125–136. https://doi.org/10.1007/s11920-019-1120-2

Ben-Porath, Y. S., & Tellegen, A. (2008). *The Minnesota Multiphasic Personality Inventory–2 Restructured Form (RF): Manual for administration, scoring and interpretation.* University of Minnesota Press.

Ben-Porath, Y. S., & Tellegen, A. (2020). *The Minnesota Multiphasic Personality Inventory–3: Manual for administration, scoring and interpretation.* University of Minnesota Press.

Blais, M. A., & Sinclair, S. J. (2018). *SPECTRA: Indices of psychopathology: Professional manual.* Psychological Assessment Resources.

Blais, M. A., Sinclair, S. J., Richardson, L. A., Massey, C., & Stein, M. B. (2021). External correlates of the SPECTRA: Indices of Psychopathology (SPECTRA) in a clinical sample. *Clinical Psychology & Psychotherapy, 28*(4), 929–938. https://doi.org/10.1002/cpp.2546

Blais, M. A., Stein, M. B., Sinclair, S. J., & Ruchensky, J. (2021). Initial validation of the SPECTRA: Indices of Psychopathology's (SPECTRA) hierarchical dimensional measurement model. *Personality and Individual Differences, 179*, Article 110946. https://doi.org/10.1016/j.paid.2021.110946

Caspi, A., Houts, R. M., Belsky, D. W., Goldman-Mellor, S. J., Harrington, H., Israel, S., Meier, M. H., Ramrakha, S., Shalev, I., Poulton, R., & Moffitt, T. E. (2014). The p factor: One general psychopathology factor in the structure of psychiatric disorders? *Clinical Psychological Science, 2*(2), 119–137. https://doi.org/10.1177/2167702613497473

Cuthbert, B. N., & Morris, S. E. (2021, February). Evolving concepts of the schizophrenia spectrum: A research domain criteria perspective. *Frontiers in Psychiatry, 12*, Article 641319. https://doi.org/10.3389/fpsyt.2021.641319

Forbes, M. K., Sunderland, M., Rapee, R. M., Batterham, P. J., Calear, A. L., Carragher, N., Ruggero, C., Zimmerman, M., Baillie, A. J., Lynch, S. J., Mewton, L., Slade, T., & Krueger, R. F. (2021). A detailed hierarchical model of psychopathology: From individual symptoms up to the general factor of psychopathology. *Clinical Psychological Science, 9*(2), 139–168. https://doi.org/10.1177/2167702620954799

Fried, E. I., Greene, A. L., & Eaton, N. R. (2021). The p factor is the sum of its parts, for now. *World Psychiatry, 20*(1), 69–70. https://doi.org/10.1002/wps.20814

Ghaemi, S. N., Hsu, D. J., Soldani, F., & Goodwin, F. K. (2003). Antidepressants in bipolar disorder: The case for caution. *Bipolar Disorders, 5*(6), 421–433. https://doi.org/10.1046/j.1399-5618.2003.00074.x

Hafeman, D. M., Merranko, J., Axelson, D., Goldstein, B. I., Goldstein, T., Monk, K., Hickey, M. B., Sakolsky, D., Diler, R., Iyengar, S., Brent, D., Kupfer, D., & Birmaher, B. (2016). Toward the definition of a bipolar prodrome: Dimensional predictors of bipolar spectrum disorders in at-risk youths. *The American Journal of Psychiatry, 173*(7), 695–704. https://doi.org/10.1176/appi.ajp.2015.15040414

Hyman, S. E. (2011). Diagnosing the *DSM*: Diagnostic classification needs fundamental reform. *Cerebrum: The Dana Forum on Brain Science, 2011,* 6.

Kotov, R., Ruggero, C. J., Krueger, R. F., Watson, D., Yuan, Q., & Zimmerman, M. (2011). New dimensions in the quantitative classification of mental illness. *Archives of General Psychiatry, 68*(10), 1003–1011. https://doi.org/10.1001/archgenpsychiatry.2011.107

Kraepelin, E. (1921). *Manic-depressive insanity and paranoia* (G. M. Robertson, Ed., R. M. Barclay, Trans.). E and S Livingstone. https://doi.org/10.1097/00005053-192104000-00057 (Original work published 1886)

Krueger, R. F. (1999). The structure of common mental disorders. *Archives of General Psychiatry, 56*(10), 921–926. https://doi.org/10.1001/archpsyc.56.10.921

Krueger, R. F., & Markon, K. E. (2006). Understanding psychopathology: Modeling behavior genetics, personality, and quantitative psychology to develop an empirically based model. *Current Directions in Psychological Science, 15*(3), 113–117. https://doi.org/10.1111/j.0963-7214.2006.00418.x

Lahey, B. B., Applegate, B., Hakes, J. K., Zald, D. H., Hariri, A. R., & Rathouz, P. J. (2012). Is there a general factor of prevalent psychopathology during adulthood? *Journal of Abnormal Psychology, 121*(4), 971–977. https://doi.org/10.1037/a0028355

Morey, L. C. (1991). *Personality assessment inventory professional manual.* Psychological Assessment Resources.

Perlis, R. H. (2010). Rating scales for bipolar disorder. In L. Baer & M. A. Blais (Eds.), *Handbook of clinical rating sales and assessment in psychiatry* (pp. 73–86). Humana Press–Springer.

Phelps, J. (2016). *A spectrum approach to mood disorders: Not fully bipolar but not unipolar–practical management.* W. W. Norton.

Ringwald, W. R., Forbes, M. K., & Wright, A. G. C. (2021). Meta-analysis of structural evidence for the hierarchical taxonomy of psychopathology (HiTOP) model. *Psychological Medicine.* Advance online publication. https://doi.org/10.1017/S0033291721001902

Ro, E., & Clark, L. A. (2009). Psychosocial functioning in the context of diagnosis: Assessment and theoretical issues. *Psychological Assessment, 21*(3), 313–324. https://doi.org/10.1037/a0016611

Sinclair, S. J., McRitchie, A., DeFilippo, S., Blais, M. A., Toomey, J., Colby, K. A., Goldsmith, G., Antonius, D., Laguerre, J., & Haggerty, G. (2022). The SPECTRA: Indices of Psychopathology: Construct validity and sensitivity to change in an inpatient psychiatric sample. *Journal of Psychopathology and Behavioral Assessment, 44,* 286–296. https://doi.org/10.1007/s10862-021-09885-0

Smith, G. T., Atkinson, E. A., Davis, H. A., Riley, E. N., & Oltmanns, J. R. (2020). The general factor of psychopathology. *Annual Review of Clinical Psychology, 16*(1), 75–98. https://doi.org/10.1146/annurev-clinpsy-071119-115848

Snyder, H. R., Young, J. F., & Hankin, B. L. (2017). Strong homotypic continuity in common psychopathology-, internalizing- and externalizing-specific factors over time in adolescents. *Clinical Psychological Science, 5*(1), 98–110. https://doi.org/10.1177/2167702616651076

Spearman, C. (1904). "General intelligence," objectively determined and measured. *The American Journal of Psychology, 15*(2), 201–292. https://doi.org/10.2307/1412107

Wright, A. G. C., Krueger, R. F., Hobbs, M. J., Markon, K. E., Eaton, N. R., & Slade, T. (2013). The structure of psychopathology: Toward an expanded quantitative empirical model. *Journal of Abnormal Psychology, 122*(1), 281–294. https://doi.org/10.1037/a0030133

7

Rating Scales and Screening Assessment of Bipolar Spectrum Disorders

James H. Kleiger

Using rating scales in psychological assessment can be a quick and economical way to screen for diagnostic conditions of interest. Why are screening measures for bipolar disorders important? Research has shown that incorrect or delayed diagnosis of bipolar spectrum disorders frequently occurs (Hirschfeld et al., 2003). Even among individuals with a history of major depression, many clinicians do not routinely screen for bipolarity (Brickman et al., 2002). The consequences of missed or delayed diagnosis are immense (Conus et al., 2014; see also the Introduction in this volume) and may result in poor outcomes, including persistent symptoms, symptom relapse, educational and occupational impairment, comorbidities, and increased suicidality (McIntyre et al., 2021).

An increasing number of bipolar screening instruments have appeared in the literature (Sajatovic et al., 2015), many of which are available as free downloads (e.g., https://www.sciencedirect.com/topics/psychology/mania-scale).

The scales and instruments selected for this chapter by no means exhaust the inventory of screening measures that currently exist. Commonly used interview–clinician rated measures are discussed first, followed by self-report scales. Within each category, measures that focus solely on manic/hypomanic symptoms, general depression, bipolar depression, and bipolar II disorder are distinguished

https://doi.org/10.1037/0000356-008
Psychological Assessment of Bipolar Spectrum Disorders, J. H. Kleiger and I. B. Weiner (Editors)

from those that focus on both depressive and manic/hypomanic features. Whether the instruments are used only with adults, children and adolescents, or all ages is also specified. Finally, limitations and cautions for using screening assessment instruments are discussed.

INTERVIEW–CLINICIAN RATED MEASURES

Clinician-rated scales include gold standard instruments often used as criterion measures in clinical and pharmacological investigations. Many are based on semistructured interviews and some on clinician judgment alone.

Structured Clinical Interview for *DSM-5* Disorders

The Structured Clinical Interview for *DSM-5* Disorders (SCID-5) includes a research version (RV) and a clinical version (CV; First et al., 2016). Module A in both versions covers current and past mood episodes (major depression, manic and hypomanic episodes, substance/medication-induced bipolar and depressive disorders), and persistent depressive disorder. The RV also has ratings for current cyclothymic disorders. The SCID-CV may be used in diagnostic consultations to target specific disorders. SCID modules contain probes to target core symptoms. Interviewers rely on their clinical judgment to gather additional information to assess target symptoms. The bipolar module in an earlier version, the SCID-IV for Axis I disorders (First et al., 1996), demonstrated adequate reliability in large international and multisite trials (Williams et al., 1992). The SCID appears to be significantly more reliable than other structured interviews, such as the Diagnostic Interview Schedule (Robins et al., 1981), the Composite International Diagnostic Interview (Andrews & Peters, 1998), and more standard clinical interviews (Miller et al., 2009; Ramirez Basco et al., 2000). The SCID Mood Module is used primarily with adult disorders. Routine use by clinicians is probably uncommon, due to the time it takes and the training required to develop proficiency.

Schedule for Affective Disorders and Schizophrenia

The Schedule for Affective Disorders and Schizophrenia (SADS; Endicott & Spitzer, 1978) was constructed to assist with Axis I diagnostic decision making. The psychometric properties have been established for both symptoms and diagnoses (Andreasen et al., 1981; Rogers et al., 2001). Mania symptom ratings achieved good reliability (interrater and test–retest) from 5 to 10 years with young adults (Coryell et al., 1995; Rice et al., 1986). The SADS was also shown to correlate significantly with other measures of mania (Secunda et al., 1985). The SADS-C (Change Version) mania subscale is a five-item interview that assesses the severity of current dimensions of mania (Spitzer & Endicott, 1977).

Spitzer and Endicott (1977) developed the SADS-C into an 11-item Mania Rating Scale (MRS), which was found to have strong psychometric properties.

The Kiddie Schedule for Affective Disorders and Schizophrenia for School Aged Children, Present and Lifetime Version

The Kiddie Schedule for Affective Disorders and Schizophrenia for School Aged Children, Present and Lifetime Version (KSADS-PL) was developed (Kaufman et al., 2000) for the *Diagnostic and Statistical Manual of Mental Disorders* (5th ed.; *DSM-5*; American Psychiatric Association, 2013). Like the SADS, the KSADS-PL provides a reliable and valid diagnostic assessment of *DSM* disorders. The MRS (Axelson et al., 2003) is based on items from the WASH-U-KSADS (Geller et al., 2001). The interviewer rates the presence of 15 symptoms of mania or hypomania over the past 2 months. Some symptoms, such as a need for sleep, racing thoughts, hyperactivity, grandiosity, and increased energy are also rated if they fluctuate with an expansive or irritable mood. It is important that raters can clearly demarcate the beginning and end of manic and hypomanic episodes. The rater also needs to establish whether multiple symptoms occurred at the same time. If any items are judged to be present, the interviewer inquires into how the child was behaving at the time.

Like the SCID and SADS, the KSADS-PL can be time-consuming to learn and administer. Psychologists in general outpatient settings may not have the time to conduct gold standard interview scales, not to mention the excessive demands that lengthy interviews may place on children with limited tolerance for sitting and focusing.

KSADS-PL materials are available for clinical use with permission from the authors at the website of the University of Pittsburgh Center for Childhood Bipolar Spectrum Services. The KSADS-PL is available online from the Kennedy Krieger Institute (https://www.kennedykrieger.org/sites/default/files/library/documents/faculty/ksads-dsm-5-screener.pdf). Focal assessment with the Manic or Depression Rating Scales of the KSADS may also be downloaded from the University of Pittsburgh website (https://www.pediatricbipolar.pitt.edu/resources/instruments).

Bipolar Depression Rating Scale

The Bipolar Depression Rating Scale (BDRS) was developed as an interview-based scale to identify symptom severity in bipolar depression (Berk et al., 2007). Raters complete a 20-item scale following a clinical interview to rate the severity of depression, as well as mixed symptoms over the past several days. The BDRS has been shown to be sensitive to symptoms characteristic of bipolar depression, such as hyperphagia and hypersomnia, which may be overlooked by standard depression rating scales. The measure was also shown to differentiate bipolar from unipolar depression (Galvão et al., 2013), which is a frequent differential diagnostic question. The scale developers demonstrated that the BDRS had good psychometric properties with acceptable levels of reliability and validity. Exploratory factor analysis revealed three factors corresponding to psychological depression, somatic depression, and mixed symptom clusters (e.g., increased motor drive, sleep disturbance, agitation). The scale and scoring manual can be downloaded for free from https://www.barwonhealth.org.au/health-professionals/bipolar-depression-rating-scale-bdrs.

Young Mania Rating Scale

One of the oldest and most frequently used MRSs is the Young Mania Rating Scale (YMRS), an 11-item clinician-rated instrument (Young et al., 1978). Modeled on the Hamilton Depression Scale (Hamilton, 1960), the YMRS is based on a 15- to 30-minute interview conducted by a trained clinician. The YMRS integrates clinician observations with patient self-report of manic symptoms over the previous 2 days. The 11 items cover core symptoms of a manic episode pertaining to mood, activity level, sexual interest, sleep, irritability, speech, grandiosity, flight of ideas, aggressive behavior, appearance, and insight. One of the items combines symptoms of grandiosity with psychotic symptoms, such as paranoia, ideas of reference, hyper-religiosity, delusions, and hallucinations. The items have five defined grades of severity. Four items are double-weighted (irritability, speech, thought content, and disruptive/aggressive behavior). Factor analytic studies showed factors of thought disturbance, overactive/aggressive behavior, elevated mood, and psychomotor symptoms (Double, 1990). Psychometric properties were shown to be excellent (Young et al., 1978). Young et al. (1978) found adequate interrater reliability ranging from .93 for the total score and .67 to .95 for individual items. The time required to complete YMRS is about 15 minutes. It also contains a parent-rating version. The scale is available as a free download at https://dcf.psychiatry.ufl.edu/files/2011/05/Young-Mania-Rating-Scale-Measure-with-background.pdf.

Mania Scale

Like the YMRS, the Mania Scale (MAS; Bech et al., 1979) is used in both clinical and research settings. Also known as the Bech–Rafaelsen Scale, the MAS covers the same dimensions of mania as the YMRS and has been shown to have excellent psychometric properties. The MAS consists of 11 items assessing motor activity, verbal activity, flight of thoughts, voice/noise level, hostility/destructiveness, mood (feelings of well-being), self-esteem, contact with others, sleep changes, sexual interest, and work activities. Each item is rated on a 5-point scale with 0 indicating normal mood and behavior and 4 indicating severe impairment. The total score can be used to reflect the severity of mania as mild (15–20), moderate (21–28), marked (29–32), severe (33–43), or extreme (≥44). Behavioral anchors are provided for each rating. Ratings are made for symptoms that occur over the past 3 days, based on a clinical interview with the client which takes 15 to 30 minutes to complete.

Bipolarity Index

The Bipolarity Index (Phelps, 2016; Sachs, 2004) is a clinician-rated measure that is not based on a semistructured interview. The Index rates key aspects of bipolarity, including nonmanic markers across five domains, which include (a) signs and symptoms, (b) family history, (c) age of onset, (d) course of illness and associated features, and (e) response to treatment. There are a total of 24 features that are weighted within each domain from 2 to 20 points. A cutoff of 50 has good sensitivity and specificity for identifying bipolar spectrum disorders (Aiken et al., 2015). The Bipolarity Index is an excellent diagnostic aid and can be downloaded from https://www.moodtreatmentcenter.com/wp-content/uploads/2021/01/bipolarityindex.pdf.

Pediatric Behavior Rating Scale

The Pediatric Behavior Rating Scale (PBRS; Marshall & Wilkerson, 2008) is a commercially published parent- and teacher-rated scale for identifying early-onset bipolar disorders in children aged 3 to 18. Norm-referenced scores are computed for Symptom Scales and a Total Bipolar Index. A Validity Scale (inconsistent responses) and Critical Items are also reported. Symptom scales include Atypicality (psychotic symptoms), Grandiosity, Aggression, Irritability, Hyperactivity, Inattention, Affective Disturbance, and Social Interactions. The parent scale contains 102 items and the teacher scale has 95 items. *T* scores above 70 reflect emotional dysregulation, and scores above 80 suggest the presence of early-onset bipolar disorder. The manual contains information on psychometric features. Validity studies mostly consist of correlations with other screening measures like the Child Mania Rating Scale (CMRS), Behavioral Assessment System for Children, and Clinical Assessment of Behavior.

Bipolar Prodrome Symptom Interview and Scale

The Bipolar Prodrome Symptom Interview and Scale (BPSS) is a retrospective measure developed to assess subthreshold symptoms of mania, depression, and psychosis (Correll et al., 2014). Correll et al. (2014) found that in the 52 subjects with either child- or adolescent-onset mania, all had experienced at least one manic symptom before demonstrating a full-blown manic episode. Roughly half of the subjects experienced an insidious progression at least a year prior to the onset of their more severe symptoms. The remainder demonstrated a subacute onset of symptoms from 1 month to a year prior to displaying a full range of manic symptomatology. Among the subthreshold symptoms, racing thoughts, depressed mood, irritability, and increased energy level marked the most frequent subthreshold symptoms. As part of their study, Correll et al. developed a prospective version of the BPSS (BPSS-P). The scale discriminated between individuals with bipolar disorders, nonclinical controls, and subjects with other disorders. Although the

BPSS-P correlated with other scales measuring depressive and manic symptoms, its use in prospective studies has not been demonstrated.

SELF-REPORT SCALES

Whereas gold standard measures like the SCID, SADS, and KSADS-PL are diagnostic in scope, self-report scales are screening instruments that, if positive, suggest the need for a more comprehensive evaluation. Self-report scales are appealing for clinicians or researchers looking for diagnostic support from user-friendly, evidence-based instruments. Scales are grouped in terms of (a) symptom-specific measures (mania, depression, and bipolar II disorder), (b) biphasic symptoms of bipolar spectrum disorders, and (c) prodromal symptoms of bipolar disorders.

Mania-Specific Scales

Altman Self-Rating Mania Scale
The Altman Self-Rating Mania Scale (ASRM; Altman et al., 1997) was developed initially as a brief, five-item scale in which subjects were asked to identify 11 characteristics of mania over a 7-day time frame. Items addressed elevated mood, increased self-esteem, decreased need for sleep, pressured speech, and psychomotor retardation. Items are rated on a 5-point scale. Scores of 6 or above indicate a higher greater chance of manic or hypomanic symptoms. The scale was expanded to 11- and 14-item versions, with added items to assess psychotic features (Altman & Østergaard, 2019). Psychometric properties and major studies involving the ASRM are described by Meyer et al. (2020).

Hypomania Checklist
The Hypomania Checklist (HCL-32) is a questionnaire consisting of 32 items developed for identifying hypomanic features in patients presenting with a depressive episode (Meyer et al., 2007). Angst et al. (2005) described HCL-32 as a sensitive but less specific measure for distinguishing major depression from bipolar disorders.

Self-Report Mania Inventory
The Self-Report Mania Inventory (SRMI) is a 47-item true-or-false instrument focusing on hypomanic symptoms (Shugar et al., 1992). A total score of 14 or more provided optimal sensitivity and specificity for identifying acutely manic inpatients (see Meyer et al., 2020). The SRMI successfully distinguished mania from other diagnoses. It takes roughly 15 minutes to complete.

Mood Disorder Questionnaire
Developed as a screening tool for manic symptoms based on *DSM-IV* criteria, the Mood Disorder Questionnaire (MDQ) has become a popular screening tool. It consists of 13 items relating to manic symptoms, plus additional items asking if

symptoms co-occurred and whether the endorsed symptoms caused at least a moderate level of impairment (Hirschfeld et al., 2000). A score of 7 indicates a positive screen. Studies have demonstrated varying levels of sensitivity and specificity, with some research showing relatively low coefficients (see Meyer et al., 2020). The MDQ also has a parent-rated version.

Child Mania Rating Scale–Parent Rating

The Child Mania Rating Scale–Parent Rating (CMRS-P) is frequently used in clinical assessment and research. It was developed to address the need for a brief, easily administered parent-reporting measure for pediatric mania (Pavuluri et al., 2006). The 21-item version demonstrated excellent psychometric properties and accuracy in distinguishing pediatric mania from attention-deficit/hyperactivity disorder (ADHD). A briefer 10-item version showed comparable accuracy in differentiating youth with bipolar disorders from children with other psychiatric disorders, including ADHD (Henry et al., 2008). The CMRS-P is in the public domain and can be downloaded from https://brainandwellness.com/accordian/upload_file/CMRS-P_followup.pdf.

Depression Rating Scales

Hamilton Depression Rating Scale

Developed initially as a 17-item rating scale for depression, the Hamilton Depression Rating Scale (HAM-D; Hamilton, 1960) was expanded to 21 items to assess symptom severity and change over time. The HAM-D is frequently used in clinical and research settings as a measure of depression. Three clusters include energy and activity, mood, and other symptoms.

Beck Depression Inventory

Along with the HAM-D, the Beck Depression Inventory (BDI) is considered a gold standard self-report measure to screen for depression (Beck et al., 1961). With its wide age range, the BDI has utility as both a clinical screening instrument and a criterion measure in empirical studies. The inventory contains 21 multiple-choice items and can be completed in roughly 10 minutes. The validity and reliability have been demonstrated in studies in multiple countries over more than 50 years.

PHQ-9 Depression Scale

The Patient Health Questionnaire–9 (PHQ-9) was developed as a nine-item scale based on *DSM-IV* (American Psychiatric Association, 1994) criteria for major depression in a primary-care setting (Kroenke et al., 2001). The PHQ-9 can be used in both clinical and research settings for a quick and valid measure of the severity of depression.

The most commonly used depression screening measures are in the public domain: https://www.apa.org/depression-guideline/assessment.

Bipolar-II-Specific Scales

Bipolar-II Diagnostic Questionnaire

The Bipolar-II Diagnostic Questionnaire (BPIIDQ) was constructed to fill a diagnostic void: distinguishing unipolar from bipolar depression (Leung et al., 2016). Based on a study with 298 subjects, the questionnaire was developed from multiple factors, including (a) positive family history, (b) age of onset, (c) presence of postpartum depression, (d) episodic course, (e) panicky feelings, (f) social phobia, (g) hypersomnia, and (h) agoraphobia. The questionnaire differentiated unipolar depression from bipolar II disorder with a sensitivity/specificity of .75/.63 and a slightly high rate for females who had given birth.

Biphasic Hypomania/Depression and Mixed Symptom Scales

General Behavior Inventory

The General Behavior Inventory (GBI) was developed to assess core symptoms of bipolarity, including both depressive and manic symptoms (Depue et al., 1981). It has become one of the most popular self-report measures for identifying broad symptoms of bipolarity. There are self- and parent-report scales with versions ranging from the original 72 items down to 14 (Youngstrom et al., 2013). The GBI not only has value in identifying manic/hypomanic, depressive, and mixed symptoms but can also be used as a screener for prodromal bipolar features. Both the original and brief versions have excellent psychometric properties and have become valuable screening tools in clinical assessments. The full version of the GBI is a free download from https://cls.unc.edu/wp-content/uploads/sites/3019/2014/06/GBI_self_English_v1a.pdf. A 10-item parent-report version (Youngstrom et al., 2001) can be downloaded from https://moodcenter.org/wp-content/uploads/2015/08/PGBI-Clinical-Version-.pdf.

Bipolar Spectrum Diagnostic Scale

The Bipolar Spectrum Diagnostic Scale (BSDS; Nassir Ghaemi et al., 2005) was designed to identify patients falling along a broader bipolar spectrum. It is a widely used and well-validated measure that performs as well as other more established scales (Phelps, 2016). Part A is presented as a paragraph about mood-related experiences. The respondent reads through the paragraph and then checks statements referring to hypomanic/manic symptoms and depressive experiences that apply to them. Part B has questions pertaining to how well the statements in Part A describe the individual. One point is given for each sentence checked, and additional points are given for how well the story fits with the respondent's experience. The BSDS has shown good sensitivity for bipolar I, bipolar II, and not otherwise specified bipolar disorders, and identified a large percentage of unipolar patients (85%) as not having a bipolar spectrum disorder. The BSDS is available at https://www.healthline.com/health/bipolar-disorder/bipolar-spectrum.

MoodCheck

MoodCheck is a self-report scale that combines questions from the BSDS with the Bipolarity Index described previously (Phelps, 2014). Parts A and B are the original items in the BSDS. Part C screens for a family of possible bipolar spectrum conditions. Part D consists of 13 questions that form the basis of the Bipolarity Index. MoodCheck is a quick and cost-effective way to screen for bipolarity, including nonmanic and mixed features, in patients presenting with depression. The instrument is simple to score and interpret. The MoodCheck can be downloaded for free from https://psycheducation.org/blog/moodcheck-bipolar-screening.

Rapid Mood Screener

The Rapid Mood Screener (RMS) consists of questions developed to decrease the likelihood of misdiagnosing adult patients with bipolar I features as having major depressive disorder (McIntyre et al., 2021). Three questions pertain to hypomanic/manic symptoms and three to bipolar risk factors like activation and irritability after taking an antidepressant, early onset depression, and multiple depressive episodes. The RMS is a simple and effective screener with easily understood questions, which can be completed in less than 2 minutes. The RMS, scoring guide, and psychometric properties are in the public domain and may be downloaded from https://howdenmedicalclinic.com/wp-content/uploads/2021/03/RMS-scale.pdf.

Scales for Predicting Bipolar Disorders

Bipolar Prodrome Symptom Scale, Abbreviated Screen for Patients

A self-report version of the BPSS was developed to identify patients who should be further evaluated with the full BPSS interview scale (Van Meter et al., 2019). The initial validation showed that the Bipolar Prodrome Symptom Scale, Abbreviated Screen for Patients (BPSS-A-SP) correlated well with the interview-based BPSS and other measures of mania and depression. However, as promising as developing a predictive measure might be, the predictive validity of BPSS-A-SP has yet to be established.

Hypomanic Personality Scale

The Hypomanic Personality Scale (HPS; Eckblad & Chapman, 1986) measures an extroversive style of social interaction. Originally designed to assess predisposition to bipolar disorders, questions surfaced on whether the scale measured personality style or bipolarity. Of most interest was whether the HPS could be used to predict the risk of developing bipolar disorders. Early studies found that high scores on the HPS were associated with elevated lifetime rates of mood, disruptive behavior, and substance use problems but was not predictive of future development of bipolar disorders (Klein et al., 1996). Nonetheless, this research found that subjects with a past history of major depression and hypomanic traits had increased levels of depression at the time of assessment, along with higher rates of attempted suicide, concurrent disruptive behavior disorders, and recurrent major depressive episodes. However, Kwapil et al. (2000) found high scores on the HPS predicted bipolar disorders at 13-year follow-up, but only 25% of high-scoring subjects actually developed bipolar disorders. More recent research showed that the HPS was highly confounded by correlations with other measures of bipolar disorders, casting further doubt on using the HPS as a measure of bipolar risk or prodrome (Parker et al., 2014).

Child Behavior Checklist Subscales

The Child Behavior Checklist (CBCL; Achenbach & Rescorla, 2000) is a commonly used, broadband parent-reporting measure for children and adolescents. Longitudinal research found that high scores on the sum of subscales of attention, aggression, and anxiety/depression predicted new-onset bipolar disorder in youth with ADHD (Biederman et al., 2009). As a result, they termed this profile "the pediatric bipolar disorder phenotype" or CBCL-PBD. However, Diler et al. (2009) found that the profile also predicted conduct disorders and depression. Thus, the CBCL-PBD became regarded as an indicator of general psychopathology, predicting the severity of the disorder and poor functioning. A 19-item mania scale developed from CBCL (CBCL-MS; Papachristou et al., 2013) was found to have acceptable psychometric properties. Internal consistency was high, and the scale effectively differentiated young people with Type I bipolar disorder (BD-I) from nonclinical controls. Young subjects with BD-I were also found to score higher on the CBCL-MS than those subjects diagnosed with anxiety (*p* .004) and major depression (*p* .002). However, high scores on the CBCL-MS did not discriminate between BD-I and ADHD or oppositional defiant disorder. Finally, a longitudinal study of youth in the Netherlands found that 11-year-olds who had mild to higher levels of symptoms on the CBCL-MS were 2–5 times more prone to be diagnosed with bipolar disorders by the age of 19 (Papachristou et al., 2017).

CAVEATS AND LIMITATIONS

Providing that they have good psychometric properties and are sensitive and specific to the groups being studied, rating scales are easy-to-administer tools that can save clinicians time. Scales with acceptable psychometric properties can add evidence-based support for clinical inferences and also indicate the need to delve more deeply into the nature and severity of symptoms.

Screening scales are helpful for clinicians in general practice for treatment decision making, primarily as it relates to prescribing medication and tracking symptoms to gauge change or response to treatment. Screening measures can also be used productively in psychological assessment, provided that psychodiagnosticians remember that most such measures are what the name implies: screening tools that help determine whether more in-depth assessment instruments are indicated.

Despite their utility in mental-health and primary-care settings, evaluators need to be aware of the limited scope of screening measures and rating scales (Kleiger & Khadivi, 2015). Rating scales are principally symptom- or diagnosis-focused, whereas multimethod psychological assessment has a broader focus in identifying, describing, and organizing a narrative regarding dimensions of psychological functioning and implications for treatment.

From this review, it is clear that not all screening measures are of equal value. Gold standard interview-based scales like the SCID, SADS, and KSADS-PL may be diagnostic themselves, but they tend to be time-consuming and require significant time and training to learn. The SADS and SCID have also been less useful in assessing bipolar II disorder (Miller et al., 2009). Some that focus narrowly on the presence and severity of discrete symptoms of mania, like the YMRS, ASRM, MDQ, and CMRS-P, are simple screening tools that are easy to administer and can be useful diagnostic aids to include in one's assessment battery. However, the usefulness of scales also depends on the prevalence of the disorder in the population of interest (Phelps & Ghaemi, 2006; Youngstrom & Van Meter, 2016).

Busy clinicians will find three simple self-report scales of great value. The GBI and P-GBI are easily obtainable as free downloads. They are well-constructed, with solid research supporting their use as assessment screening measures. The GBI is also useful in assessing depressive, hypomanic/manic, and mixed features.

The Bipolarity Index includes assessments of episodic symptoms, family history, age of onset, course, and response to treatment in a single scale. Clinicians can also use both the BSDS and MoodCheck, which have all the information to compute the Bipolarity Index to help gauge the presence of nonmanic features and the ultimate likelihood of a bipolar spectrum disorder. Given the high number of patients with underlying bipolarity who initially present with depression, accurate diagnosis is of critical importance for treatment planning.

A final note regarding the use of rating scales is important. Although screening measures with sound psychometric properties have a role in assessing psychopathology, restricting assessment practice to self-report and structured-interview scales may lead clinicians to focus too much on manifest symptoms and move away from traditional methods designed to assess psychological functioning and personality structure and dynamics. Rating scales may provide information about symptoms but tell us little about the person with the symptoms, which is often what referral sources are seeking to understand about those whom they refer for psychological assessment.

REFERENCES

Achenbach, T. M., & Rescorla, L. A. (2000). *Manual for the ASEBA preschool forms and profiles*. University of Vermont Department of Psychiatry.

Aiken, C. B., Weisler, R. H., & Sachs, G. S. (2015). The Bipolarity Index: A clinician-rated measure of diagnostic confidence. *Journal of Affective Disorders, 177*, 59–64. https://doi.org/10.1016/j.jad.2015.02.004

Altman, E. G., Hedeker, D., Peterson, J. L., Davis, J. M. (1997). The Altman Self-Rating Mania Scale. *Biological Psychiatry, 42*(10), 948–955. https://doi.org/10.1016/S0006-3223(96)00548-3

Altman, E. G., & Østergaard, S. D. (2019). The 11-item and 14-item versions of the Altman Self-Rating Mania Scale. *Acta Psychiatrica Scandinavica, 139*(3), 292–293. https://doi.org/10.1111/acps.12988

American Psychiatric Association. (1994). *Diagnostic and statistical manual of mental disorders* (4th ed.).

American Psychiatric Association. (2013). *Diagnostic and statistical manual of mental disorders* (5th ed.).

Andreasen, N. C., Grove, W. M., Shapiro, R. W., Keller, M. B., Hirschfeld, R. M., & McDonald-Scott, P. (1981). Reliability of lifetime diagnosis. A multicenter collaborative perspective. *Archives of General Psychiatry, 38*(4), 400–405. https://doi.org/10.1001/archpsyc.1981.01780290034003

Andrews, G., & Peters, L. (1998). The psychometric properties of the Composite International Diagnostic Interview. *Social Psychiatry and Psychiatric Epidemiology, 33*(2), 80–88. https://doi.org/10.1007/s001270050026

Angst, J., Adolfsson, R., Benazzi, F., Gamma, A., Hantouche, E., Meyer, T. D., Skeppar, P., Vieta, E., & Scott, J. (2005). The HCL-32: Towards a self-assessment tool for hypomanic symptoms in outpatients. *Journal of Affective Disorders, 88*(2), 217–233. https://doi.org/10.1016/j.jad.2005.05.011

Axelson, D., Birmaher, B. J., Brent, D., Wassick, S., Hoover, C., Bridge, J., & Ryan, N. (2003). A preliminary study of the Kiddie Schedule for Affective Disorders and Schizophrenia for School-Age Children mania rating scale for children and adolescents. *Journal of Child and Adolescent Psychopharmacology, 13*(4), 463–470. https://doi.org/10.1089/104454603322724850

Bech, P., Bolwig, T. G., Kramp, P., & Rafaelsen, O. J. (1979). The Bech–Rafaelsen Mania Scale and the Hamilton Depression Scale. *Acta Psychiatrica Scandinavica, 59*(4), 420–430. https://doi.org/10.1111/j.1600-0447.1979.tb04484.x

Beck, A. T., Ward, C. H., Mendelson, M., Mock, J., & Erbaugh, J. (1961). An inventory for measuring depression. *Archives of General Psychiatry, 4*(6), 561–571. https://doi.org/10.1001/archpsyc.1961.01710120031004

Berk, M., Malhi, G. S., Cahill, C., Carman, A. C., Hadzi-Pavlovic, D., Hawkins, M. T., Tohen, M., Mitchell, P. B., & Mitchell, P. B. (2007). The Bipolar Depression Rating Scale (BDRS): Its development, validation and utility. *Bipolar Disorders, 9*(6), 571–579. https://doi.org/10.1111/j.1399-5618.2007.00536.x

Biederman, J., Petty, C. R., Monuteaux, M. C., Evans, M., Parcell, T., Faraone, S. V., & Wozniak, J. (2009). The Child Behavior Checklist–Pediatric Bipolar Disorder profile predicts a subsequent diagnosis of bipolar disorder and associated impairments in ADHD youth growing up: A longitudinal analysis. *The Journal of Clinical Psychiatry, 70*(5), 732–740. https://doi.org/10.4088/JCP.08m04821

Brickman, A. L., LoPiccolo, C. J., & Johnson, S. L. (2002). Screening for bipolar disorder. *Psychiatric Services, 53*(3), Article 349. https://doi.org/10.1176/appi.ps.53.3.349

Conus, P., Macneil, C., & McGorry, P. D. (2014). Public health significance of bipolar disorder: Implications for early intervention and prevention. *Bipolar Disorders, 16*(5), 548–556. https://doi.org/10.1111/bdi.12137

Correll, C. U., Olvet, D. M., Auther, A. M., Hauser, M., Kishimoto, T., Carrión, R. E., Snyder, S., & Cornblatt, B. A. (2014). The Bipolar Prodrome Symptom Interview and Scale–Prospective (BPSS-P): Description and validation in a psychiatric sample and healthy controls. *Bipolar Disorders, 16*(5), 505–522. https://doi.org/10.1111/bdi.12209

Coryell, W., Endicott, J., Maser, J. D., Keller, M. B., Leon, A. C., & Akiskal, H. S. (1995). Long-term stability of polarity distinctions in the affective disorders. *The American Journal of Psychiatry, 152*(3), 385–390. https://doi.org/10.1176/ajp.152.3.385

Depue, R. A., Slater, J. F., Wolfstetter-Kausch, H., Klein, D., Goplerud, E., & Farr, D. (1981). A behavioral paradigm for identifying persons at risk for bipolar depressive disorder: A conceptual framework and five validation studies. *Journal of Abnormal Psychology, 90*(5), 381–437. https://doi.org/10.1037/0021-843X.90.5.381

Diler, R. S., Birmaher, B., Axelson, D., Goldstein, B., Gill, M., Strober, M., Kolko, D. J., Goldstein, T. R., Hunt, J., Yang, M., Ryan, N. D., Iyengar, S., Dahl, R. E., Dorn, L. D., & Keller, M. B. (2009). The Child Behavior Checklist (CBCL) and the CBCL–Bipolar Phenotype are not useful in diagnosing pediatric bipolar disorder. *Journal of Child and Adolescent Psychopharmacology, 19*(1), 23–30. https://doi.org/10.1089/cap.2008.067

Double, D. B. (1990). The factor structure of manic rating scales. *Journal of Affective Disorders, 18*(2), 113–119. https://doi.org/10.1016/0165-0327(90)90067-I

Eckblad, M., & Chapman, L. J. (1986). Development and validation of a scale for hypomanic personality. *Journal of Abnormal Psychology, 95*(3), 214–222. https://doi.org/10.1037//0021-843x.95.3.214

Endicott, J., & Spitzer, R. L. (1978). A diagnostic interview: The schedule for affective disorders and schizophrenia. *Archives of General Psychiatry, 35*(7), 837–844. https://doi.org/10.1001/archpsyc.1978.01770310043002

First, M. B., Spitzer, R. L., Gibbon, M., & Williams, J. B. W. (1996). *Structured Clinical Interview for* DSM-IV *Axis I Disorders–Clinician Version (SCID-CV)*. American Psychiatric Press.

First, M. B., & Williams, J. B., Karg, R. S., & Spitzer, R. L. (2016). *Structured Clinical Interview for* DSM-5 *Disorders–Clinician Version (DSM-5-CV)*. American Psychiatric Press.

Galvão, F., Sportiche, S., Lambert, J., Amiez, M., Musa, C., Nieto, I., Dubertret, C., & Lepine, J. P. (2013). Clinical differences between unipolar and bipolar depression: Interest of BDRS (Bipolar Depression Rating Scale). *Comprehensive Psychiatry, 54*(6), 605–610. https://doi.org/10.1016/j.comppsych.2012.12.023

Geller, B., Zimerman, B., Williams, M., Bolhofner, K., Craney, J. L., DelBello, M. P., & Soutullo, C. (2001, April). Reliability of the Washington University in St. Louis Kiddie Schedule for Affective Disorders and Schizophrenia (WASH-U-KSADS) mania and rapid cycling sections. *Journal of the American Academy of Child and Adolescent Psychiatry, 40*(4), 450–455. https://doi.org/10.1097/00004583-200104000-00014

Hamilton, M. (1960). The Hamilton Depression Scale—Accelerator or break on antidepressant drug discovery? *Psychiatry, 23*(1), 56–62. https://doi.org/10.1136/jnnp-2013-306984

Henry, D. B., Pavuluri, M. N., Youngstrom, E., & Birmaher, B. (2008). Accuracy of brief and full forms of the child mania rating scale. *Journal of Clinical Psychology, 64*(4), 368–381. https://doi.org/10.1002/jclp.20464

Hirschfeld, R. M., Calabrese, J. R., Weissman, M. M., Reed, M., Davies, M. A., Frye, M. A., Kleck, P. E., Lewis, L., McElroy, S. L., McNulty, J. P, & Wagner, K. D. (2003). Screening for bipolar disorder in the community. *Journal of Clinical Psychology, 64*(1), 53–59. https://doi.org/10.4088/jcp.v64n0111

Hirschfeld, R. M., Williams, J. B. W., Spitzer, R. L., Calabrese, J. R., Flynn, L., Keck, P. E., Jr., Lewis, L., McElroy, S. L., Post, R. M., Rapport, D. J., Russell, J. M., Sachs, G. S., & Zajecka, J. (2000). Development and validation of a screening instrument for bipolar spectrum disorder: The Mood Disorder Questionnaire. *The American Journal of Psychiatry, 157*(11), 1873–1875. https://doi.org/10.1176/appi.ajp.157.11.1873

Kaufman, J., Birmaher, B., Brent, D. A., Ryan, N. D., & Rao, U. (2000). K-SADS-PL. *Journal of the American Academy of Child and Adolescent Psychiatry, 39*(10), Article 1208. https://doi.org/10.1097/00004583-200010000-00002

Kleiger, J. H., & Khadivi, A. (2015). *Assessing psychosis: A clinician's guide*. Routledge; Taylor & Francis Group.

Klein, D. N., Lewinsohn, P. M., & Seeley, J. R. (1996). Hypomanic personality traits in a community sample of adolescents. *Journal of Affective Disorders, 38*(2–3), 135–143. https://doi.org/10.1016/0165-0327(96)00005-5

Kroenke, K., Spitzer, R. L., & Williams, J. B. W. (2001). The PHQ-9: Validity of a brief depression severity measure. *Journal of General Internal Medicine, 16*(9), 606–613. https://doi.org/10.1046/j.1525-1497.2001.016009606.x

Kwapil, T. R., Miller, M. B., Zinser, M. C., Chapman, L. J., Chapman, J., & Eckblad, M. (2000). A longitudinal study of high scorers on the Hypomanic Personality Scale. *Journal of Abnormal Psychology, 109*(2), 222–226. https://doi.org/10.1037/0021-843X.109.2.222

Leung, C. M., Yim, C. L., Yan, C. T. Y., Chan, C. C., Xiang, Y.-T., Mak, A. D. P., Fok, M. L., & Ungvari, G. S. (2016). The bipolar II depression questionnaire: A self-report tool for detecting bipolar II depression. *PLOS ONE, 11*(3), Article e0149752. https://doi.org/10.1371/journal.pone.0149752

Marshall, R. M., & Wilkerson, B. J. (2008). *Pediatric Bipolar Rating Scale (PBRS)*. Psychological Assessment Resources.

McIntyre, R. S., Patel, M. D., Masand, P. S., Harrington, A., Gillard, P., McElroy, S. L., Sullivan, K., Montano, C. B., Brown, T. M., Nelson, L., & Jain, R. (2021). The Rapid Mood Screener (RMS): A novel and pragmatic screener for bipolar I disorder. *Current Medical Research and Opinion, 37*(1), 135–144. https://doi.org/10.1080/03007995.2020.1860358

Meyer, T. D., Crist, N., La Rosa, N., Ye, B., Soares, J. C., & Bauer, I. E. (2020). Are existing self-ratings of acute manic symptoms in adults reliable and valid?—A systematic review. *Bipolar Disorders, 22*(6), 558–568. https://doi.org/10.1111/bdi.12906

Meyer, T. D., Hammelstein, P., Nilsson, L. G., Skeppar, P., Adolfsson, R., & Angst. J. (2007). The HCL-32: Its factorial structure and association to indices of impairment in a German and Swedish non-clinical sample. *Comprehensive Psychiatry, 48*, 79–87. https://doi.org/10.1016/j.comppsych.2006.07.001

Miller, C. J., Johnson, S. L., & Eisner, L. (2009). Assessment tools for adult bipolar disorder. *Clinical Psychology: Science and Practice, 16*(2), 188–201. https://doi.org/10.1111/j.1468-2850.2009.01158.x

Nassir Ghaemi, S., Miller, C. J., Berv, D. A., Klugman, J., Rosenquist, K. J., & Pies, R. W. (2005). Sensitivity and specificity of a new bipolar spectrum diagnostic scale. *Journal of Affective Disorders, 84*(2–3), 273–277. https://doi.org/10.1016/S0165-0327(03)00196-4

Papachristou, E., Oldehinkel, A. J., Ormel, J., Raven, D., Hartman, C. A., Frangou, S., & Reichenberg, A. (2017). The predictive value of childhood subthreshold manic symptoms for adolescent and adult psychiatric outcomes. *Journal of Affective Disorders, 212*, 86–92. https://doi.org/10.1016/j.jad.2017.01.038

Papachristou, E., Ormel, J., Oldehinkel, A. J., Kyriakopoulos, M., Reinares, M., Reichenberg, A., & Frangou, S. (2013). Child Behavior Checklist–Mania Scale (CBCL-MS): Development and evaluation of a population-based screening scale for bipolar disorder. *PLOS ONE, 8*(8), Article e69459. https://doi.org/10.1371/journal.pone.0069459

Parker, G., Fletcher, K., McCraw, S., & Hong, M. (2014). The Hypomanic Personality Scale: A measure of personality and/or bipolar symptoms? *Psychiatry Research, 220*(1–2), 654–658. https://doi.org/10.1016/j.psychres.2014.07.040

Pavuluri, M. N., Henry, D. B., Devineni, B., Carbray, J. A., & Birmaher, B. (2006). Child Mania Rating Scale: Development, reliability, and validity. *Journal of the American Academy of Child & Adolescent Psychiatry, 45*(5), 550–560. https://doi.org/10.1097/01.chi.0000205700.40700.50

Phelps, J. (2014). *MoodCheck: Bipolar screening.* https://psycheducation.org/blog/moodcheck-bipolar-screening/

Phelps, J. (2016). *A spectrum approach to mood disorders. Not fully bipolar but not unipolar—Practical management.* W. W. Norton.

Phelps, J. R., & Ghaemi, S. N. (2006). Improving the diagnosis of bipolar disorder: Predictive value of screening tests. *Journal of Affective Disorders, 92*(2–3), 141–148. https://doi.org/10.1016/j.jad.2006.01.029

Ramirez Basco, M., Bostic, J. Q., Davies, D., Rush, A. J., Witte, B., Hendrickse, W., & Barnett, V. (2000). Methods to improve diagnostic accuracy in a community mental health setting. *The American Journal of Psychiatry, 157*(10), 1599–1605. https://doi.org/10.1176/appi.ajp.157.10.1599

Rice, J. P., McDonald-Scott, P., Endicott, J., Coryell, W., Grove, W. M., Keller, M. B., & Altis, D. (1986). The stability of diagnosis with an application to bipolar II disorder. *Psychiatry Research, 19*(4), 285–296. https://doi.org/10.1016/0165-1781(86)90121-6

Robins, L. N., Helzer, J. E., Croughan, J., & Ratcliff, K. S. (1981). National Institute of Mental Health diagnostic interview schedule: Its history, characteristics, and validity. *Archives of General Psychiatry, 38*(4), 381–389. https://doi.org/10.1001/archpsyc.1981.01780290015001

Rogers, R., Jackson, R. L., & Cashel, M. (2001). The Schedule for Affective Disorders and Schizophrenia (SADS). In R. Rogers (Ed.), *Handbook of diagnostic and structured interviewing* (pp. 84–102). Guilford Press.

Sachs, G. S. (2004). Strategies for improving treatment of bipolar disorder: Integration of measurement and management. *Acta Psychiatrica Scandinavica. 110*(422), 7–17. https://doi.org/10.1111/j.1600-0447.2004.00409.x

Sajatovic, M., Chen, P., & Young, R. (2015). Rating scales in bipolar disorders. In M. Tohen, C. L. Bowden, A. A. Nierenberg, & J. R. Geddes (Eds.), *Clinical trial design challenges in mood disorders* (pp. 105–136). Academic Press. https://doi.org/10.1016/B978-0-12-405170-6.00009-9

Secunda, S. K., Katz, M. M., Swann, A., Koslow, S. H., Maas, J. W., Chuang, S., & Croughan, J. (1985). Mania: Diagnosis, state measurement and prediction of treatment response. *Journal of Affective Disorders, 8*(2), 113–121. https://doi.org/10.1016/0165-0327(85)90033-3

Shugar, G., Schertzer, S., Toner, B. B., & Di Gasbarro, I. (1992). Development, use, and factor analysis of a self-report inventory for mania. *Comprehensive Psychiatry, 33*(5), 325–331. https://doi.org/10.1016/0010-440X(92)90040-W

Spitzer, R. A., & Endicott, J. (1977). *Schedule for affective disorders and schizophrenia–change version*. Biometrics Research, State Psychiatric Institute.

Van Meter, A., Guinart, D., Bashir, A., Sareen, A., Cornblatt, B. A., Auther, A., Carrión, R. E., Carbon, M., Jiménez-Fernández, S., Vernal, D. L., Walitza, S., Gerstenberg, M., Saba, R., Cascio, N. L., & Correll, C. U. (2019). Bipolar Prodrome Symptom Scale–Abbreviated Screen for Patients: Description and validation. *Journal of Affective Disorders, 249*, 357–365. https://doi.org/10.1016/j.jad.2019.02.040

Williams, J. B. W., Gibbon, M., First, M. B., Spitzer, R. L., Davies, M., Borus, D. M., Borus, J., Howes, M. J., Kane, J., Pope, H. G., Rounsaville, B., & Wittchen, H. U. (1992). The Structured Clinical Interview for the *DSM-III-R* (SCID). II. Multisite test–retest. *Archives of General Psychiatry, 9*(8), 630–636. https://doi.org/10.1001/archpsyc.1992.01820080038006

Young, R. C., Biggs, J. T., Ziegler, V. E., & Meyer, D. A. (1978). A rating scale for mania: Reliability, validity and sensitivity. *The British Journal of Psychiatry, 133*(5), 429–435. https://doi.org/10.1192/bjp.133.5.429

Youngstrom, E. A., Findling, R. L., Danielson, C. K., & Calabrese, J. R. (2001). Discriminative validity of parent report of hypomanic and depressive symptoms on the General Behavior Inventory. *Psychological Assessment, 13*(2), 267–276. https://doi.org/10.1037/1040-3590.13.2.267

Youngstrom, E. A., Murray, G., Johnson, S. L., & Findling, R. L. (2013). The 7 Up 7 Down Inventory: A 14-item measure of manic and depressive tendencies carved from the General Behavior Inventory. *Psychological Assessment, 25*(4), 1377–1383. https://doi.org/10.1037/a0033975

Youngstrom, E. A., & Van Meter, A. (2016). Empirically supported assessment of children and adolescents. *Clinical Psychology: Science and Practice, 23*(4), 327–347. https://doi.org/10.1037/h0101738

III

PERFORMANCE-BASED METHODS

8

Rorschach Comprehensive System (RCS) Assessment of Bipolar Spectrum Disorders

Irving B. Weiner

The Rorschach is a multifaceted personality assessment method in which respondents are shown 10 inkblots, one at a time, and asked, "What might this be?" Of the 10 blots, five are in shades of black and gray; two are in shades of red, black, and gray; and the other three are in shades of pastel colors. Should respondents be uncertain how to answer, they are asked further, "What does it look like to you?" or "What do you see in it?" After the 10 blots have been administered, for each reported percept, its location in the blot (e.g., whole, detail) and what determined its content (e.g., form, color) are inquired into. As elaborated in texts by Exner (2003), Weiner (2013), and Choca (2013), summaries of these scores and the thematic imagery in response content provide information about a person's cognitive functioning, affective disposition, self-perception, and interpersonal relatedness.

The Rorschach Comprehensive System (RCS) is a contemporary guideline for administering, scoring, and interpreting the Rorschach method, which was created by Swiss psychiatrist Hermann Rorschach and first published in the 1921 book *Psychodiagnostics: A Diagnostic Test Based on Perception*. Rorschach had spent several years showing inkblots in a variety of shapes and colors to 288 mental hospital patients and 117 nonpatients, asking what they saw in them. From among the blots that elicited particularly interesting responses, he selected the 10 blots that became the standard test stimuli that have been used since then in Rorschach assessments around the world. An English translation of Rorschach's monograph first appeared in 1942, and more recently

https://doi.org/10.1037/0000356-009

Psychological Assessment of Bipolar Spectrum Disorders, J. H. Kleiger and I. B. Weiner (Editors)

Keddy et al. (2021) published a newly translated and annotated 100th-anniversary edition of the text.

Whereas Rorschach's 10 chosen inkblots have continued in the United States and abroad to constitute the test stimuli, clinicians and scholars began in the 1930s to introduce modifications in the administration and scoring of the measure and to elaborate varying interpretive guidelines for using it as a personality assessment instrument. Five such modified Rorschach systems were formulated in the United States by Samuel Beck, Bruno Klopfer, Zygmunt Piotrowski, Marguerite Hertz, and David Rapaport/Roy Schafer (see Weiner, in press). These five systems differed in their terminology and in their approach to interpretation. Some favored an empirical focus on the quantitative features of a Rorschach protocol (i.e., its scores), while others favored a conceptual focus on its qualitative features (i.e., its thematic imagery).

The differences among these five systems in their terminology and interpretive focus had the regrettable consequence of impeding communication among their adherents and limiting cumulative research on the meaning, implications, and psychometric properties of Rorschach variables. Weiner (1993) likened this circumstance to the Tower of Babel, a biblical symbol of poor communication among people whose language differences prevented them from understanding each other.

This problematic circumstance began to change when Rapaport advised one of his trainees, John Exner, to become familiar with all five of the U.S. Rorschach systems. Exner did so, including in-person interviews with each of the five system authors, and in 1969 he published *The Rorschach Systems*, an extensive review and comparison of the five systems. His work on this book led Exner to begin in the 1970s to combine features of the systems into what he decided to call the RCS. He hoped that this new system would become widely used and thereby foster improved communication and cumulative research among Rorschach scholars and clinicians.

The first edition of Exner's landmark book, *The Rorschach: A Comprehensive System*, appeared in 1974 and was followed by revised editions in 1986, 1993, and 2003. The RCS did indeed facilitate constructive communication among Rorschach practitioners and promote data-sharing among Rorschach researchers. Exner also addressed the RCS assessment of younger people in *The Rorschach: Assessment of Children and Adolescents*, which was published in two editions, in 1982 and 1995, with Irving Weiner as coauthor (Exner & Weiner, 1995).

In the subsequent editions of his 1974 text, Exner enriched the RCS with several new scores and indices that play a prominent part in the interpretive process These new scores and indices included the critical special scores of Deviant Verbalization (DV), Incongruous Combination (INCOM), Deviant Response (DR), Fabulized Combination (FABCOM), and Contamination (CONTAM); the Suicide Constellation (S-CON); the Perceptual Thinking Index (PTI); the Coping Deficit Index (CDI); and the Hypervigilance Index (HVI).

Following the appearance of Exner's fourth and final edition in 2003, other innovators continued the evolution of the present-day RCS with such new scales as the Ego Impairment Index (EII; Viglione et al., 2003); the Rorschach Oral Dependency Scale (ROD; Bornstein & Masling, 2005); the Rorschach Prognostic Rating Scale (RPRS; Handler & Clemence, 2005); the Rorschach Extended Aggression Scores (Gacono et al., 2005); and, more recently, the Rorschach Reality Fantasy Scale (RFS; Tibon-Czopp et al., 2016), the Rorschach Developmental Index (RDI; Resende et al., 2019), the Rorschach Hope Index (Scioli et al., 2018), and the Rorschach Omnipotence Scale (Homann, 2018). Other contemporary publications have elaborated on considerations in the RCS assessment of adolescents (Tibon-Czopp & Weiner, 2016) and senior adults (Weiner et al., 2019), and the utility of the RCS in evaluating disordered thinking and perception (Weiner, 2021).

Also of note is the continued international presence of Rorschach research and practice. The International Society of the Rorschach (ISR) was founded in 1933 and has expanded over the years to now include member societies from 21 countries. The ISR publishes a journal, *Rorschachiana*, which appears annually in book form with articles in English and summaries in French, Spanish, and Japanese.

The Comprehensive International Reference Values (CIRV) data consist of the mean frequency of occurrence and standard deviation (*SD*) of each of the coded RCS variables and the percent of this normative population who showed certain levels of RCS ratios and indices. These normative data can help examiners determine whether a particular finding falls within the normative range or deviates sufficiently from normative expectations to suggest the presence of some type of psychological disorder.

For example, the mean X-% score in the CIRV nonpatient population was .19 with an *SD* of .11. Using 1 *SD* as a criterion score would make .30 the upper limit of the normative range of X-%. Of the CIRV nonpatients, 41% had an X-% more than .20, but only 14% had an X-% more than .30. These frequencies would be consistent with suggesting that an X-% in the .20's would indicate an occasional tendency to misperceive people and events but would not document psychopathology, whereas the more an X-% rises above .30, the more likely it is to identify a diagnostically significant breakdown in reality testing.

Turning to bipolar spectrum disorders, the Rorschach assessment of these conditions has received scant attention in the research literature. The few published studies in this area have consisted of empirical comparisons of the Rorschach protocols of small groups of mental health patients diagnosed with unipolar depression, bipolar depression, or bipolar mania (see Khadivi et al., 1997; Kimura et al., 2013; Le Chevanton et al., 2020; Singer & Brabender, 1993). These studies found little difference in the Rorschach scores of the three groups, except for the patients with mania being more likely than the patients with depression to show signs of cognitive slippage, which may be attributable to their having given longer and more complex responses.

The present chapter addresses the Rorschach assessment of bipolar spectrum disorders from a conceptual rather than an empirical perspective. To this end, the text reviews the defining psychological characteristics of bipolar spectrum disorders and then elaborates on how Rorschach scores, thematic imagery, and test behavior can assist in identifying these characteristics.

CHARACTERISTICS OF BIPOLAR SPECTRUM DISORDERS

Bipolar spectrum disorders, as described in the *Diagnostic and Statistical Manual of Mental Disorders* (5th ed., text rev.; *DSM-5-TR*; American Psychiatric Association, 2022) and the *International Statistical Classification of Diseases and Related Health Problems* (11th ed.; *ICD-11*; World Health Organization, 2018), are mood disorders characterized by marked shifts in (a) emotional state, (b) level of energy and activity, (c) tone of attitudes and expectations, (d) quality of self-perception and self-regard, and (e) extent of social and interpersonal interest and involvement. With respect to their emotional state, persons with a bipolar spectrum disorder typically vacillate between feeling happy or sad and seeming to be elated or dejected. In their level of activity, they sometimes have abundant energy at their disposal, in which case they think, talk, and move rapidly, and at other times can call on only limited energy, in which case their behavior is lethargic rather than accelerated.

In their attitudes and expectations, persons with bipolar spectrum disorders alternate between positive and negative perspectives on their current circumstances and between optimistic and pessimistic anticipation of what the future will bring. As for their self-perception and self-regard, bipolar individuals sometimes consider themselves to be attractive, worthy, and able, in which case they are quite self-assured, while at other times they disparage themselves as being unappealing, unworthy, and inept, in which case they have little confidence in themselves.

In their social and interpersonal lives, bipolar individuals in a manic phase typically seek out and enjoy the company of other people, whom they expect to impress with their self-perceived worthiness and, by doing so, affirm their elevated self-esteem. When depressed, by contrast, people with a bipolar disorder tend to avoid or at least limit their involvement with other people, in whose presence their feelings of inadequacy are exacerbated by perceiving them as more able, appealing, and accomplished than they are.

The obtained scores, thematic imagery, and test behavior in a Rorschach examination provide diagnostically relevant information about each of these five dimensions of bipolar spectrum disorder: emotional state, energy level, attitudes and expectations, self-perception and self-regard, and interpersonal interest and involvement. The diagnostic utilization of this information is facilitated by conceiving of bipolar disorder as consisting of depressing concerns and defensive efforts to minimize or deny these concerns by means of an exaggerated sense of well-being. The Rorschach assessment of a possible bipolar spectrum disorder can accordingly begin with examining the test data for indications of depression and then, if such indications are present, determining whether there are indications of mania as well, in which case the respondent is likely to have a bipolar spectrum disorder.

RORSCHACH ASSESSMENT OF EMOTIONAL STATE

Bipolar spectrum disorders are basically affective disorders, which makes emotional state the most telling indicator of whether a person has some type of this disorder. On the Rorschach, emotional state is measured largely by how people use color in formulating their responses, both chromatic colors and shades of gray and black. The interpretive implications of chromatic and achromatic color use are captured by the emotional tone of such expressions as "dark clouds" or a "sunny sky."

With respect to responses of the "dark clouds" variety, the use of black and gray as determinants in formulating Rorschach responses is indicated by the Sum Shading variable, which is the total number of T (texture), V (vista), Y (diffuse shading), and C' (achromatic color) determinants in the record. In the CIRV nonpatient population, the Sum Shading variable had a mean frequency of 4.29 with an SD of 3.48. Using one SD above or below the mean as the boundaries of the normative range, a Sum Shading > 7 is likely to identify depressing feelings of gloom, with the extent of depression increasing as the frequency of Sum Shading increases.

As for responses of the "sunny sky" variety, the use of chromatic color as a determinant in formulating Rorschach responses is coded by the WSumC variable, which consists of the sum of 0.5 points for each form color (FC), 1 point for each color form (CF), and 1.5 points for each pure color (C). The CIRV mean for WSumC was 3.11 with an SD of 2.71, which would suggest that a WSumC > 6 would exceed normative expectations and indicate an above-average level of emotional experience and expression. This implication of an elevated WSumC for heightened emotionality increases when the frequency of $CF + C$ responses in a record exceeds the frequency of FC responses by more than one (i.e., $CF + C > FC + 1$). Only 24% of the CIRV nonpatients showed this predominance of color-form over form-color responses, and it usually indicates a considerable extent of emotional intensity and lability. Such prominent emotional intensity and lability is not necessarily diagnostic of affective disorder, but it is a common feature of mania and disposes people to alternating episodes of euphoria and dysphoria.

Color use can provide two other indications of a respondent's susceptibility to mood swings and possible bipolar disorder. One of these indications is a Color Shading Blend, which is a percept that includes both color and shading determinants, as in seeing the upper red details on Card II as "Red party hats, but they're sort of fuzzy looking." Color Shading Blends are quite rare in nonpatients, with a mean CIRV frequency of just 0.6, and even one such response in a record is likely to indicate ambivalent emotionality and a proclivity to attach both pleasant and unpleasant connotations to experiences and events.

The other additional color use indicator of susceptibility to mood swings is color projection (CP), which is coded when a respondent maintains that a black and gray inkblot is chromatic, as in seeing Card V as "A colorful butterfly." Such CP responses are a transparent attempt to transform an affectively unpleasant impression (represented by something gray and black) into a pleasant one (represented by chromatic colors). People who give even one CP response are inclined in their daily lives to mute unpleasant affect by using denial to contravene it, which results in a forced gaiety that often characterizes a manic episode.

In addition to these RCS color use indicators of emotional state, the thematic imagery in respondents' percepts can provide a clue to how they are feeling. Movement responses are particularly likely to mirror a person's emotional state. Seeing human figures as laughing can be a projection of feelings of happiness and a sense of well-being, for example, whereas seeing people as crying is likely a projection of feelings of sadness and a sense of despair.

The nature of the objects people see in the blots can also be a window into their emotional state. Consider, for example, the contrasting implications of whether a blot detail is seen as a crib or as a coffin, as an angel or as a devil, or as a sports car or as a hearse. An abundance of such bright side imagery as a crib, angel, or sports car would suggest that the respondent is in a good mood, whereas recurrence of such dark side imagery as a coffin, devil, or hearse would suggest instead that the respondent is feeling blue. The presence of both notably bright side and notably dark side imagery in a record, in common with Color Shading Blends and CP, is likely to indicate a susceptibility to the alternating episodes of gay and somber emotionality that characterize bipolar spectrum disorders.

RORSCHACH ASSESSMENT OF ENERGY LEVEL

The main indications of energy level in Rorschach responses are productivity, speed, and complexity. Productivity is indexed by the number of responses given to the inkblots (R). The CIRV mean for R is 22.31 with a suggested normative range of 17–27 responses. In this population, 25% gave a relatively short record with fewer than 17 responses, and 20% gave a relatively long record with more than 27 responses. A long record has few if any implications for psychopathology, except perhaps in helping to infer mania or rule out depression. A short record, on the other hand, speaks diagnostically to the limited level of energy that characterizes depression.

Given a short record, however, the possibility should be considered that it is a product of guardedness rather than depression. This distinction can usually be made by noting the speed and manner with which responses are delivered. Guarded respondents tend to make short shrift of their task, delivering their responses rapidly and emphatically in a few words and quickly handing the card back or laying it face down, as if satisfied with what they have said. Motivated but depressed respondents, by contrast, are likely to speak slowly and haltingly and dwell on the cards, as if struggling to find percepts and concerned about not performing well on their tasks.

Complexity in Rorschach responses is measured by blended responses and by the constriction ratio. Blended responses are percepts with more than one determinant, as in seeing on Card II "Some bears fighting, and there's blood all around" (coded FMa.*CF*) or on Card III "Two men in black suits bowing to each other" (coded Ma.*FC'*). The previously mentioned Color Shading Blends are one type of such multiply determined responses. Blended responses had a mean CIRV frequency of 4.01 and accounted on average for 18% of the responses given by the nonpatients. A record without any blended responses can be an indication of the respondent having limited energy available for investment in the Rorschach task.

The constriction ratio is the percentage of responses having no determinant other than form, which is scored as PureF% in the RCS. PureF% had a mean CIRV frequency of 0.39 and an *SD* of 0.17. Again using a one *SD* criterion for establishing a normative range, a Rorschach record with a PureF% more than 60%, like the absence of Blends, shows limited energy being devoted to formulating the more complex movement, color, and shading percepts. An above-average frequency of blended responses and a PureF% less than 20%, on the other hand, would indicate energetic involvement in the Rorschach task. Abundant energy, like a joyful emotional tone, is a common characteristic of mania but does not by itself document psychopathology. However, a high-energy person who shows signs of depression as well is likely to be susceptible to the mood swings that typify bipolar spectrum disorders.

RORSCHACH ASSESSMENT OF ATTITUDES AND EXPECTATIONS

Respondents' attitudes and expectations are captured in Rorschach responses by the flavor of their thematic imagery. Some percepts have an upbeat flavor by virtue of depicting, predicting, or symbolizing successful striving (as in "animals climbing a mountain"), worthy accomplishments (as in "a medal" or "a trophy"), or pleasant events (as in "flowers growing" or "people dancing"). Other percepts may have a downside flavor, pointing in the opposite direction to failed effort (as in "animals falling off a cliff"), limited ability (as in "a dunce cap"), or gloomy events (as in "a person dying").

Should respondents give more downside than upbeat answers, their imagery is a likely indicator of the pessimistic attitudes and gloomy expectations that characterize a state of depression. In the other direction, however, a prepon-derance of upbeat responses and the optimistic attitudes and expectations they suggest do not necessarily identify mania. Rather, like a joyful emotional state and abundant energy, prevalent optimism may speak to being in good spirits, within the normal range, and not necessarily to a psychological disorder. Another possibility to consider, however, is that emphatically positive attitudes and expectations may be serving as a manic defense against underlying depressive concerns, in which case they would be masking a susceptibility to the alternating mood states that characterize bipolar spectrum disorders.

RORSCHACH ASSESSMENT OF SELF-PERCEPTION AND SELF-REGARD

How people are likely to perceive and regard themselves is assessed in the Rorschach by the frequency of Reflection and Morbid (MOR) responses. Reflection responses symbolize people looking at themselves in a mirror and admiring what they see there. Such responses are normatively infrequent, with a CIRV mean of less than one (0.41) and with only 25% of these nonpatients giving any Reflection responses at all. When they do occur, Reflection responses are commonly associated with self-satisfaction, self-confidence, and a self-centered focus on one's own needs and concerns with little attention to the needs and concerns of other people. The more numerous their Reflection responses, the more likely respondents are to overvalue their personal assets and embrace an egocentric sense of superiority.

Such egocentricity is characteristic of mania but, like a joyful mood and an optimistic perspective, is not by itself diagnostic of an affective disorder. On the other hand, once more with regard to the implications of maladaptive combinations, the presence of Reflection responses in a record that includes indications of depression as well raises the possibility of a bipolar spectrum disorder.

Morbid responses describe people and objects as dead, damaged, injured, broken, or in some other way dysfunctional. Percepts of this kind suggest that respondents regard themselves in a similarly negative way, as being physically impaired or vulnerable to becoming so. Morbid responses occur somewhat more frequently than Reflection responses, with a mean CIRV frequency of 1.26 such responses per record and with only 16% of this nonpatient population giving more than two Morbid responses. Accordingly, respondents with MOR > 2 should be considered likely to devalue their personal appeal, doubt their capabilities, and harbor a depressing sense of inferiority. Similarly, multiple Morbid responses in a record that includes Reflection responses as well suggest a propensity for the mood swings that typify bipolar spectrum disorders.

RORSCHACH ASSESSMENT OF SOCIAL AND INTERPERSONAL INTEREST AND INVOLVEMENT

The Rorschach is rich in scores and imagery relevant to assessing a respondent's interpersonal interest and involvement. Interpersonal interest is measured on the Rorschach by the number of whole human figures seen (SumH) and by the RCS Isolation Index (ISOL). The CIRV mean for SumH is 2.43 responses, which suggests that two or more *H* responses in a record is likely to indicate an adaptive extent of interpersonal interest. At the opposite end, only 35% of these nonpatients gave fewer than two *H* responses, and all of them gave at least one.

These normative data suggest that respondents who have just one *H* in their record, especially when their SumH = 0, are giving evidence of the limited interpersonal interest that characterizes a state of depression.

The ISOL consists of the weighted sum of five nonhuman contents (2 points for each Clouds and Nature content plus 1 point for each Botany, Geography, and Landscape content) divided by the total number of responses (*R*). ISOL scores were not included in the CIRV data report, but survey data presented by Exner (2007) showed a mean ISOL of .19 in nonpatient adults. An ISOL much above this average expectation, in common with SumH = 0, is likely to identify disinterest in other people and limited involvement with them.

An additional Rorschach variable indicative of interpersonal disengagement and social withdrawal is the affective ratio (Afr), which consists of the number of responses to Cards VIII–X (the multicolored cards) divided by the number of responses to Cards I–VII (the black, gray, and red cards). The CIRV mean for Afr was .53, indicating that these nonpatients gave on average twice as many responses to the three multicolored and relatively affect-arousing blots than to the seven black, gray, and red cards. Only 27% of this nonpatient population had an Afr below .40, and the farther an Afr falls below this point, the more likely it is to indicate withdrawal from interpersonal interactions, especially those involving an exchange of feelings.

Whereas a low Afr points to detachment from other people, an Afr elevated above .60 suggests considerable openness to interpersonal involvement and shared emotional experience. Such social enthusiasm is characteristic of a manic condition, but in common with the four previously noted features of mania— elated affect, abundant energy, prevailing optimism, and egocentricity—it can fall within the normal range without being by itself diagnostic of a manic condition. In combination, however, the more of these five features of mania there are in a record, the more likely it is to indicate the manic phase of a bipolar spectrum disorder.

Of further note, however, the social enthusiasm that typically characterizes mania can in some instances be tempered by interpersonal discomfort generated by the manic person's emotional intensity. Adults who have difficulty modulating affect in moderation—as evidenced by the previously mentioned *CF* + *C* > *FC* + 1—often find that other adults do not respond favorably to their childlike intensity and excitability. Being shunned or criticized for their emotionality (as in "Calm down!," "Don't be that way!," or "What's the matter with you?") can be an unpleasant experience that puts a damper on social enthusiasm and may lead a manic individual to avoid people rather than seek them out.

SUMMARY

Bipolar spectrum disorders consist of mood swings between being happy or sad and between having abundant or limited energy, an optimistic or pessimistic frame of mind, a positive or negative self-image, and an engaged or detached social life. Rorschach indices are presented for each of these personality characteristics, with attention to normative expectations for the RCS established by the CIRV. Rorschach scores, imagery, and test behavior that suggest gloom, lethargy, pessimism, self-doubt, and social withdrawal point to a diagnostic inference of depression. Mania is somewhat more difficult to diagnose than depression because its chief characteristics—namely, being in good spirits and an energetic, optimistic, self-confident, and socially active person—can fall within the normative range and not separately warrant inferring an affective disorder. Taken together, however, multiple manic characteristics in a Rorschach record do point to psychopathology, and a record containing indications of depression as well does indicate a likelihood of mood swings that, when marked, identify a bipolar spectrum disorder.

REFERENCES

American Psychiatric Association. (2022). *Diagnostic and statistical manual of mental disorders: DSM-5-TR* (5th ed., text rev.).

Bornstein, R. F., & Masling, J. M. (2005). The Rorschach Oral Dependency Scale. In R. F. Bornstein & J. M. Masling (Eds.), *Scoring the Rorschach: Seven validated systems* (pp. 135–157). Lawrence Erlbaum. https://doi.org/10.4324/9781410612526

Choca, J. P. (2013). *The Rorschach Inkblot Test: An interpretive guide for clinicians.* American Psychological Association. https://doi.org/10.1037/14039-000

Exner, J. E., Jr. (2003). *The Rorschach: A comprehensive system* (4th ed.). Wiley.

Exner, J. E., Jr. (2007). A new U.S. adult nonpatient sample. *Journal of Personality Assessment, 89*(Suppl. 1), S154–S158. https://doi.org/10.1080/00223890701583523

Exner, J. E., Jr., & Weiner, I. B. (1995). *The Rorschach: A comprehensive system: Vol. 3. Assessment of children and adolescents* (2nd ed.). Wiley.

Gacono, C. B., Gacono-Ballantyne, L., Meloy, J. R., & Baity, M. (2005). The Rorschach extended aggression scores. *Rorschachiana, 27*(1), 164–190. https://doi.org/10.1027/1192-5604.27.1.164

Handler, L., & Clemence, A. J. (2005). The Rorschach Prognostic Rating Scale. In R. F. Bornstein & J. M. Masling (Eds.), *Scoring the Rorschach: Seven validated systems* (pp. 1–24). Lawrence Erlbaum.

Homann, E. (2018). The Rorschach Omnipotence Scale and closed-system processing. *Psychoanalytic Psychology, 35*(4), 454–461. https://doi.org/10.1037/pap0000193

Keddy, P. J., Signer, R., Erdberg, P., & Schneider-Stocking, A. (2021). *Hermann Rorschach's psychodiagnostics.* Hogrefe.

Khadivi, A., Wetzler, S., & Wilson, A. (1997). Manic indices on the Rorschach. *Journal of Personality Assessment, 69*(2), 365–375. https://doi.org/10.1207/s15327752jpa6902_8

Kimura, H., Osaki, A., Kawashima, R., Inoue, T., Nakagawa, S., Suzuki, K., Asakura, S., Tanaka, T., Kitaichi, Y., Masui, T., Kitagawa, N., Kako, Y., Abekawa, T., Kusumi, I., Yamanaka, H., Denda, K., & Koyama, T. (2013). Differences between bipolar and unipolar depression on Rorschach testing. *Neuropsychiatric Disease and Treatment, 9,* 619–627. https://doi.org/10.2147/NDT.S42702

Le Chevanton, T., Fouques, D., Julien-Sweerts, S., Petot, D., & Polosan, M. (2020). Differentiating unipolar and bipolar depression: Contribution of the Rorschach Test (comprehensive system). *Journal of Clinical Psychology, 76*(4), 769–777. https://doi.org/10.1002/jclp.22912

Resende, A. C., Viglione, D. J., Martins, L. D., & Yazigi, L. (2019). Criterion validity of the Rorschach Developmental Index with children. *Journal of Personality Assessment, 101*(2), 191–198. https://doi.org/10.1080/00223891.2017.1368021

Scioli, A., Cofrin, M., Aceto, F., & Martin, T. (2018). Toward a Rorschach Hope Index. *Rorschachiana Journal of the International Society for the Rorschach, 39*(2), 157–177. https://doi.org/10.1027/1192-5604/a000110

Singer, H. K., & Brabender, V. (1993). The use of the Rorschach to differentiate unipolar and bipolar disorders. *Journal of Personality Assessment, 60*(2), 333–345. https://doi.org/10.1207/s15327752jpa6002_10

Tibon-Czopp, S., Appel, L., & Zeligman, R. (2016). Assessing personality patterns of functioning in a decision-making ambiguous task: The Rorschach Reality–Fantasy Scale (RFS-2). *Group Decision and Negotiation, 25*(1), 65–73. https://doi.org/10.1007/s10726-015-9432-z

Tibon-Czopp, S., & Weiner, I. B. (2016). *Rorschach assessment of adolescents.* Springer. https://doi.org/10.1007/978-1-4939-3151-4

Viglione, D. J., Perry, W., & Meyer, G. (2003). Refinements in the Rorschach Ego Impairment Index incorporating the human representational variable. *Journal of Personality Assessment, 81*(2), 149–156. https://doi.org/10.1207/S15327752JPA8102_06

Weiner, I. B. (1993). Speaking Rorschach: A tower of Babel no longer. *Rorschachiana, 1*(1), 1–6. https://doi.org/10.1027/1192-5604.18.1.1

Weiner, I. B. (2013). *Principles of Rorschach interpretation* (2nd ed.). Lawrence Erlbaum.

Weiner, I. B. (2021). Rorschach Comprehensive System (RCS) for assessing disordered thought and perception. In I. B. Weiner & J. H. Kleiger (Eds.), *Psychological assessment of disordered thinking and perception* (pp. 137–150). American Psychological Association. https://doi.org/10.1037/0000245-009

Weiner, I. B. (in press). Rorschach systems in the United Sates. *Rorschachiana.*

Weiner, I. B., Appel, L., & Tibon-Czopp, S. (2019). *Rorschach assessment of senior adults.* Routledge. https://doi.org/10.4324/9780429282171

World Health Organization. (2018). *International Statistical Classification of Diseases and Related Health Problems* (11th ed.).

Rorschach Performance Assessment System (R-PAS) Assessment of Bipolar Spectrum Disorders

Joni L. Mihura and Kim J. Görner

This chapter provides guidance on using the Rorschach Performance Assessment System (R-PAS; Meyer et al., 2011) in the assessment of bipolar disorders. It is important to note that neither R-PAS nor self-report questionnaires are designed to make formal *Diagnostic and Statistical Manual of Mental Disorders* (*DSM*) or *International Statistical Classification of Diseases and Related Health Problems* (*ICD*) diagnoses. However, as described in what follows, R-PAS data can aid diagnosis by informing the decision process in a multimethod assessment.

THE RORSCHACH PERFORMANCE ASSESSMENT SYSTEM

R-PAS is currently the most contemporary Rorschach system (Meyer et al., 2011; Meyer & Mihura, 2021). R-PAS improves upon the previous popular system, the Rorschach Comprehensive System (RCS; Exner, 2003), by addressing the major criticisms of it (see Mihura & Meyer, 2022). After John Exner's death in 2006, R-PAS was developed by members of Exner's Rorschach Research Council (Gregory J. Meyer, Donald J. Viglione, Joni L. Mihura, and Philip Erdberg) and a prominent forensic psychologist (Robert E. Erard) to replace the RCS. The RCS, first published in 1974 (Exner, 1974), was designed as a replacement for five Rorschach systems in the United States (Beck, 1937; Hertz, 1936;

https://doi.org/10.1037/0000356-010
Psychological Assessment of Bipolar Spectrum Disorders, J. H. Kleiger and I. B. Weiner (Editors)

Klopfer et al., 1954; Piotrowski, 1957; Rapaport et al., 1946) that were designed as extensions of and replacements for Rorschach's (1921) original test.

R-PAS includes four major alterations of the RCS to resolve problems that Exner's Research Council had identified. First, its development was guided by extensive systematic reviews and meta-analyses by two R-PAS developers and their students that examined the construct validity of 65 RCS variables (Mihura et al., 2013) as well as by meta-analyses of other non-RCS variables (Bornstein, 1999; Diener et al., 2011; Graceffo et al., 2014; Monroe et al., 2013).[1] The results of the pivotal study by Mihura et al. (2013) terminated the Rorschach critics' recommendation of a full-scale embargo on the use of the Rorschach in clinical and forensic practice (Mihura et al., 2015; Wood et al., 2015). R-PAS development was also informed by a large sample of experienced clinicians who rated test variables' clinical utility (Meyer et al., 2013).

The second improvement on previous Rorschach systems was reducing variability in the number of responses (R) that test-takers report to the 10 inkblots. This has been referred to as the "problem of R" and can interfere with test reliability (Sultan & Meyer, 2009). In addition, high R can result in over-pathologizing respondents plus long administration and scoring times, whereas low R can lead to an insufficient behavioral sample to assess pertinent psychological attributes (Meyer, 1993). To solve this problem, R-PAS uses "R-Optimization" or "R-Opt," which asks respondents to provide two to three responses per card. If only one response is given, the administrator encourages an additional response. If the respondent provides a fourth response, the assessor gives a reminder of "2 . . . maybe 3 responses" and asks for the card back. R-Opt significantly decreases the variance in R and the associated problems (Hosseininasab et al., 2019; Meyer et al., 2011; Pianowski et al., 2016, 2021).

The third R-PAS objective was collecting normative samples to improve the accuracy of interpretation. Evidence that Exner's RCS norms deviated significantly from other nonpatient samples has accrued over the years, with his child and adolescent norms being even more problematic than the adult norms (Meyer et al., 2007; Shaffer et al., 1999; Viglione & Hilsenroth, 2001; Wood et al., 2001). At the time of writing, examiners proficient in R-PAS administration and coding are collecting adult international norms. In the transition, statistically modeled norms are being used (see Meyer et al., 2011). The transitional norms for youth use 346 protocols mostly from Brazil and the United States, as well as some from Italy. Because the age-based subsamples (ages 6–17) are small, R-PAS used two statistical procedures to target true developmental changes: (a) continuous inferential norming (Zachary & Gorsuch, 1985; Zhu & Chen, 2011) and (b) bootstrap resampling procedures (Efron & Tibshirani, 1993; Howell, 2010; see Meyer & Erdberg, 2018).

The fourth alteration to developing R-PAS was reducing the time and effort needed to learn how to use the test. Free teaching aids support supervisors and

---

[1] A *meta-analysis* is a statistical summary of the strength of research findings in a particular area.

instructors. In contrast to the RCS, instead of requiring assessors to look up the descriptive statistics for each test variable to determine where the scores are high, average, or low, R-PAS plots the results in Standard Scores (SS) with a mean of 100 and *SD* of 15, like intelligence tests such as the Wechsler Adult Intelligence Scale, Fourth Edition (WAIS-IV; Wechsler, 2008). The test results are plotted on two separate pages; the Page 1 variables are more strongly supported empirically than those on Page 2.

ASSESSING BIPOLAR DISORDER

Historically, the activation, irritability, and psychosis dimensions of bipolar disorder have been emphasized (Benazzi & Akiskal, 2005; Cassidy et al., 1998; Hanwella & de Silva, 2011; Serretti et al., 1999; Topor et al., 2013). However, more contemporary research finds that the *positive activation symptoms*—euphoric mood, grandiosity, and increased energy (and related increase in activities)—form the dimension unique to bipolar disorder, whereas irritability, racing thoughts, and impaired concentration are transdiagnostic dimensions not specific to mania (Stanton et al., 2019). In the contemporary Hierarchical Taxonomy of Psychopathology (Kotov et al., 2017), the placement of bipolar disorder continues to be unresolved (Ringwald et al., 2021).

Most bipolar I patients experience the *positive symptoms of psychosis* (Tillman et al., 2008; van Bergen et al., 2019)[2]—delusions, hallucinations, and disorganized speech—which must be accurately assessed due to their predictive ability of functional impairment (Bonnín et al., 2019). The most common delusions in bipolar disorder are grandiose and occur in the manic phase (Canuso et al., 2008; Smith et al., 2017; Tillman et al., 2008). In contrast, persecutory delusions most commonly occur in the depressed phase and are, along with auditory hallucinations, significantly associated with a childhood adversity history (van Bergen et al., 2019). Research suggests that, compared with those experienced by patients with schizophrenia, hallucinations are less severe for bipolar patients and more likely to be visual rather than auditory (Baethge et al., 2005). Auditory hallucinations rarely, if ever, occur during the grandiose delusions of bipolar disorder (Smith et al., 2017; Toh et al., 2015). Finally, bipolar patients often exhibit disorganized speech; however, compared with schizophrenia, in which it is more chronic or stable, disorganized speech is more likely to occur mainly during an acute manic episode (Yalincetin et al., 2017).

In general, the bipolar condition can result in significant cognitive impairment. Systematic reviews and meta-analyses of cognitive studies with bipolar patients show problems in working memory, set-shifting, fluency, attention, and response inhibition (Abramovitch et al., 2021; East-Richard et al., 2020)—even in samples

---

[2] By definition, in the *Diagnostic and Statistical Manual of Mental Disorders* (5th ed., text rev.; *DSM-5-TR*) and *International Statistical Classification of Diseases and Related Health Problems* (11th ed.; *ICD-11*), the presence of psychosis disqualifies a patient for hypomania/bipolar II disorder and requires a bipolar I diagnosis.

largely consisting of patients in euthymic bipolar and bipolar II states (see Abramovitch et al., 2021). The overall cognitive dysfunction of bipolar patients was $d = 0.60$ compared with 0.43 for patients with attention-deficit/hyperactivity disorder. Research suggests that this cognitive impairment is stable rather than mood-episode dependent (Easter et al., 2022).

USING R-PAS TO ASSESS BIPOLAR DISORDER

The following sections provide general considerations and empirical guidance for using R-PAS when assessing for bipolar disorder. Our primary goal is to provide clinicians guidance for two common challenges in the differential diagnosis of bipolar disorder in which R-PAS can assist. The first is the differential diagnosis for patients in a depressive episode and whether they meet the criteria for major depressive disorder (MDD) or bipolar disorder. The second is the differential diagnosis of bipolar mania versus schizophrenia for patients who present with disorganized speech (see also Chapter 16 in this volume).[3]

First, we address the nature of the Rorschach task and compare it with the clinical interview to understand how patients with bipolar disorder may perform differently in each situation in the number of responses and their reaction time (RT) in providing them. Then we review the contemporary Rorschach system (RCS, R-PAS) test variables that are most often studied for patients with bipolar disorders. The R-PAS variables are number of *R*, emotional reactivity (Color), reality testing (Form Quality), and the disordered and disorganized thinking (Cognitive Codes) variables.

Positive Activation Symptoms: Behaviors

Number of R

At the very core of the test, coded in every popular Rorschach system, is the number of *R* that a respondent produces.[4] Given the high energy of persons with mania that includes talkativeness driven by the pressure to speak, clinical lore (and a reasonable expectation) is that patients experiencing a manic episode will produce a high number of responses compared with the norms as well as with depressed patients. However, research does not support this assumption (Ilonen et al., 1999; Mishra et al., 2010). While increased verbal productivity propelled by pressured speech and disinhibition is common in the clinical interview during a manic episode, it does not result in an elevated number of responses to the Rorschach inkblots.[5] Perhaps even more surprisingly, research has also not

---

[3] At the time of writing, R-PAS is in the process of preparing a second edition of its test manual. None of the anticipated modifications should change the interpretations and conclusions in this empirical section.

[4] All the studies that follow, except reaction time (RT), use *DSM-III* criteria or more recent.

[5] Patients who are too manic or agitated to follow test instructions are likely the very patients for whom formal testing procedures to diagnose mania is not required because the symptoms are extreme and obvious.

found that patients in a manic state give more responses to the inkblots than patients with MDD (Ilonen et al., 1999; Singer & Brabender, 1993). An exception is a study that found patients with MDD who had psychosis gave fewer Rorschach responses than patients experiencing a manic episode; however, this was not because patients experiencing mania gave more responses, but rather because patients with MDD who had psychosis gave fewer responses than patients with mania and schizophrenia and nonpatients (Ilonen et al., 1999).

Why would patients with mania not produce more responses to Rorschach's inkblots? We must consider the task. The Rorschach is a performance-based task that requires the respondent to follow the rules and attend to the task at hand rather than talk to the examiner. The patient is asked to solve the problem of "What might this be?" because the inkblots do not look exactly like any one thing and conflicting perceptual components exist (e.g., a bear on Card VIII, but it is pink). This performance task is different from simply talking to a clinical interviewer. As previously noted, bipolar patients have significant problems with performance tasks due to cognitive deficits (Abramovitch et al., 2021; East-Richard et al., 2020). The manic patient may be very talkative, but they will find focusing their attention on any extended performance task to be challenging.

Reaction Time

Studies have consistently found that patients with mania have faster RT in responding to the inkblots than controls. Patients with mania had faster RT compared with nonpatients (Pratap & Kapur, 1984; Schmidt & Fonda, 1954), patients with depression (Chaudhury et al., 2007), and patients with schizophrenia (Chaudhury et al., 2007; Schmidt & Fonda, 1954), and when comparing the same patients experiencing a manic versus a depressed episode (Wagner & Heise, 1981). As a caveat, we found no RT studies using contemporary Rorschach administration or diagnoses using the *Diagnostic and Statistical Manual of Mental Disorders* (3rd ed.; *DSM-III*) or after. However, the findings are highly consistent and fit what a clinician would expect given high activation and response inhibition deficits in mania.

Reactivity to Chromatic Color

Research has found support for the hypothesis that patients with bipolar disorders are more reactive to the chromatic color in the inkblots. This included those in the manic (Mishra et al., 2010) as well as the depressed phase (Kimura et al., 2013). However, these studies used different chromatic color variables ((*CF* + *C*):*FC*, Kimura et al., 2013; WSumC, Mishra et al., 2010). Therefore, caution should be used in applying these study findings in clinical practice until they can be replicated.

Positive Symptoms of Psychosis

Visual Misperceptions

Given the visual hallucinations in bipolar disorder, we would expect elevations on the R-PAS measure of visual misperceptions. The meta-analytically supported variable (Mihura et al., 2013) in R-PAS is a measure of visual misperception called Form Quality minus (FQ–).[6] In R-PAS, FQ– is defined by both a very low frequency of occurrence of people reporting the object to the particular blot location ($\leq 1.5\%$ of the sample) plus ratings of poor fit to that blot area based on an average of 9.9 raters per blot location (see Chapter 13 in Meyer et al., 2011). Research using functional magnetic resonance imaging shows that when such responses are given to the Rorschach inkblots, the portions of the brain with emotional memories override the external stimuli's impact on the occipital lobes, which leads to visual misperceptions (Asari et al., 2008, 2010a, 2010b). Patients with psychosis give significantly more of these responses than patients without psychosis, with a large effect size difference ($d = 1.065$,[7] Mihura et al., 2013).

Bipolar, Depressed Versus MDD. We found two studies comparing patients with bipolar disorders in the depressed phase with those with MDD. Those with bipolar disorders had more visual misperceptions on the Rorschach than those with MDD (Kimura et al., 2013; Singer & Brabender, 1993). Patients with bipolar disorders also showed visual misperceptions both within and between episodes (Osher & Bersudsky, 2007), whereas this was not the case for patients with unipolar MDD (Hartmann et al., 2003). Therefore, a particularly high FQ–% for a patient with depression showing no symptoms of psychosis is more consistent with a bipolar rather than MDD diagnosis.

Disorganized Thinking

A systematic review and meta-analysis shows that disordered thinking can be as elevated for persons experiencing a manic episode as it is for persons diagnosed with schizophrenia (Yalincetin et al., 2017). R-PAS contains six types of variables called Cognitive Codes that are well-validated to assess disordered thinking (Biagiarelli et al., 2015; Eblin et al., 2018; Mihura et al., 2013). Four Cognitive Codes (Deviant Response [DR], Deviant Verbalization [DV], Incongruous Combination [INC], Fabulized Combination [FAB]) have two severity levels (Levels 1 and 2). The other two (Peculiar Logic [PEC], Contamination) are considered severe on their own. The Cognitive Codes are further differentiated as either (a) linguistic codes that involve language and reasoning or (b) perceptual visual codes that involve images. Table 9.1 illustrates how the R-PAS linguistic codes overlap with the interview-based measure of disorganized thinking called The Scale for the Assessment of Thought, Language, and Communication (Andreasen, 1986) and provides examples of the visual combinatory imagery-based codes. The Cognitive Codes are aggregated to form summary variables, of which the most common type in the bipolar studies weights the individual Cognitive Codes for their level of severity called the Weighted Sum of Cognitive Codes (WSumCog).

---

[6] Note that Exner's (2003) norms for the FQ variables overpathologize respondents on this measure of psychosis, particularly of misperceptions (Meyer et al., 2007).
[7] Converted from the *r* metric reported in Table 4 in Mihura et al. (2013).

TABLE 9.1. Comparing Positive Thought Disorder Scores on the R-PAS and the TLC

Rorschach variable	Definition and associated TLC category
Linguistic codes	
Deviant Responses (DR)	Communication either deviates two or more steps away from the task of describing what the inkblot might be and why, or the verbiage is so odd and inappropriate that it need not meet the two-step rule (e.g., "I saw the spiders, they were in a spider war, like the government. I got some me some new boots, and the psychologists were angry").
TLC categories	Derailment, tangentiality, loss of goal, incoherence. Possibly relevant: Distractible speech and circumstantiality
Deviant Verbalizations (DV)	Broad category of using the wrong word or phrase, using either a real or a made-up word (e.g., a "paperskate" for the word pen; "globulasanamous," unclear what it means)
TLC categories	Neologisms, word-approximations, clanging, semantic paraphasia, phonemic paraphasia
Peculiar Logic (PEC)	Illogical or problematic reasoning is used to justify the response (e.g., "It's a king because he isn't moving").
TLC categories	Illogicality
Perceptual codes	
Combinatory responses (FAB, INC, CON)	Unrealistic or impossible visual combinations between separate objects (e.g., "a woman eating a spaceship"; Fabulized Combinations [FAB]), between components or attributes of a single object (e.g., "a man's head with feet for ears"; Incongruous Combinations [INC]), or overlapping images (e.g., seeing a bat superimposed on an angel; Contaminations [CON])
TLC categories	None

Note. R-PAS = Rorschach Performance Assessment System; TLC = Scale for the Assessment of Thought, Language, and Communication.

Bipolar, Mania Versus Schizophrenia. The previous meta-analysis by Yalincetin et al. (2017) that found disorganized thinking equally elevated for patients with mania and those with schizophrenia included a clinical interview and Rorschach-based measures. Most interesting for our purposes is that the type of disordered thinking that differentiated mania from schizophrenia were Rorschach imagery-based perceptual variables (e.g., "a beetle crying," "neon pink bears") that cannot be derived from the clinical interview. Specifically, the Rorschach studies by Yalincetin et al. (2017) used an aggregate of three visual combinatory scores from the Thought Disorder Index (Holzman et al., 2005; Johnston & Holzman, 1979) that overlap with the R-PAS INC and FAB scores (incongruous combinations, fabulized combinations, playful confabulations). Daniels et al. (1988) and Shenton et al. (1987) found that patients with mania scored significantly higher on these visual combinatory scores than patients with schizophrenia (see also Chapter 16 in this volume). Mishra et al. (2009) used the INC and FAB variables coded in R-PAS and found patients with mania scored higher on these scores than patients with schizophrenia.

Bipolar, Depressed Versus MDD. Patients with bipolar depression and MDD are both likely to have elevations on disordered thinking on R-PAS (Hartmann et al., 2003; Kimura et al., 2013; Mason et al., 1985). This disordered thinking is more likely to persist between mood episodes for patients with bipolar disorders but not for those with MDD (Hartmann et al., 2003; Meyer et al., 2007; Osher & Bersudsky, 2007). Yet patients with bipolar depression show even more disordered thinking on the Rorschach than those with MDD (Kimura et al., 2013; Le Chevanton et al., 2020; Singer & Brabender, 1993)—in particular, on derailed or tangential speech (DRs) and more benign levels of the imagery-based combinatory thinking variables (INC1; Le Chevanton et al., 2020; Singer & Brabender, 1993). Therefore, a high WSumCog scale that includes DR and/or INC elevations is more consistent with a patient with a bipolar disorder in a depressed state than a patient with MDD.

Clinical Implications

When patients present for treatment in a depressed state, unless the clinician is familiar with the patient's history, it can be unclear whether the patient meets the criteria for MDD or bipolar depression. It is crucial to identify assessment tools that can alert the clinician to the possibility of a bipolar rather than MDD diagnosis. Prescribing monotherapy antidepressants to depressed patients with even minimal manic symptoms at the baseline can result in the emergence of hypomania or mania (Barbuti et al., 2017; Bhowmik et al., 2014; Frye et al., 2009).

The unique visual nature of the Rorschach can make it a useful tool to add to the clinical interview when assessing for bipolar disorder. Research shows that patients with bipolar disorders are more likely than those with schizophrenia to have visual rather than auditory hallucinations. The Rorschach, not the clinical interview, can behaviorally assess visual misperceptions (FQ−%) and unrealistic visual combinations (INC, FAB). Specifically, compared with patients with MDD, those with bipolar depression are likely to have elevated FQ−% and WSumCog on R-PAS. Further, the WSumCog elevation is most likely to include the visual combinatory scores. In fact, INC is likely to be elevated throughout the bipolar spectrum, during depressed, manic, and even stable or euthymic states. Both types of visual combinatory scores (INC, FAB) are more likely to be elevated in bipolar, mania.

CASE ILLUSTRATION WITH A MULTIMETHOD FOCUS

Ms. CD was a 26-year-old cisgender White female law student seeking accommodations for her upcoming bar exam, because she claimed that anxiety interfered with her test performance by affecting her attention and concentration.[8] She had taken the Law School Admission Test (LSAT) twice without

---

[8] The identity of this individual has been carefully disguised to protect their identity.

accommodations and had obtained modest scores of 140 and 145. She was accepted to a provisionally accredited law school that shut down before she graduated. She transferred to an accredited but low-ranked law school. Ms. CD carried a diagnosis of bipolar II disorder, for which she was taking Wellbutrin and an atypical antipsychotic. She said the medications were effective, except for her continued difficulties falling and staying asleep. Her primary concern was anxiety impairing her ability to perform well on exams.

Consistent with Ms. CD's self-reported anxiety in the clinical interview, her highest Personality Assessment Inventory (PAI) scores were on the anxiety scales (Anxiety [ANX], Anxiety-Related Disorders [ARD]). On the Anxiety-Related Disorders Obsessive-Compulsive subscale, she reported extreme perfectionism and keeping herself and her impulses under very tight control. On the PAI and Minnesota Multiphasic Personality Inventory–2 (MMPI-2), her anxiety symptoms were mainly physiological. On the depression scales, she reported physiological symptoms including sleep problems as well as a lack of energy and a sense of psychomotor slowness. She also described social anxiety and a tendency to avoid social situations in a clinical interview, which was also indicated on the MMPI-2 Social Discomfort and PAI Schizophrenia-Social Detachment scales. On R-PAS, the measure of implicit distress (Sum of Shading + Achromatic Color [YTVC']) was moderately elevated. Behaviorally, she frequently criticized her performance and worried aloud what the examiner would think of it.

Positive Activation Symptoms

Despite Ms. CD's subjective sense of psychomotor slowness and her self-criticism, she had elevated PAI scales assessing positive activation, including mania activity level (MAN-A), grandiosity (MAN-G), impulsive acts (Borderline-Self-Harm [BOR-S]), and affective instability related to rapidly shifting and intense moods (BOR-Affective Instability [BOR-A]). She reported racing thoughts, speaking so quickly that people often cannot keep up, possessing special talents, and accomplishing remarkable things. During the assessment, she was constantly moving (shaking her leg, tapping fingers, talking, moving in her seat) and spoke with pressured speech. She approached each task with notable urgency to complete it as quickly as possible. She completed the PAI, MMPI-2, and R-PAS in half the time that is typical in clinical settings. On the Conners' Continuous Performance Test II (CPT-II), her RT was very fast, and she made numerous commission errors. When the CPT-II was readministered emphasizing accuracy rather than speed, her commission errors reduced. Although Ms. CD could slow down and improve her accuracy, this took a toll; she appeared exhausted after the cognitive testing.

Positive Symptoms of Psychosis

Ms. CD's PAI grandiosity scale was elevated, but not at delusional levels. On R-PAS, her visual misperceptions scale was entirely average (FQ−%, SS = 100); instead, her perceptions were unconventional (Popular, SS = 88). Therefore, testing did not support perceptual anomalies or delusion thinking. However, her self-view was somewhat inflated, given she equated her school performance with having special talents even though she had mediocre LSAT scores and difficulty getting into a good law school.

In the clinical interview, she was very talkative, but her thoughts were linear, simple, and easy to follow. Consistent with the interview, her R-PAS results also did not indicate disorganized thinking (DRs = 0), neologisms (DV2 = 0), or illogical thinking (PEC = 0). Like the content of her speech in the clinical interview, the content of her R-PAS imagery was quite simple. For example, of her 23 responses, she saw seven bugs, three leaves, a big cloud of gas, a cloud of "something exploding," and seven animals (a bird, two crabs, two iguanas, and two seahorses). Her Content Complexity score was very low (SS = 79). Seven of her images included benign visual combinatory thinking scores (INC1s), which is extremely high (SS = 146). These were entirely due to identifying "antlers" or "arms" on bugs or animals: a bug with antler-like arms and a stinger, a bug with arms, two bugs with antlers, a face with an antler sticking from the forehead, an iguana with arms, and a crab with arms.

Symptom Impact on Cognitive Impairment

Ms. CD's Wechsler Abbreviated Scale Intelligence, Second Edition Full Scale IQ was average with little variability across subscale scores. Her Wechsler Memory Scale, Fourth Edition auditory memory was in the high average range; her WAIS-IV Digit Span and her Wechsler Memory Scale, Fourth Edition visual, visual working, immediate, and delayed memory scores were average. Arithmetic was her only low working memory score; Ms. CD told the assessor that she was just "bad at math." On R-PAS, Ms. CD's Complexity score was low (SS = 85), consistent with the simple content of her imagery. Persons with higher IQs tend to have higher Complexity scores (e.g., Meyer, 2016). Therefore, although anxiety could have interfered with her overall cognitive performance, there was no evidence that it specifically affected attention and concentration.

Conclusion and Recommendations

Ms. CD self-reported high levels of anxiety, as is common in patients with bipolar disorders, particularly those with bipolar II (Akiskal et al., 2006; Rihmer et al., 2001; Spoorthy et al., 2019). Yet, strikingly, across all methods of assessment, Ms. CD was clearly negatively impacted by positive activation symptoms. Her benign visual combinatory thinking and rapid response on R-PAS also suggested a tendency for impulsively disregarding realistic perceptions of the world. A pressured sense of urgency pervaded her performance, resulting in impulsivity and difficulty thinking things through. When she exerted effort to slow down and concentrate, she could perform less impulsively. However, doing so exhausted her psychological resources.

Ms. CD was already taking medication to address her bipolar II symptoms; however, results of the multimethod assessment showed that she was exerting a significant amount of energy trying to slow down in order to concentrate on tests. Therefore, her psychiatrist was provided with these assessment findings, which suggested that a medication adjustment to address her level of activation might be beneficial. Ms. CD's psychiatrist started by reducing her Wellbutrin from 300 mg to 150 mg given its energizing effects.

LIMITATIONS

The biggest limitation of this chapter is the limited number of relevant empirical studies with different study designs. For example, some studies included patients with bipolar disorders when depressed, others when manic, and still others when in a euthymic state. Some studies reported that the bipolar sample had psychotic features while for other studies it was unclear. The comparison samples ranged from nonpatients to those with MDD or schizophrenia, and sometimes a sample design comparing the depressed with the manic phase. Another limitation was the lack of pure bipolar II samples. Arguably, unless the patient is hospitalized due to mania, other bipolar presentations can require additional testing for differential diagnosis. Accurate diagnosis of bipolar disorder is crucial, as it is delayed up to 10 or more years after the onset of symptoms (Hirschfeld et al., 2003; Yatham et al., 2018; see also the Introduction in this volume). Visual combinatory thinking cannot be assessed in the clinical interview; therefore, in this way, R-PAS can add to the evidence of a bipolar spectrum diagnosis. We provided an actual case of bipolar II for illustration of how the R-PAS visual combinatory scores were elevated even when the patient was medicated.

CONCLUSION AND FUTURE DIRECTIONS

As discussed, patients with bipolar disorders in acute manic states are as likely to show disorganized speech as those with schizophrenia (DR2 in R-PAS). However, research indicates that those with bipolar disorders display more visual combinatory thinking on the Rorschach—incongruous combinations (INC) and fabulized combinations (FAB)—than patients with schizophrenia or MDD (for additional discussion, see Kleiger, 2017). Consistent with the increased chance of visual hallucinations in bipolar I disorder, the R-PAS visual misperception variable (FQ−%) is also likely to be elevated. We caution clinicians against expecting manic or hypomanic patients to produce an elevated number of responses as research does not support this.

 There is a need for Rorschach research targeting patients with bipolar II disorder. For clinical illustration, we provided multimethod assessment results that included R-PAS for a young woman diagnosed with bipolar II disorder. Finally, we encourage R-PAS researchers to replicate the findings with patients with bipolar I described in this chapter. The visual aberrations in mania and the visual nature of the Rorschach can provide incremental diagnostic validity to the clinical interview and self-report measures like the PAI and MMPI-3.

REFERENCES

Abramovitch, A., Short, T., & Schweiger, A. (2021). The C factor: Cognitive dysfunction as a transdiagnostic dimension in psychopathology. *Clinical Psychology Review, 86*, Article 102007. https://doi.org/10.1016/j.cpr.2021.102007

Akiskal, H. S., Akiskal, K. K., Perugi, G., Toni, C., Ruffolo, G., & Tusini, G. (2006). Bipolar II and anxious reactive "comorbidity": Toward better phenotypic characterization suitable for genotyping. *Journal of Affective Disorders, 96*(3), 239–247. https://doi.org/10.1016/j.jad.2006.08.010

Andreasen, N. C. (1986). Scale for the assessment of thought, language, and communication (TLC). *Schizophrenia Bulletin, 12*(3), 473–482. https://doi.org/10.1093/schbul/12.3.473

Asari, T., Konishi, S., Jimura, K., Chikazoe, J., Nakamura, N., & Miyashita, Y. (2008). Right temporopolar activation associated with unique perception. *NeuroImage, 41*(1), 145–152. https://doi.org/10.1016/j.neuroimage.2008.01.059

Asari, T., Konishi, S., Jimura, K., Chikazoe, J., Nakamura, N., & Miyashita, Y. (2010a). Amygdalar enlargement associated with unique perception. *Cortex, 46*(1), 94–99. https://doi.org/10.1016/j.cortex.2008.08.001

Asari, T., Konishi, S., Jimura, K., Chikazoe, J., Nakamura, N., & Miyashita, Y. (2010b). Amygdalar modulation of frontotemporal connectivity during the inkblot test. *Psychiatry Research, 182*(2), 103–110. https://doi.org/10.1016/j.pscychresns.2010.01.002

Baethge, C., Baldessarini, R. J., Freudenthal, K., Streeruwitz, A., Bauer, M., & Bschor, T. (2005). Hallucinations in bipolar disorder: Characteristics and comparison to unipolar depression and schizophrenia. *Bipolar Disorders, 7*(2), 136–145. https://doi.org/10.1111/j.1399-5618.2004.00175.x

Barbuti, M., Pacchiarotti, I., Vieta, E., Azorin, J.-M., Angst, J., Bowden, C. L., Mosolov, S., Young, A. H., Perugi, G., & the BRIDGE-II-Mix Study Group. (2017). Antidepressant-induced hypomania/mania in patients with major depression: Evidence from the BRIDGE-II-MIX study. *Journal of Affective Disorders, 219*, 187–192. https://doi.org/10.1016/j.jad.2017.05.035

Beck, S. J. (1937). *Introduction to the Rorschach method: A manual of personality study.* American Orthopsychiatric Association. https://doi.org/10.1037/12226-000

Benazzi, F., & Akiskal, H. (2005). Irritable-hostile depression: Further validation as a bipolar depressive mixed state. *Journal of Affective Disorders, 84*(2–3), 197–207. https://doi.org/10.1016/j.jad.2004.07.006

Bhowmik, D., Aparasu, R. R., Rajan, S. S., Sherer, J. T., Ochoa-Perez, M., & Chen, H. (2014). Risk of manic switch associated with antidepressant therapy in pediatric bipolar depression. *Journal of Child and Adolescent Psychopharmacology, 24*(10), 551–561. https://doi.org/10.1089/cap.2014.0028

Biagiarelli, M., Roma, P., Comparelli, A., Andraos, M. P., Di Pomponio, I., Corigliano, V., Curto, M., Masters, G. A., & Ferracuti, S. (2015). Relationship between the Rorschach Perceptual Thinking Index (PTI) and the Positive and Negative Syndrome Scale (PANSS) in psychotic patients: A validity study. *Psychiatry Research, 225*(3), 315–321. https://doi.org/10.1016/j.psychres.2014.12.018

Bonnín, C. M., Jiménez, E., Solé, B., Torrent, C., Radua, J., Reinares, M., Grande, I., Ruíz, V., Sánchez-Moreno, J., Martínez-Arán, A., & Vieta, E. (2019). Lifetime psychotic symptoms, subthreshold depression and cognitive impairment as barriers to functional recovery in patients with bipolar disorder. *Journal of Clinical Medicine, 8*(7), Article E1046. https://doi.org/10.3390/jcm8071046

Bornstein, R. F. (1999). Criterion validity of objective and projective dependency tests: A meta-analytic assessment of behavioral prediction. *Psychological Assessment, 11*(1), 48–57. https://doi.org/10.1037/1040-3590.11.1.48

Canuso, C. M., Bossie, C. A., Zhu, Y., Youssef, E., & Dunner, D. L. (2008). Psychotic symptoms in patients with bipolar mania. *Journal of Affective Disorders, 111*(2–3), 164–169. https://doi.org/10.1016/j.jad.2008.02.014

Cassidy, F., Forest, K., Murry, E., & Carroll, B. J. (1998). A factor analysis of the signs and symptoms of mania. *Archives of General Psychiatry, 55*(1), 27–32. https://doi.org/10.1001/archpsyc.55.1.27

Chaudhury, S., Saldanha, D., Srivastava, K., Jyothi, S. G., Sundari, G. S., & Augustine, M. (2007). Rorschach responses of Indian children and adolescents with psychiatric disorders. *Journal of Projective Psychology & Mental Health, 14*(2), 150–161. https://2d-crowd.com/sisJournal/abstracts/27

Daniels, E. K., Shenton, M. E., Holzman, P. S., Benowitz, L. I., Coleman, M., Levin, S., & Levine, D. (1988). Patterns of thought disorder associated with right cortical damage, schizophrenia, and mania. *The American Journal of Psychiatry, 145*(8), 944–949. https://doi.org/10.1176/ajp.145.8.944

Diener, M. J., Hilsenroth, M. J., Shaffer, S. A., & Sexton, J. E. (2011). A meta-analysis of the relationship between the Rorschach Ego Impairment Index (EII) and psychiatric severity. *Clinical Psychology & Psychotherapy, 18*(6), 464–485. https://doi.org/10.1002/cpp.725

Easter, R. E., Ryan, K. A., Estabrook, R., Marshall, D. F., McInnis, M. G., & Langenecker, S. A. (2022). Limited time-specific and longitudinal effects of depressive and manic symptoms on cognition in bipolar spectrum disorders. *Acta Psychiatrica Scandinavica, 146*(5), 430–441. https://doi.org/10.1111/acps.13436

East-Richard, C., R. -Mercier, A., Nadeau, D., & Cellard, C. (2020). Transdiagnostic neurocognitive deficits in psychiatry: A review of meta-analyses. *Canadian Psychology, 61*(3), 190–214. https://doi.org/10.1037/cap0000196

Eblin, J. J., Meyer, G. J., Mihura, J. L., Viglione, D. J., & O'Gorman, E. T. (2018). Development and preliminary validation of a brief behavioral measure of psychotic propensity. *Psychiatry Research, 268*, 340–347. https://doi.org/10.1016/j.psychres.2018.08.006

Efron, B., & Tibshirani, R. J. (1993). *An introduction to the bootstrap (monographs on statistics and applied probability)* (Vol. 57). Chapman and Hall. https://doi.org/10.1007/978-1-4899-4541-9

Exner, J. E. (1974). *The Rorschach: A comprehensive system.* Wiley.

Exner, J. E. (2003). *The Rorschach: A comprehensive system* (4th ed.). Wiley.

Frye, M. A., Helleman, G., McElroy, S. L., Altshuler, L. L., Black, D. O., Keck, P. E., Jr., Nolen, W. A., Kupka, R., Leverich, G. S., Grunze, H., Mintz, J., Post, R. M., & Suppes, T. (2009). Correlates of treatment-emergent mania associated with antidepressant treatment in bipolar depression. *The American Journal of Psychiatry, 166*(2), 164–172. https://doi.org/10.1176/appi.ajp.2008.08030322

Graceffo, R. A., Mihura, J. L., & Meyer, G. J. (2014). A meta-analysis of an implicit measure of personality functioning: The Mutuality of Autonomy Scale. *Journal of Personality Assessment, 96*(6), 581–595. https://doi.org/10.1080/00223891.2014.919299

Hanwella, R., & de Silva, V. A. (2011). Signs and symptoms of acute mania: A factor analysis. *BMC Psychiatry, 11*(1), Article 137. https://doi.org/10.1186/1471-244X-11-137

Hartmann, E., Wang, C. E., Berg, M., & Saether, L. (2003). Depression and vulnerability as assessed by the Rorschach method. *Journal of Personality Assessment, 81*(3), 242–255. https://doi.org/10.1207/S15327752JPA8103_07

Hertz, M. R. (1936). *Frequency tables for scoring responses to the Rorschach Inkblot Test.* Western Reserve University Press.

Hirschfeld, R. M., Lewis, L., & Vornik, L. A. (2003). Perceptions and impact of bipolar disorder: How far have we really come? Results of the national depressive and manic-depressive association 2000 survey of individuals with bipolar disorder. *The Journal of Clinical Psychiatry, 64*(2), 161–174. https://doi.org/10.4088/JCP.v64n0209

Holzman, P. S., Levy, D. L., & Johnston, M. H. (2005). The use of the Rorschach technique for assessing formal thought disorder. In R. F. Bornstein & J. M. Masling (Eds.), *Scoring the Rorschach: Seven validated systems* (pp. 55–95). Lawrence Erlbaum.

Hosseininasab, A., Meyer, G. J., Viglione, D. J., Mihura, J. L., Berant, E., Resende, A. C., Reese, J., & Mohammadi, M. R. (2019). The effect of RCS administration or an R-optimized alternative on R-PAS variables: A meta-analysis of findings from six studies. *Journal of Personality Assessment, 101*(2), 199–212. https://doi.org/10.1080/00223891.2017.1393430

Howell, D. C. (2010). *Statistical methods for psychology* (8th ed.). Cengage Learning.

Ilonen, T., Taiminen, T., Karlsson, H., Lauerma, H., Leinonen, K. M., Wallenius, E., Tuimala, P., & Salokangas, R. K. R. (1999). Diagnostic efficiency of the Rorschach schizophrenia and depression indices in identifying first-episode schizophrenia and severe depression. *Psychiatry Research, 87*(2–3), 183–192. https://doi.org/10.1016/S0165-1781(99)00061-X

Johnston, M. H., & Holzman, P. S. (1979). *Assessing schizophrenic thinking: A clinical and research instrument for measuring thought disorder* (1st ed.). Jossey-Bass.

Kimura, H., Osaki, A., Kawashima, R., Inoue, T., Nakagawa, S., Suzuki, K., Asakura, S., Tanaka, T., Kitaichi, Y., Masui, T., Kitagawa, N., Kako, Y., Abekawa, T., Kusumi, I., Yamanaka, H., Denda, K., & Koyama, T. (2013). Differences between bipolar and unipolar depression on Rorschach testing. *Neuropsychiatric Disease and Treatment, 9*, 619–627. https://doi.org/10.2147/NDT.S42702

Kleiger, J. H. (2017). *Rorschach assessment of psychotic phenomena: Clinical, conceptual, and empirical developments*. Routledge/Taylor & Francis. https://doi.org/10.4324/9781315271385

Klopfer, B., Ainsworth, M. D., Klopfer, W. G., & Holt, R. R. (1954). *Developments in the Rorschach technique: Vol. 1. Technique and theory*. World Book.

Kotov, R., Krueger, R. F., Watson, D., Achenbach, T. M., Althoff, R. R., Bagby, R. M., Brown, T. A., Carpenter, W. T., Caspi, A., Clark, L. A., Eaton, N. R., Forbes, M. K., Forbush, K. T., Goldberg, D., Hasin, D., Hyman, S. E., Ivanova, M. Y., Lynam, D. R., Markon, K., . . . Zimmerman, M. (2017). The Hierarchical Taxonomy of Psychopathology (HiTOP): A dimensional alternative to traditional nosologies. *Journal of Abnormal Psychology, 126*(4), 454–477. https://doi.org/10.1037/abn0000258

Le Chevanton, T., Fouques, D., Julien-Sweerts, S., Petot, D., & Polosan, M. (2020). Differentiating unipolar and bipolar depression: Contribution of the Rorschach test (Comprehensive System). *Journal of Clinical Psychology, 76*(4), 769–777. https://doi.org/10.1002/jclp.22912

Mason, B. J., Cohen, J. B., & Exner, J. E., Jr. (1985). Schizophrenic, depressive, and nonpatient personality organizations described by Rorschach factor structures. *Journal of Personality Assessment, 49*(3), 295–305. https://doi.org/10.1207/s15327752jpa4903_16

Meyer, G. J. (1993). The impact of response frequency on the Rorschach constellation indices and on their validity with diagnostic and MMPI-2 criteria. *Journal of Personality Assessment, 60*(1), 153–180. https://doi.org/10.1207/s15327752jpa6001_13

Meyer, G. J. (2016). Neuropsychological factors and Rorschach performance in children. *Rorschachiana, 37*(1), 7–27. https://doi.org/10.1027/1192-5604/a000074

Meyer, G. J., & Erdberg, P. (2018). Using R-PAS norms with an emphasis on children and adolescents. In J. L. Mihura & G. J. Meyer (Eds.), *Using the Rorschach Performance Assessment System® (R-PAS®)* (pp. 46–61). Guilford Press.

Meyer, G. J., Erdberg, P., & Shaffer, T. W. (2007). Toward international normative reference data for the comprehensive system. *Journal of Personality Assessment, 89*(Suppl. 1), S201–S216. https://doi.org/10.1080/00223890701629342

Meyer, G. J., Hsiao, W.-C., Viglione, D. J., Mihura, J. L., & Abraham, L. M. (2013). Rorschach scores in applied clinical practice: A survey of perceived validity by experienced clinicians. *Journal of Personality Assessment, 95*(4), 351–365. https://doi.org/10.1080/00223891.2013.770399

Meyer, G. J., & Mihura, J. L. (2021). Rorschach Performance Assessment System (R-PAS) for assessing disordered thought and perception. In I. B. Weiner & J. H. Kleiger (Eds.), *Psychological assessment of disordered thinking and perception* (pp. 151–168). American Psychological Association. https://doi.org/10.1037/0000245-010

Meyer, G. J., Viglione, D. J., Mihura, J. L., Erard, R. E., & Erdberg, P. (2011). *Rorschach Performance Assessment System: Administration, coding, interpretation, and technical manual.* Rorschach Performance Assessment System.

Mihura, J. L., & Meyer, G. J. (2022). The Rorschach Performance Assessment System (R-PAS) in multimethod assessment. In J. L. Mihura (Ed.), *The Oxford handbook of personality and psychopathology assessment* (2nd ed.). Oxford University Press.

Mihura, J. L., Meyer, G. J., Bombel, G., & Dumitrascu, N. (2015). Standards, accuracy, and questions of bias in Rorschach meta-analyses: Reply to Wood, Garb, Nezworski, Lilienfeld, and Duke (2015). *Psychological Bulletin, 141*(1), 250–260. https://doi.org/10.1037/a0038445

Mihura, J. L., Meyer, G. J., Dumitrascu, N., & Bombel, G. (2013). The validity of individual Rorschach variables: Systematic reviews and meta-analyses of the comprehensive system. *Psychological Bulletin, 139*(3), 548–605. https://doi.org/10.1037/a0029406

Mishra, D., Khalique, A., & Kumar, R. (2010). Rorschach profile of manic patients. *Journal of Projective Psychology & Mental Health, 17*(2), 158–164. https://2d-crowd.com/sisJournal/abstracts/33

Mishra, D., Kumar, R., & Prakash, J. (2009). Rorschach thought disorders in various psychiatric conditions. *Journal of Projective Psychology & Mental Health, 16*(1), 8–12. https://2d-crowd.com/sisJournal/abstracts/30

Monroe, J. M., Diener, M. J., Fowler, J. C., Sexton, J. E., & Hilsenroth, M. J. (2013). Criterion validity of the Rorschach Mutuality of Autonomy (MOA) scale: A meta-analytic review. *Psychoanalytic Psychology, 30*(4), 535–566. https://doi.org/10.1037/a0033290

Osher, Y., & Bersudsky, Y. (2007). Thought disorder in euthymic bipolar patients: A possible endophenotype of bipolar affective disorder? *Journal of Nervous and Mental Disease, 195*(10), 857–860. https://doi.org/10.1097/NMD.0b013e318156832d

Pianowski, G., Meyer, G. J., & de Villemor-Amaral, A. E. (2016). The impact of R-optimized administration modeling procedures on Brazilian normative reference values for Rorschach scores. *Journal of Personality Assessment, 98*(4), 408–418. https://doi.org/10.1080/00223891.2016.1148701

Pianowski, G., Meyer, G. J., de Villemor-Amaral, A. E., Zuanazzi, A. C., & do Nascimento, R. S. G. F. (2021). Does the Rorschach Performance Assessment System (R-PAS) differ from the Comprehensive System (RCS) on variables relevant to interpretation? *Journal of Personality Assessment, 103*(1), 132–147. https://doi.org/10.1080/00223891.2019.1677678

Piotrowski, Z. A. (1957). *Perceptanalysis; a fundamentally reworked, expanded, and systematized Rorschach method.* Macmillan.

Pratap, S., & Kapur, M. (1984). Rorschach study of literate manics. *Indian Journal of Clinical Psychology, 11*(2), 29–34.

Rapaport, D., Gill, M., & Schafer, R. (1946). *Diagnostic psychological testing: The theory, statistical evaluation, and diagnostic application of a battery of tests* (Vol. II). The Year Book Publishers.

Rihmer, Z., Szádóczky, E., Füredi, J., Kiss, K., & Papp, Z. (2001). Anxiety disorders comorbidity in bipolar I, bipolar II and unipolar major depression: Results from a population-based study in Hungary. *Journal of Affective Disorders, 67*(1–3), 175–179. https://doi.org/10.1016/S0165-0327(01)00309-3

Ringwald, W. R., Forbes, M. K., & Wright, A. G. C. (2021). Meta-analysis of structural evidence for the Hierarchical Taxonomy of Psychopathology (HiTOP) model. *Psychological Medicine.* Advance online publication. https://doi.org/10.1017/S0033291721001902

Rorschach, H. (1921). *Psychodiagnostics: A diagnostic test based on perception.* Hans Huber.

Schmidt, H. O., & Fonda, C. P. (1954). Rorschach scores in the manic state. *The Journal of Psychology, 38*(2), 427–437. https://doi.org/10.1080/00223980.1954.9712949

Serretti, A., Rietschel, M., Lattuada, E., Krauss, H., Held, T., Nöthen, M. M., & Smeraldi, E. (1999). Factor analysis of mania. *Archives of General Psychiatry, 56*(7), 671–672. https://doi.org/10.1001/archpsyc.56.7.671

Shaffer, T. W., Erdberg, P., & Haroian, J. (1999). Current nonpatient data for the Rorschach, WAIS-R, and MMPI-2. *Journal of Personality Assessment, 73*(2), 305–316. https://doi.org/10.1207/S15327752JPA7302_8

Shenton, M. E., Solovay, M. R., & Holzman, P. (1987). Comparative studies of thought disorders. II. Schizoaffective disorder. *Archives of General Psychiatry, 44*(1), 21–30. https://doi.org/10.1001/archpsyc.1987.01800130023004

Singer, H. K., & Brabender, V. (1993). The use of the Rorschach to differentiate unipolar and bipolar disorders. *Journal of Personality Assessment, 60*(2), 333–345. https://doi.org/10.1207/s15327752jpa6002_10

Smith, L. M., Johns, L. C., & Mitchell, R. (2017). Characterizing the experience of auditory verbal hallucinations and accompanying delusions in individuals with a diagnosis of bipolar disorder: A systematic review. *Bipolar Disorders, 19*(6), 417–433. https://doi.org/10.1111/bdi.12520

Spoorthy, M. S., Chakrabarti, S., & Grover, S. (2019). Comorbidity of bipolar and anxiety disorders: An overview of trends in research. *World Journal of Psychiatry, 9*(1), 7–29. https://doi.org/10.5498/wjp.v9.i1.7

Stanton, K., Khoo, S., Watson, D., Gruber, J., Zimmerman, M., & Weinstock, L. M. (2019). Unique and transdiagnostic symptoms of hypomania/mania and unipolar depression. *Clinical Psychological Science, 7*(3), 471–487. https://doi.org/10.1177/2167702618812725

Sultan, S., & Meyer, G. J. (2009). Does productivity impact the stability of Rorschach scores? *Journal of Personality Assessment, 91*(5), 480–493. https://doi.org/10.1080/00223890903088693

Tillman, R., Geller, B., Klages, T., Corrigan, M., Bolhofner, K., & Zimerman, B. (2008). Psychotic phenomena in 257 young children and adolescents with bipolar I disorder: Delusions and hallucinations (benign and pathological). *Bipolar Disorders, 10*(1), 45–55. https://doi.org/10.1111/j.1399-5618.2008.00480.x

Toh, W. L., Thomas, N., & Rossell, S. L. (2015). Auditory verbal hallucinations in bipolar disorder (BD) and major depressive disorder (MDD): A systematic review. *Journal of Affective Disorders, 184*, 18–28. https://doi.org/10.1016/j.jad.2015.05.040

Topor, D. R., Swenson, L., Hunt, J. I., Birmaher, B., Strober, M., Yen, S., Hoeppner, B. B., Case, B. G., Hower, H., Weinstock, L. M., Ryan, N., Goldstein, B., Goldstein, T., Gill, M. K., Axelson, D., & Keller, M. (2013). Manic symptoms in youth with bipolar disorder: Factor analysis by age of symptom onset and current age. *Journal of Affective Disorders, 145*(3), 409–412. https://doi.org/10.1016/j.jad.2012.06.024

van Bergen, A. H., Verkooijen, S., Vreeker, A., Abramovic, L., Hillegers, M. H.,
Spijker, A. T., Hoencamp, E., Regeer, E. J., Knapen, S. E., Riemersma-van der Lek, R. F.,
Schoevers, R., Stevens, A. W., Schulte, P. F. J., Vonk, R., Hoekstra, R.,
van Beveren, N. J., Kupka, R. W., Sommer, I. E. C., Ophoff, R. A., . . . Boks, M. P. M.
(2019). The characteristics of psychotic features in bipolar disorder. *Psychological
Medicine, 49*(12), 2036–2048. https://doi.org/10.1017/S0033291718002854

Viglione, D. J., & Hilsenroth, M. J. (2001). The Rorschach: Facts, fictions, and future.
Psychological Assessment, 13(4), 452–471. https://doi.org/10.1037/1040-3590.13.4.452

Wagner, E. E., & Heise, M. R. (1981). Rorschach and Hand Test data comparing bipolar
patients in manic and depressive phases. *Journal of Personality Assessment, 45*(3),
240–249. https://doi.org/10.1207/s15327752jpa4503_3

Wechsler, D. (2008). *Wechsler Adult Intelligence Scale–Fourth Edition (WAIS-IV)* [Database
record]. APA PsycTests. https://doi.org/10.1037/t15169-000

Wood, J. M., Garb, H. N., Nezworski, M. T., Lilienfeld, S. O., & Duke, M. C. (2015).
A second look at the validity of widely used Rorschach indices: Comment on Mihura,
Meyer, Dumitrascu, and Bombel (2013). *Psychological Bulletin, 141*(1), 236–249. https://
doi.org/10.1037/a0036005

Wood, J. M., Nezworski, M. T., Garb, H. N., & Lilienfeld, S. O. (2001). The misperception of
psychopathology: Problems with the norms of the Comprehensive System for the
Rorschach. *Clinical Psychology: Science and Practice, 8*(3), 350–373. https://doi.org/10.
1093/clipsy.8.3.350

Yalincetin, B., Bora, E., Binbay, T., Ulas, H., Akdede, B. B., & Alptekin, K. (2017). Formal
thought disorder in schizophrenia and bipolar disorder: A systematic review and meta-
analysis. *Schizophrenia Research, 185*, 2–8. https://doi.org/10.1016/j.schres.2016.12.015

Yatham, L. N., Kennedy, S. H., Parikh, S. V., Schaffer, A., Bond, D. J., Frey, B. N.,
Sharma, V., Goldstein, B. I., Rej, S., Beaulieu, S., Alda, M., MacQueen, G.,
Milev, R. V., Ravindran, A., O'Donovan, C., McIntosh, D., Lam, R. W., Vazquez, G.,
Kapczinski, F., . . . Berk, M. (2018). Canadian Network for Mood and Anxiety
Treatments (CANMAT) and International Society for Bipolar Disorders (ISBD) 2018
guidelines for the management of patients with bipolar disorder. *Bipolar Disorders,
20*(2), 97–170. https://doi.org/10.1111/bdi.12609

Zachary, R. A., & Gorsuch, R. L. (1985). Continuous norming: Implications for the
WAIS-R. *Journal of Clinical Psychology, 41*(1), 86–94. https://doi.org/10.1002/1097-
4679(198501)41:1<86::AID-JCLP2270410115>3.0.CO;2-W

Zhu, J., & Chen, H.-Y. (2011). Utility of inferential norming with smaller sample sizes.
Journal of Psychoeducational Assessment, 29(6), 570–580. https://doi.org/10.1177/
0734282910396323

10

Thematic Apperception Test (TAT) and Other Narrative Assessments of Bipolar Spectrum Disorders

Sharon Rae Jenkins

The Thematic Apperception Test (Morgan & Murray, 1935; Murray, 1943) is only one of several picture sets with a supportive research literature, which I identify collectively as thematic apperceptive techniques (TATs) throughout this chapter. TATs are projective stimuli in that what is seen in a client's story originates in the cognitive structure and intentions of the clinician. What is the clinician looking for? I say this to highlight the importance of the clinician's purpose in an assessment including a TAT. There have been numerous empirically supported scoring systems that can be applied to stories or other narrative material, including early memories and other autobiographical texts. All can be used to better understand the client, so priorities for choosing a scoring system must be guided by the value of each for addressing referral questions. For bipolar spectrum disorders (BPSDs), this chapter prioritizes questions about the failures of regulation that are prominent in diagnosing BPSDs: regulation of mood, energy, emotions, and behaviors, including aggression. These are often sequelae of childhood trauma, especially attachment-related trauma. Assessment for treatment planning can benefit from choosing TAT picture stimuli for their value in identifying triggering situations.

Further, the stories as interpreted by the client in a collaborative therapeutic assessment (CTA; Finn, 2007; Fischer, 1994) can yield important self-understanding for a client beginning treatment. As clients compare and

https://doi.org/10.1037/0000356-011
Psychological Assessment of Bipolar Spectrum Disorders, J. H. Kleiger and I. B. Weiner (Editors)

contrast the emotional responses and implicit assumptions in their fictional or autobiographical stories with an empathic assessor, they may rewrite their personal story to a favored outcome. Since lack of insight is known to be a challenge for those diagnosed with BPSD, this latter application might be especially useful.

In this chapter, I first discuss the conceptualization of TATs as narrative construction tasks, including their psychometric properties; I then review the picture sets and scoring systems that are most relevant for appraising the problems characteristic of people with BPSD; finally, I present empirical support for such appraisal, organized by referral question.

CONCEPTUAL BASIS

Any theoretical orientation in the eye of the clinician can be applied to story analysis, from psychoanalytic (see Jenkins, 2008a) to behaviorist (e.g., McClelland, 1980; Ronan & Gibbs, 2008). Although historically TATs have been classified as "projective" and can certainly be approached that way, Meyer and Kurtz's (2006) critique of that classification as simplistic supports some reconceptualizations. Bornstein (2011) grouped TATs with the Rorschach inkblots as "stimulus attribution tests" in that both involve the client making more of the stimulus than is actually present in the visual display presented, with the "more" being treated as data.

However, with the exception of the Popular percepts, the Rorschach blots are mostly too under-structured to be representational. In contrast, TATs use pictures that are designed to represent people with familiar characteristics in identifiable situations that might elicit thoughts, emotions, and actions from story characters. The task of making a story from this raw material makes TATs "narrative construction tasks," with the stimulus properties of the picture becoming the background and the storyteller's job being to transcend the stimulus (Weisskopf, 1950) and produce a plot and characters. When structured scoring systems are used to quantify certain features of the narrative, stimuli other than pictures can serve that purpose, such as early memories, expressive writing essays, and other autobiographical material (e.g., Jenkins et al., 2022), even musical passages (van den Daele, 2014). In this chapter, these are denoted collectively as "narrative methods," reserving "TATs" for the use of picture stimuli.

One major benefit of TATs for use with BPSD is the typical lack of convergent validity of narrative measures with self-reported rating scales, which allows for incremental validity. A case in point concerns the measurement of attachment. Several studies supporting the theorized link between attachment insecurity and BPSD use self-report measures (e.g., Morriss et al., 2009). However, although attachment is theoretically a stable construct, Morriss et al. (2009) reported that patients differed in self-reported attachment style depending on whether their current episode was manic or depressed, concluding that assessments of attachment style should be scheduled only in remission! Most likely it is the social desirability systematic error variance, which is typically negatively correlated with depressed mood, that changes (see McClelland, 1980). As discussed later, the Adult Attachment Projective (AAP), which is less influenced by social desirability (George & West, 2012), would not be expected to show this effect.

Psychometric Properties

Evaluating the psychometric properties of TATs requires first a choice of stimuli and of one or more scoring systems for interpretation, because the psychometric properties of TATs and other narrative measures are specific to each scoring system and construct measured. They will also vary with the picture set, storyteller population, purpose of assessment, local cultural norms, scorers' personalities and training, and storytellers' perception of how the data will be used (Jenkins, 2017a, 2017b). What follows here are general considerations for determining validity and reliability; specifics for each scoring system are available in the core references.

Validity

In most cases, as with most content analysis systems, the primary validity of interest is content validity (Borsboom et al., 2004), resting on the assumption that stories are samples of the storyteller's internal narratives about how the world works in situations that resemble the stimulus (Jenkins, 2017b; McClelland, 1985). Thus, the best interpretation stays closest to the literal data. Most scoring systems are means of rating or classifying the literal data into low-inference categories or dimensions following the rules set forth in the scoring manual.

To the extent that scorable text transcends the stimulus (Weisskopf, 1950), story content and likely scores will be influenced by the storyteller's immediate and enduring preoccupations, along with prevailing cultural, historical, and local norms. Thus, the best normative data available to the practicing clinician for interpretation come from the clinician's own practice gathered over time, and those of colleagues in the same cultural location (Jenkins, 2017a). Convergent validity with other measures can be challenging to establish; TAT scores seldom correlate more than modestly with self-report scales (e.g., Köllner & Schultheiss, 2014).

In this chapter, I focus on structured scoring systems because they are most amenable to the collection of validity evidence. However, in the search for scientific objectivity and presumed generalizability (see Sue, 1999), there is necessarily a loss of the individuality that is often what gets our clients in trouble (Jenkins, 2014). Literal interpretation preserves that individuality and is justified by its low inference content validity. The best example of productive literal interpretation is that practiced in collaborative (Fischer, 1994) and therapeutic assessment (Finn, 2007). These intervention approaches rely on using assessment data as a shared focus to collaborate with the client in making interpretations that are consistent with the client's worldview and individuality. The assessor remains free to apply any of the formal scoring systems to the stories to better understand and empathize with the client's problems, and to address the storyteller's assessment questions.

Reliability

The essential reliability for narrative methods is interscorer agreement, which is the criterion for scientific objectivity. Disagreement is the major source of both random and systematic error variance in scores. Interscorer agreement is a product of the clarity and precision of the manual and is specific to the scorers in question; their skills, training, and diligence; and the match between the cultural backgrounds of the scorers and the storytellers. Thus, for structured scoring systems, individual study of the manual and practice scoring with expert-scored materials (Jenkins, 2008b) or supervised training in a credentialing workshop is essential to reduce controllable sources of error.

Other forms of reliability (test–retest, internal consistency, alternate forms) depend on the theoretical properties of the construct being measured. Personality traits and styles are theoretically stable across time and situations; states and motives are responsive to the immediate situation and to the storyteller's changing life circumstances (e.g., Jenkins, 1987, 2017a). The construct's sensitivity to situational arousal and to the content of the story told just prior (e.g., Atkinson, 1981) will perturb internal consistency reliability across a series of stories and test–retest reliability across time. Thus, these reliabilities are usually inappropriate for evaluating TATs (Jenkins, 2017b). Real change in the storyteller can be a main source of "unreliability."

THE SYSTEMS

The following sections describe each of the most relevant picture sets (Table 10.1) and scoring systems (Table 10.2) for assessing questions of bipolar spectrum, followed by its fundamental validity evidence. Because all of these have demonstrated that adequate interscorer agreement is attainable, further evidence of reliability is not presented here since ensuring adequate reliability for individual studies and for clinical use is the responsibility of the user. Empirical support for

TABLE 10.1. Picture Sets and Constructs Assessed

Name of test	Construct(s) assessed	Fundamental validity evidence	Major references
Thematic Apperception Test	Depends on scoring system	Depends on scoring system	Morgan and Murray (1935) and Murray (1943)
Adult Attachment Projective	Attachment	George and West (2012)	George and West (2012)
Tell-Me-A-Story (TEMAS)	Comprehensive	Costantino et al. (2014) and Fantini et al. (2017)	Costantino et al. (2007)
Roberts Apperception Test, Roberts-2	Comprehensive	Parolin et al. (2020)	Roberts and Gruber (2005)

TABLE 10.2. Scoring Systems and Constructs Assessed

Name of system	Construct(s) assessed	Fundamental validity evidence	Author(s) of major references
Defense Mechanisms Manual (DMM)	Denial, Projection, Identification	Cramer (2012, 2015, 2020), Hibbard et al. (2010), and Hibbard and Porcerelli (1998)	Cramer (1991, 2006)
Social Cognition and Object Relations Scales (SCORS-G)	COM, AFF, EIR, EIM, SC, AGG, SE, & ICS	Ackerman et al. (2001) and Stein et al. (2020)	Westen et al. (1990) and Stein and Slavin-Mulford (2018)

Note. COM = Complexity of Representations of People; AFF = Affect–Tone of Relationship Paradigms; EIR = distinguishes investments in Relationships; EIM = Values and Moral Standards; SC = Understanding of Social Causality; AGG = Experience and Management of Aggressive Impulses; SE = Self-Esteem; ICS = Identity and Coherence of Self.

each system's use for the most common questions in BPSD assessment is presented under the relevant problem behaviors in the next major section.

Pictures With Systems for Children and Youth

Tell-Me-A-Story

Description and Conceptual Basis. The Tell-Me-A-Story (TEMAS) test is a set of 23 brightly colored pictures (11 with gender-specific versions; a nine-card short form may be used) with a detailed scoring system. Cards are available in Black, Hispanic, White, Orthodox Jewish, and Argentinian versions (Costantino et al., 2007). Versions differ not only in characters' skin color but also cultural features of the setting, such as clothing, architectural style of buildings, and type of ball shown in children's games. Pictured scenes are more structured than those in the Roberts-2 (Roberts & Gruber, 2005); each poses a distinct problem or conflict situation that is scored as such. Stories are scored for cognitive, affective, and personality functions. Multicultural norms are available in Costantino et al. (2007).

Validity Evidence. The major resource for psychometric evidence on the TEMAS is Costantino et al. (2007). Comparing samples of Black, Hispanic, and White children in kindergarten through sixth grade using the Murray (1943) TAT and both the minority and nonminority TEMAS versions, Costantino and Malgady (1983) found that Black and Hispanic children told longer stories about both TEMAS versions than in the Murray pictures. They attributed this finding to the culturally familiar TEMAS settings rather than the characters' racial features. Fantini et al. (2017) found that children instructed to tell stories that would give the listener a positive impression of them did not differ from others on more complex scores, only the most obvious story features.

Roberts-2 (Formerly Roberts Apperception Test for Children)

Description and Conceptual Basis. The Roberts-2 (Roberts & Gruber, 2005), originally the Roberts Apperception Test for Children (RATC; McArthur & Roberts, 1982), is a set of 16 black-and-white drawings of children and adolescents alone or with their family or friends in common life situations evoking a range of emotions. Eleven of these have alternate male and female versions; there are Black, Hispanic, and White sets and norms for ages 6 to 18. The scoring system evaluates developmentally adaptive functions and clinical functions, all directed toward evaluating the storyteller's narrative expression of social understanding.

The Theme Overview Scales identify the storyteller's choice of a popular or conventional theme and the completion of a narrative that satisfies the instructions given. The Available Resources Scales identify the storyteller's awareness of available personal and environmental support systems for problem solving. The Problem Identification, Resolution, and Outcome Scales evaluate the clarity of problem definition and solution or lack of solution. The Emotion Scales (Anxiety, Aggression, Depression, and Rejection) capture content reflecting these feelings and related situations. The Unusual or Atypical Responses are rare in nonclinical samples. Stories elicited with the RATC/Roberts-2 cards can also be scored using other systems, such as the SCORS and Content Analysis of Verbal Explanations.

Validity Evidence. A recent American Psychological Association PsycInfo search showed that most of the publications for the Roberts-2 or RATC were in dissertations, case studies, or books for clinicians, with less validational research. However, Parolin et al. (2020) examined two samples, reporting psychometric information, factor structure and developmental trends, and comparing clinically referred children ($N = 86$) to a community sample. The Roberts-2 indexes differentiated among the developmental groups and between clinical and nonclinical samples.

Age-Flexible Scoring Systems

Cramer's Defense Mechanisms Manual
Description and Conceptual Basis. Derived from the psychoanalytic conceptualization of defense mechanisms as ego functions that protect against anxiety (Cramer, 1991, 2006), the Defense Mechanisms Manual (DMM) scoring categories measure three: Denial, Projection, and Identification. They are organized as a developmental hierarchy that theoretically changes with maturation. Denial, the most primitive, predominates in early childhood. Projection becomes ascendant in middle childhood through late childhood, and is superseded by Identification, the most mature, which normally dominates adulthood. Each has seven categories that are scored if present.

Validity Evidence. Good evidence supports the theorized developmental hierarchy of the DMM categories (Porcerelli et al., 1998) and its validity (Hibbard & Porcerelli, 1998; Hibbard et al., 2010).

Social Cognition and Object Relations
Description and Conceptual Basis. What has become the Social Cognition and Object Relations Scale–Global Rating Method (SCORS-G; Stein & Slavin-Mulford, 2018) began as the Object Relations and Social Cognition scales

(Westen et al., 1990), which were developed based on object relations theory concepts and social cognition literature to distinguish patients with borderline personality disorder from those with major depression and nonpatients. To the original four categories, Complexity of Representations of People (COM), Affect–Tone of Relationship Paradigms (AFF), Capacity for Emotional Investment in Relationships and Moral Standards (EI), and Understanding of Social Causality (SC), the present-day SCORS-G adds scores for Experience and Management of Aggressive Impulses (AGG), Self-Esteem (SE), and Identity and Coherence of Self (ICS) and distinguishes investments in Relationships (EIR) and Values and Moral Standards (EIM).

These eight categories are rated globally for each story on a 7-point scale by trained clinicians (Stein & Slavin-Mulford, 2018). High scores are more adaptive. From the beginning, though originally based on TATs (e.g., Westen et al., 1990), the SCORS literature has evolved using a variety of narratives, including interviews, psychotherapy transcripts, early memories, and interpersonal anecdotes.

Validity Evidence. Ackerman et al. (2001) reported convergent validities between the SCORS variables and Mutuality of Autonomy from the Rorschach. The strongest were for Affect, Relationships, Morals, Aggression, and Self-Esteem.

The Adult Attachment Projective
Description and Conceptual Basis. The AAP is based on Bowlby's (1969) and Ainsworth's (2015) developmental attachment theory. It is composed of eight theory-driven line drawings of attachment situations that increase in attachment stress related to separation, aloneness, and loss to activate the attachment system. These are used to elicit a series of stories that are coded by experienced clinicians who have been trained to meet the criterion level of interscorer reliability to identify story content, unconscious defensive processes, and self–other boundary challenges. Some of these are indicators of attachment disorganization and trauma. Storytellers are classified as secure, dismissing, preoccupied, and unresolved (George & West, 2012). The last category is associated with affective (medial temporal activation; Buchheim et al., 2006) and interpersonal (low baseline oxytocin levels; Jobst et al., 2016) dysregulation.

Validity Evidence. Extensive and detailed psychometric information was given by George and West (2012) and by Buchheim and George (2011). Criterion validity studies have produced findings consistent with theory, and it has been widely used in published CTA case studies. In a series of important and well-designed studies in patient and nonpatient women, Buchheim and colleagues connected AAP unresolved status to escalating activation of the amygdala and hippocampus across the series of increasingly attachment-stressing pictures, validating the theory used to create and order the AAP pictures (Buchheim et al., 2006, 2016).

EMPIRICAL SUPPORT FOR USING TATs AND OTHER NARRATIVE ASSESSMENTS WITH BIPOLAR SPECTRUM DISORDERS

Studies of BPSD Samples

Few studies have applied any of the TATs to BPSD samples. In one such study, Row (2008) used Roberts-2 to differentiate children diagnosed with BPSD from those diagnosed with attention-deficit/hyperactivity disorder (ADHD) and normative data. In this small sample ($N = 29$, 8 with BPSD), Roberts-2 scales did not differentiate BPSD and ADHD, but the group with BPSD differed from the normative data by having lower scores on completion of a meaningful story, Support Other-Feel (positive social environment), Resolution-2 (simple positive outcome without explanation), Resolution-4 (constructive outcome with process given), and Resolution-5 (elaborated constructive resolution with insight). They scored higher than the norms on Rejection (REJ), Unusual (UNUSL), and Atypical (ATYP). Compared with the norms, the children with BPSD found relating a meaningful narrative challenging, saw their social environment as negative and rejecting, had difficulty understanding social problem solving, and gave more pathological responses.

In adult clinical samples, Sharma and Sinha (2010) used the DMM to compare defense patterns between three groups: bipolar manic, bipolar depressed, and unipolar depressed. Denial was significantly higher in both bipolar groups than in the unipolar group. The Denial related to the severity of manic symptoms. The unipolar patients scored higher in Identification than the manic patients, and their more severe depression symptoms correlated negatively with Identification.

Studies of Bipolar Spectrum Disorder Characteristics

Taking a dimensional spectrum approach to BPSD allows for organizing this section by referral question; that is, clinicians' observations that raise questions about possible BPSD and generate assessment consultation. Arguably the most common feature of BPSD is failure to regulate mood, energy, emotions, and impulses, including aggression, which may manifest in disordered perceptions/cognitions or reactivity to stress. The most common source of dysregulation across the literature is childhood psychological trauma, of which the most common and serious type for BPSD is attachment-related trauma (see Chapter 15 in this volume) and failure of defenses against its sequelae. Many contextual elements and sequelae of trauma are social cognitive and relational and are well captured by TATs. I organize these developmentally in Table 10.3.

For children and adolescents who may struggle with accuracy on self-report scales, extreme scores on the Roberts-2 Depression Scale might be helpful for BPSD diagnosis. Comparing the RATC Depression score with the Children's Depression Inventory, the Reynolds Child Depression Scale, and the Child Behavior Checklist, Mijal (1995) reported that the RATC appeared to be the

TABLE 10.3. Assessment Referral Questions Matched to TAT Suggested Indicators

System suggested	Childhood trauma	Impulsivity/ poor controls	Emotional dysregulation	Grandiosity	Reality testing problems	Aggression
TEMAS	Interpersonal Relations, Self-Concept, card comparisons[a]	Delay of Gratification	Anxiety/Depression	Achievement Motivation, Reality Testing	Reality Testing	Aggression, Interpersonal Relations, Moral Judgment, Angry
Roberts-2 (RATC)	Sexual Abuse Scoring Profile	Low RES-2, RES-4, RES-5	Low Support, Other-Feel		REJ, UNUSL, ATYP, less meaningful story	ATYP
Defense Mechanisms Manual		High Denial, Low Identification	High Denial, Low Identification		High Projection	High Denial, High Projection, Low Identification
SCORS-G	Lower scores for all scales, card comparisons[a]	Low AFF, EIR, EIM	Low EIR, EIM, ICS	SE	Lower scores for all scales	Lower scores for all scales
AAP	Unresolved attachment status, card comparisons[a]		Unresolved attachment status, card comparisons[a]			

Note. TAT = Thematic Apperception Test; TEMAS = Tell-Me-A-Story; RATC = Roberts Apperception Test for Children; RES-2 = simple positive outcome without explanation; RES-4 = constructive outcome with process given; RES-5 = elaborated constructive resolution with insight; REJ = rejection; UNUSL = unusual; ATYP = atypical; SCORS-G = Social Cognition and Object Relations Scales; AFF = Affect–Tone of Relationship Paradigms; EIR = distinguishes investments in Relationships; EIM = Values and Moral Standards; ICS = Identity and Coherence of Self; SE = Self-Esteem; AAP = Adult Attachment Projective.
[a] To identify trigger situations.

most comprehensive measure of children's depression in a sample of children who were depressed or oppositional.

Impulsivity/Poor Controls: DMM

A common reaction to abuse among children is acting out, including impulsivity. The best-known regulatory psychological construct is defense mechanisms, for which Cramer firmly established the DMM as the preeminent measure. The acquisition of increasingly mature defenses is an important developmental task that should improve regulatory processes in general, and particularly self-control processes that reduce the impulsivity and emotional dysregulation of BPSD. In a series of important developmental papers from the archival data of the Institute of Human Development longitudinal studies at the University of California, Berkeley, Cramer related the use of different defense mechanisms to different aspects of psychological development and boundary regulation. The findings of these papers align well with Miklowitz and Cicchetti's (2010) BPSD developmental model.

Cramer (2015) examined children's DMM scores and mothers' reports of children's behavior problems at ages 9 and 12, finding that children whose stories manifested more projection showed less internalizing. Children who used more identification, which Cramer tied to self-regulation, showed decreasing externalization over this period. In a different article on a related sample, Cramer (2009) found that early adolescents who more often used the defense of denial increased in ego under-control and externalizing behavior problems over time. In a sample of young adults, men's use of projection was related to externalizing, but not women's. For both genders, identification was negatively related to internalizing, suggesting that using the more mature defense of identification might be protective against depression (Cramer, 2020). Early diagnosis of BPSD should attend to extremes of internalizing and externalizing disorders in children and adolescents and the defenses that attend them.

Adults' impulsivity can be viewed as residual immaturity and the failure to acquire the skills for self-control that come with mature integration of cognition and affect. In the adulthood series of Institute of Human Development studies, Cramer and Jones (2007) examined changes in self-control related to the use of defense mechanisms over decades. Participants who used more Identification in the stories around age 30 had more stable self-control scores relative to those who used less Identification, who showed either larger increases or larger decreases in self-control over the decades.

Emotional Dysregulation: AAP and Social Cognition and Object Relations

Emotional dysregulation has been identified as a common sequela of an unresolved attachment status, which in turn is a common sequela of childhood relational trauma, including abuse and neglect. In a sample of 25 nonpatient adults who reported a childhood trauma history, Jacques (2002) found that more than half were classified as AAP Unresolved attachment status, and those scored higher than others on the Rorschach Pure Color, Depression Index, and Perceptual-Thinking Index. In a study by Buchheim et al. (2016), the unresolved nonpatients showed additional activation in brain areas associated with cognitive control over emotions and the planning of context-appropriate actions. The authors interpreted this activation difference as suggesting a mechanism that might explain the emotional dysregulation common with borderline personality disorder (and by extension, perhaps in BPSD) when the control-related activation seen in the nonpatients is not present.

Emotion regulation can also be assessed using the SCORS. In a psychophysiological study of the SCORS and emotion regulation, Desatnik et al. (2021) studied an adolescent nonpatient sample who engaged in a task that measured emotion regulation while data on event-related potentials were collected. SCORS from an early memories protocol explained 48% of the variance in late positive potential, an indicator of activated emotional processes that is decreased with successful emotion-regulation strategies, specifically expressive suppression. EIR predicted a lack of suppression and EIM and ICS predicted suppression, all at moderate effect sizes. The authors explained that this parallels the normal developmental transition from reliance on external regulation to internalized, intrinsic, and less effortful internal regulation.

Aggression: DMM

In a study of college men, Porcerelli et al. (2004) found that men who used more Denial reported the most extreme violence toward strangers. Men who used relatively more Projection reported the most extreme violence toward partners. Men who used relatively more Identification used the least extreme violence toward both strangers and partners.

Use of Card Comparisons to Identify Triggering Situations

Flexibility of stimulus selection is a strength for TATs because the clinician typically selects a few cards from a larger set. This flexibility is particularly useful for trauma-related disorders, for which a referral question might concern the identification of situational stimuli that might trigger episodes. In BPSD, for example, upstream of impulsive acting out is the trigger that might set it off. Is the impulsivity due to immaturity and failed self-control or residual trauma? Especially with childhood traumatic abuse, patients may vary in their ability to verbalize the specific features of a situation that function as triggers, since lack of insight is a known complication of BPSD.

A second asset given by TAT's flexibility is that many of the scoring systems reviewed here can be applied to narratives elicited by any set of picture stimuli as well as autobiographical material. The older psychoanalytic interpretive approaches and the newer thought sampling ones agree on the importance of considering normative themes that pictures elicit, a feature called "card pull." However, the latter allows for card selection by applying strategic situation sampling principles (Jenkins, 2017b) to organize cards to parallel the client's various life situations that inspire problematic or benign behavior. Rather than relying on norms for interpretation, this approach capitalizes on the client's individuality by using within-person comparisons to identify the distinguishing features of the storyteller's experiences in triggering versus benign situations.

To identify triggers, clinicians may begin by devising a stimulus sampling frame (Jenkins, 2017b) that organizes stimuli relevant to the client's life situation, comparing situations that might contain triggers to neutral situations that have never elicited a trigger response. The Jenkins frame used three dimensions—role-relationships of characters, interpersonal versus task activity, and affective tone—but dimensions should be designed purposefully to make strategic choices that best fit the client's range of troublesome experiences (e.g., work situation, family setting, competitive). The resulting stories may be scored using any relevant system; analyses are within-person, comparing stories to identify which dimensions appear most relevant. With this strategy, the story-teller may be the most helpful interpreter within a CTA intervention process.

For example, among college men who did or did not report committing violence, Kim et al. (2005) reported that the violent group scored higher on DMM Denial, which the authors interpreted as indicating psychological imma-turity. Given the Murray (1943) Cards 1, 2, 4, 6BM, 7BM, and 13MF, Cards 4 and 13MF pull more strongly for mention of violence, which is rare in stories about Card 1 (boy with violin), 2 (farm scene), and 6BM (old woman, young man). Violent stories about Cards 1 and 2, which have the most consistent achievement pull, and not about Cards 4 and 13MF might represent extreme reactions to familial achievement demands, a hypothesis that can be tested against the substantive story themes. Furthermore, which stories scored highest in denial? Such a pattern might support Alloy et al.'s (2010) Behavioral Approach System (BAS) sensitivity and frustrated goal pursuit model of trigger-ing, and the additional information about denial and projection (or their absence in the violent stories) could beneficially guide therapy interventions.

CONCLUSION

This chapter does not exhaust the range of potential uses of TATs for a better understanding of BPSD. For research purposes, the scoring systems for human social motives (need for Achievement—*n* Ach; need for Affiliation—*n* Aff; and need for Power, *n* Pow) were empirically derived based on McClelland's (1985) behavioral theory of human motives as learned personality dispositions to be sensitized (aroused) in response to cues about the situational availability of motive gratifications. Although these systems were never intended for clinical use, in combination they parallel Alloy et al.'s (2010) BAS dysregulation model of bipolar spectrum etiology, especially for *n* Power and the imperial motive pattern (McClelland, 1975). Although Alloy et al.'s model emphasizes achieve-ment orientation, the motives literature suggests that the more relevant motive might be *n* Power, for which the satisfying goal-state is to have an impact on people and the world, which better addresses the grandiosity associated with BPSD.

REFERENCES

Ackerman, S. J., Hilsenroth, M. J., Clemence, A. J., Weatherill, R., & Fowler, J. C. (2001). Convergent validity of Rorschach and TAT scales of object relations. *Journal of Personality Assessment, 77*(2), 295–306. https://doi.org/10.1207/S15327752JPA7702_11

Ainsworth, M. D. S. (2015). *Patterns of attachment: A psychological study of the strange situation.* Taylor and Francis. https://doi.org/10.4324/9780203758045

Alloy, L. B., Abramson, L. Y., Urosevic, S., Nusslock, R., & Jager-Hyman, S. (2010). Course of early-onset bipolar spectrum disorders during the college years: A behavioral approach system dysregulation perspective. In D. J. Miklowitz & D. Cicchetti (Eds.), *Understanding bipolar disorder: A developmental psychopathology perspective* (pp. 166–191). Guilford Press.

Atkinson, J. W. (1981). Studying personality in the context of an advanced motivational psychology. *American Psychologist, 36*(2), 117–128. https://doi.org/10.1037/0003-066X.36.2.117

Bornstein, R. F. (2011). Toward a process-focused model of test score validity: Improving psychological assessment in science and practice. *Psychological Assessment, 23*(2), 532–544. https://doi.org/10.1037/a0022402

Borsboom, D., Mellenbergh, G. J., & van Heerden, J. (2004). The concept of validity. *Psychological Review, 111*(4), 1061–1071. https://doi.org/10.1037/0033-295X.111.4.1061

Bowlby, J. (1969). *Attachment and loss.* Basic Books.

Buchheim, A., Erk, S., George, C., Kächele, H., Martius, P., Pokorny, D., Spitzer, M., & Walter, H. (2016). Neural response during the activation of the attachment system in patients with borderline personality disorder: An fMRI study. *Frontiers in Human Neuroscience, 10*, Article 389. https://doi.org/10.3389/fnhum.2016.00389

Buchheim, A., Erk, S., George, C., Kächele, H., Ruchsow, M., Spitzer, M., Kircher, T., & Walter, H. (2006). Measuring attachment representation in an fMRI environment: A pilot study. *Psychopathology, 39*(3), 144–152. https://doi.org/10.1159/000091800

Buchheim, A., & George, C. (2011). Attachment disorganization in borderline personality disorder and anxiety disorder. In J. Solomon & C. George (Eds.), *Disorganized attachment and caregiving* (pp. 343–382). Guilford Press.

Costantino, G., Dana, R. H., & Malgady, R. G. (2007). *TEMAS (Tell-Me-A-Story) assessment in multicultural societies.* Lawrence Erlbaum.

Costantino, G., Litman, L., Waxman, R., Dupertuis, D., Pais, E., Rosenzweig, C., Forti, G., Paronik, J., & Canales, M. M. F. (2014). Tell-Me-A-Story (TEMAS) assessment for culturally diverse children and adolescents. *Rorschachiana, 35*(2), 154–175. https://doi.org/10.1027/1192-5604/a000054

Costantino, G., & Malgady, R. G. (1983). Verbal fluency of Hispanic, Black and White children on TAT and TEMAS, a new Thematic Apperception Test. *Hispanic Journal of Behavioral Sciences, 5*(2), 199–206. https://doi.org/10.1177/07399863830052005

Cramer, P. (1991). *The development of defense mechanisms: Theory, research and assessment.* Springer. https://doi.org/10.1007/978-1-4613-9025-1

Cramer, P. (2006). *Protecting the self: Defense mechanisms in action.* Guilford Press.

Cramer, P. (2009). An increase in early adolescent undercontrol is associated with the use of denial. *Journal of Personality Assessment, 91*(4), 331–339. https://doi.org/10.1080/00223890902935746

Cramer, P. (2012). Psychological maturity and change in adult defense mechanisms. *Journal of Research in Personality, 46*(3), 306–316. https://doi.org/10.1016/j.jrp.2012.02.011

Cramer, P. (2015). Change in children's externalizing and internalizing behavior problems: The role of defense mechanisms. *Journal of Nervous and Mental Disease, 203*(3), 215–221. https://doi.org/10.1097/NMD.0000000000000265

Cramer, P. (2020). Externalizing/projection; internalizing/identification: An examination. *Psychoanalytic Psychology, 37*(3), 207–211. https://doi.org/10.1037/pap0000255

Cramer, P., & Jones, C. J. (2007). Defense mechanisms predict differential lifespan change in self-control and self-acceptance. *Journal of Research in Personality, 41*(4), 841–855. https://doi.org/10.1016/j.jrp.2006.10.005

Desatnik, A., Bel-Bahar, T., Taylor, L., Nolte, T., Crowley, M. J., Fonagy, P., & Fearon, P. (2021). Emotion regulation in adolescents: Influences of internal representations of relationships—An ERP study. *International Journal of Psychophysiology, 160*, 1–9. https://doi.org/10.1016/j.ijpsycho.2020.11.010

Fantini, F., Banis, A., Dell'Acqua, E., Durosini, I., & Aschieri, F. (2017). Exploring children's induced defensiveness to the Tell Me a Story test (TEMAS). *Journal of Personality Assessment, 99*(3), 275–285. https://doi.org/10.1080/00223891.2016.1261359

Finn, S. E. (2007). *In our clients' shoes: Theory and techniques of therapeutic assessment.* Lawrence Erlbaum.

Fischer, C. T. (1994). *Individualizing psychological assessment.* Lawrence Erlbaum.

George, C., & West, M. L. (2012). *The adult attachment projective picture system: Attachment theory and assessment in adults.* Guilford Press.

Hibbard, S., & Porcerelli, J. (1998). Further validation for the Cramer defense mechanism manual. *Journal of Personality Assessment, 70*(3), 460–483. https://doi.org/10.1207/s15327752jpa7003_6

Hibbard, S., Porcerelli, J., Kamoo, R., Schwartz, M., & Abell, S. (2010). Defense and object relational maturity on Thematic Apperception Test scales indicate levels of personality organization. *Journal of Personality Assessment, 92*(3), 241–253. https://doi.org/10.1080/00223891003670190

Jacques, C. A. (2002). Disorganized attachment and its relationship to disordered thinking and emotional dysregulation a study of adults with a history of childhood trauma, using the Adult Attachment Projective Test and the Rorschach Inkblot Test. In *Dissertation abstracts international: Section B. The sciences and engineering* (Vol. 63, Issue 4–B, p. 2060). ProQuest Information & Learning.

Jenkins, S. R. (1987). Need for achievement and women's careers over 14 years: Evidence for occupational structure effects. *Journal of Personality and Social Psychology, 53*(5), 922–932. https://doi.org/10.1037/0022-3514.53.5.922

Jenkins, S. R. (Ed.). (2008a). *Handbook of clinical scoring systems for thematic apperceptive techniques.* Lawrence Erlbaum.

Jenkins, S. R. (2008b). Teaching how to learn reliable scoring. In S. R. Jenkins (Ed.), *Handbook of clinical scoring systems for thematic apperceptive techniques* (pp. 39–66). Lawrence Erlbaum.

Jenkins, S. R. (2014). Thematic apperceptive techniques inform a science of individuality. *Rorschachiana, 35*(2), 92–102. https://doi.org/10.1027/1192-5604/a000065

Jenkins, S. R. (2017a). The narrative arc of TATs: Introduction to the JPA special section on thematic apperceptive techniques. *Journal of Personality Assessment, 99*(3), 225–237. https://doi.org/10.1080/00223891.2016.1244066

Jenkins, S. R. (2017b). Not your same old story: New rules for thematic apperceptive techniques (TATs). *Journal of Personality Assessment, 99*(3), 238–253. https://doi.org/10.1080/00223891.2016.1248972

Jenkins, S. R., Shamji, J. F., Straup, M. L., & Boals, A. (2022). Beyond traits and states: Interpersonal decentering is also activated social information processing. *Personality and Individual Differences, 186*(A), Article 111332. https://doi.org/10.1016/j.paid.2021.111332

Jobst, A., Padberg, F., Mauer, M.-C., Daltrozzo, T., Bauriedl-Schmidt, C., Sabass, L., Sarubin, N., Falkai, P., Renneberg, B., Zill, P., Gander, M., & Buchheim, A. (2016).

Lower oxytocin plasma levels in borderline patients with unresolved attachment representations. *Frontiers in Human Neuroscience, 10,* Article 125. https://doi.org/10. 3389/fnhum.2016.00125

Kim, M., Cogan, R., Carter, S., & Porcerelli, J. H. (2005). Defense mechanisms and self-reported violence toward strangers. *Bulletin of the Menninger Clinic, 69*(4), 305–312. https://doi.org/10.1521/bumc.2005.69.4.305

Köllner, M. G., & Schultheiss, O. C. (2014). Meta-analytic evidence of low convergence between implicit and explicit measures of the needs for achievement, affiliation, and power. *Frontiers in Psychology, 5,* Article 826. https://doi.org/10.3389/fpsyg. 2014.00826

McArthur, D. S., & Roberts, G. E. (1982). *Roberts Apperception Test for Children (RATC) manual.* Western Psychological Services.

McClelland, D. C. (1975). *Power: The inner experience.* Irvington Press.

McClelland, D. C. (1980). Motive dispositions: The merits of operant and respondent measures. In L. Wheeler (Ed.), *Review of personality and social psychology* (Vol. 1, pp. 10–41). Sage Publications.

McClelland, D. C. (1985). *Human motivation.* Scott Foresman.

Meyer, G. J., & Kurtz, J. E. (2006). Advancing personality assessment terminology: Time to retire "objective" and "projective" as personality test descriptors. *Journal of Personality Assessment, 87*(3), 223–225. https://doi.org/10.1207/s15327752jpa8703_01

Mijal, S. E. (1995). A study of the relationship of depression in children who are depressed and children with oppositional disorder. In *Dissertation abstracts international: Section B. The sciences and engineering* (Vol. 55, Issue 11–B, p. 5079). ProQuest Information & Learning.

Miklowitz, D. J., & Cicchetti, D. (Eds.). (2010). *Understanding bipolar disorder: A developmental psychopathology perspective* (pp. 166–191). Guilford Press.

Morgan, C. D., & Murray, H. A. (1935). A method for investigating fantasies: The Thematic Apperception Test. *Archives of Neurology and Psychiatry, 34*(2), 289–306. https://doi.org/ 10.1001/archneurpsyc.1935.02250200049005

Morriss, R. K., van der Gucht, E., Lancaster, G., & Bentall, R. P. (2009). Adult attachment in bipolar 1 disorder. *Psychology and Psychotherapy: Theory, Research and Practice, 82*(3), 267–277. https://doi.org/10.1348/147608309X415309

Murray, H. A. (1943). *Thematic Apperception Test manual.* Harvard University Press.

Parolin, L., De Carli, P., & Locati, F. (2020). The Roberts-2: Italian validation on a sample of children and adolescents. *Journal of Personality Assessment, 102*(3), 390–404. https:// doi.org/10.1080/00223891.2018.1546713

Porcerelli, J. H., Cogan, R., Kamoo, R., & Leitman, S. (2004). Defense mechanisms and self-reported violence toward partners and strangers. *Journal of Personality Assessment, 82*(3), 317–320. https://doi.org/10.1207/s15327752jpa8203_07

Porcerelli, J. H., Thomas, S., Hibbard, S., & Cogan, R. (1998). Defense mechanisms development in children, adolescents, and late adolescents. *Journal of Personality Assessment, 71*(3), 411–420. https://doi.org/10.1207/s15327752jpa7103_9

Roberts, G. E., & Gruber, C. (2005). *Roberts-2.* Western Psychological Services.

Ronan, G. F., & Gibbs, M. S. (2008). Scoring manual for personal problem-solving system-revised. In S. R. Jenkins (Ed.), *Handbook of clinical scoring systems for thematic apperceptive techniques* (pp. 209–228). Lawrence Erlbaum.

Row, C. S. (2008). Utility of the Roberts-2 to differentiate childhood attention deficit/ hyperactivity disorder and bipolar disorder. In *Dissertation abstracts international: Section B. The sciences and engineering* (Vol. 69, Issue 5–B, p. 3276). ProQuest Information & Learning.

Sharma, P., & Sinha, U. K. (2010). Defense mechanisms in mania, bipolar depression and unipolar depression. *Psychological Studies, 55*(3), 239–247. https://doi.org/10.1007/ s12646-010-0017-2

Stein, M. B., Calderon, S., Ruchensky, J., Massey, C., Slavin, M. J., Chung, W., Richardson, L. A., & Blais, M. A. (2020). When's a story a story? Determining interpretability of Social Cognition and Object Relations Scale–Global ratings on Thematic Apperception Test narratives. *Clinical Psychology & Psychotherapy, 27*(4), 567–580. https://doi.org/10.1002/cpp.2442

Stein, M. B., & Slavin-Mulford, J. (2018). *The Social Cognition and Object Relations Scale–Global Rating Method (SCORS-G): A comprehensive guide for clinicians and researchers.* Routledge.

Sue, S. (1999). Science, ethnicity, and bias: Where have we gone wrong? *American Psychologist, 54*(12), 1070–1077. https://doi.org/10.1037/0003-066X.54.12.1070

van den Daele, L. (2014). The Music Apperception Test: Coding, research, and application. *Rorschachiana, 35*(2), 214–235. https://doi.org/10.1027/1192-5604/a000055

Weisskopf, E. A. (1950). A transcendence index as a proposed measure in the TAT. *The Journal of Psychology, 29*(2), 379–390. https://doi.org/10.1080/00223980.1950.9916039

Westen, D., Lohr, N., Silk, K. R., Gold, L., & Kerber, K. (1990). Object relations and social cognition in borderlines, major depressives, and normals: A Thematic Apperception Test analysis. *Psychological Assessment, 2*(4), 355–364. https://doi.org/10.1037/1040-3590.2.4.355

11

Cognitive and Neuropsychological Assessment of Bipolar Spectrum Disorders

Jed Yalof

The cognitive and neuropsychological assessment of bipolar spectrum disorders poses a challenge to assessors that includes a complex symptom presentation; differential diagnostic decisions that often involve consideration of the potential use and impact of unprescribed substances; comorbid personality and symptom-based diagnoses; side effects of prescribed medications; and, when evaluating older adults, age-related issues that might complicate the clinical picture. The assessor has to select and prioritize tests and measures that assay and qualify the bipolar diagnosis while attending to sociocultural factors and patient access to psychosocial support.

The literature on bipolar spectrum disorders is steeped in psychiatric history, beginning with the classic work of Kraepelin (1904), who, in describing a patient's depressive and expansive attacks, landed on the term *maniacal-depressive insanity* (p. 71), the idea of a spectrum of mood disorders emerged gradually as a viable nosological construct. Akiskal (1983), a central figure in the development of the bipolar spectrum, included mania, hypomania or cyclothymia, antidepressant association hypomania, and hyperthymia as a grouping of soft-spectrum disorders (Akiskal, 2002) with temperamental variations (Perugi & Akiskal, 2002). Ghaemi (2013) considered the bipolar spectrum to include "those patients who fall in the middle of the mood spectrum between the classic unipolar and type I bipolar extremes" (p. 220). Although Paris (2012) challenged

https://doi.org/10.1037/0000356-012
Psychological Assessment of Bipolar Spectrum Disorders, J. H. Kleiger and I. B. Weiner (Editors)
Copyright © 2023 by the American Psychological Association. All rights reserved.

the validity of a bipolar spectrum construct as an overly inclusive classification system for adults and children, the American Psychiatric Association's (2022) *Diagnostic and Statistical Manual of Mental Disorders* (5th ed., text rev.; *DSM-5-TR*) current diagnostic nomenclature supports the bipolar spectrum as a group of related disorders that have a strong biological base.

Bipolar spectrum disorders represent "a chronic and recurrent mental illness caused by unusual mood shifts" (Sole et al., 2012, p. 194) that are highly heritable and projected to affect "about 50 million people worldwide" (O'Connell & Coombes, 2021, p. 2156). When compared with other disorders (e.g., autism spectrum, schizophrenia, attention-deficit/hyperactivity disorder [ADHD]), "BD has the greatest twin-based heritability estimate and, similar to other traits, also has a substantial proportion not captured by common variations" (O'Connell & Coombes, 2021, p. 2157). The *DSM-5-TR* recognizes the importance of assessing and classifying bipolar spectrum disorders as a spectrum group of related disorders bounded on one end by schizophrenic spectrum and other psychotic disorders, and, at the other end, by depressive disorders. Both schizophrenic spectrum and bipolar spectrum disorders have strong genetic loading. Diagnosis is organized around unstable mood but distinguished by symptom presentation and further qualified by neuropsychological assessment. Further, the diagnosis of a bipolar spectrum disorder (i.e., related disorders) often signals a lifelong diagnosis, including medication management, susceptibility to relapse, and ongoing treatment.

DIAGNOSTIC CONSIDERATIONS

Clear delineation of diagnostic criteria is essential when evaluating disorders that have overlapping symptoms; this is especially the case for bipolar spectrum disorders, where there are multiple related disorders, rule-outs for each disorder, and a pediatric spectrum that differs in some respects from adult bipolar spectrum disorders. The *DSM-5-TR* provides a comprehensive overview of diagnostic criteria, including specific symptoms, for each bipolar spectrum disorder and addresses matters related to children and youth between ages 6 and 18 in a more focused way under the category of disruptive mood dysregulation disorder. The three primary symptom clusters that require particular attention when diagnosing bipolar spectrum disorders using *DSM-5-TR* are major depression, mania, and hypomania. Disorders associated with depression and mood elevation that occur during discrete periods are diagnosed by careful qualification of symptom duration, history, and rule-outs. The reader is referred to *DSM-5-TR* for specific symptom clusters associated with various bipolar spectrum disorders. In what follows, disorders of the bipolar spectrum are summarized to provide context for the clinical case illustration.

Major depressive disorder is diagnosed when there is a period of at least 2 weeks of intensification of at least five symptoms, depression and includes either a depressed mood or an anhedonia presentation. When diagnosing major depression, the clinician is alert for changes in such areas as weight, energy, appetite, sleep disturbance, guilt, and impaired concentration. Thoughts of dying might also be present. Children and adolescents might show different symptoms (e.g., somatic, disengagement in school). Suicide risk is important to consider and assess, with risk higher for women but completion rates higher for men.

The diagnosis of bipolar I disorder is made on the basis of at least one manic episode and one major depressive episode (American Psychiatric Association, 2022). A manic episode is diagnosed following a distinct period of a notable shift in mood (e.g., elevated, expansive) in addition to various symptoms (e.g., flight of ideas, pressured speech) whose duration differentiates mania from hypomania. Symptoms include inflated self-esteem, decreased need for sleep, increased talking or pressured speech, flight of ideas or racing thoughts, distractibility, increase in goal-directed activity, and excessive involvement in high-risk activities. For bipolar I, differential diagnoses include generalized anxiety disorder, panic disorder, posttraumatic stress disorder or other anxiety disorders; substance/medication-induced bipolar disorder, attention-deficit/hyperactivity disorder, personality disorders, and disorders with prominent irritability (American Psychiatric Association, 2022).

In contrast to bipolar I, a diagnosis of bipolar II disorder requires at least one major depressive episode and at least one hypomanic episode (American Psychiatric Association, 2022). When diagnosing hypomania, the neuropsychologist evaluates the patient's clinical presentation for the heightening of mood during discrete period, decreased sleep, talkativeness, flight of ideas, or racing thoughts, distractibility, goal-directed activity, and excessive involvement in high-risk activities. The difference between manic and hypomanic is length of time of the discrete episode: at least 1 week for manic and at least 4 consecutive days for hypomanic. Differential diagnoses for bipolar II are major depressive disorder, cyclothymic disorder, schizophrenia spectrum and other related psychotic disorders, panic disorder or other anxiety disorders, substance use disorders, ADHD, personality disorders, and other bipolar spectrum disorders (American Psychiatric Association, 2022).

Other bipolar spectrum disorders reflect different mood presentations, including cyclothymia, brief hypomanic or major depressive disorders, disruptive mood regulation, and childhood bipolar spectrum disorders. Cyclothymia carries a risk of evolving into bipolar I or II disorder. Changes in mood can be caused by different factors that include medication, medical conditions, and other clinical disorders.

NEUROPSYCHOLOGICAL ASSESSMENT

Relevant Literature

A strategic approach to the neuropsychological assessment of cognitive problems associated with bipolar spectrum disorders requires a model for organizing the assessment process. As a first step, familiarity with research is important; here, the literature is extensive. For example, Sole et al. (2012) reviewed literature from 1980 to 2009 and identified neurocognitive deficits in groups with bipolar I and bipolar II across different domains, including intelligence, memory and learning, attention, executive, psychomotor, affective processing, and social cognition, concluding that "the findings so far concerning BD-II as compared to BD-I suggest that BD-II is not free of cognitive impairment and that the functional impact of cognitive disturbances may be as high as that found in BD-I" (p. 198). Lin et al. (2015) evaluated patients diagnosed with soft bipolar spectrum disorders, which captures depression with cyclothymic or hyperthymic temperament, and depression with hypomania associated with an antidepressant. They found that processing speed, visual–spatial working memory, and verbal working memory were stronger for the soft bipolar disorder spectrum group compared with those with unipolar depression. The ability to shift cognitive set and visual–spatial memory was better for the soft bipolar spectrum group compared with those with bipolar I. There were no differences between the soft bipolar spectrum and bipolar II groups. The results suggested that the neurocognitive performance of people diagnosed with a soft bipolar spectrum disorder was closer to the bipolar II group and different from strict unipolar and bipolar I depression.

Meta-analytic studies show that deficits in memory and executive functioning "are among the strongest contributors to occupational outcome in BD, with greater impact than residual mood symptoms" (Miskowiak et al., 2018, p. 185). Statistics show that "cognitive impairment in the remitted phase of BD is on average of a moderate effect size" (Miskowiak et al., 2018, p. 185). There is also considerable heterogeneity (i.e., intact, global impairment, selective impairment) among remitted patients (Miskowiak et al., 2018).

Patients with either global or selective cognitive deficits also report poor overall quality of life. De Sá Sarmento et al. (2020) used strict criteria to define impairment and found that euthymic individuals diagnosed with bipolar I disorder when compared to a control group, were more impaired on measures of processing speed, memory, and visuoconstruction. Among the group with bipolar I disorder, 82.5% were taking lithium (17.5% of these were also taking an anticonvulsant) and 37.5% were taking an antipsychotic agent in conjunction with a mood stabilizer, suggesting that even with medication, performance was not as strong for the group with bipolar I disorder compared to the euthymic group. For the group with bipolar I disorder, poorer performance (i.e., number of errors) on an executive functioning test was correlated with time since onset, late onset, and number of manic episodes. Level of education was the best predictor of performance for both groups. Varo et al. (2019) found that the diagnosis of euthymic bipolar I or bipolar II was associated with lower scores compared to healthy controls on a social intelligence measure. Lower social intelligence was associated with male gender, lower estimated intelligence, as well as poorer performance on measures of working memory, verbal learning and memory, executive functioning, attention, and processing speed.

Clinical Interview

With a working familiarity with diagnostic criteria and research, a second step in the diagnostic process is the clinical interview (see Chapter 2 in this volume). Although the context will differ depending on the patient's age and mental status, the clinical interview should be conducted with the patient, either alone or with a trusted informant (e.g., partner, parent, guardian) who can provide collateral information about the patient's history. Details that are important to clarify during the interview will vary depending on the patient's age and mental status. Important are the patient's orientation to person, place, and time; mood and affect; self-monitoring ability; insight; judgment; thought processes; potential for harm to self and others; vocational, educational, and psychosocial adjustment and support system; legal matters; substance usage; and family history of mental health. Other areas are family and peer relationships, financial situation, medications, health, and prior treatments. In addition, the clinician might request records (e.g., prior test reports, hospitalization, release to speak with current or past therapists) to have baseline information about the patient.

Screening Measures

Clinical screening measures are valuable tools when assessing patients presenting with a presumptive bipolar spectrum disorder (see also Chapter 7 in this volume). The International Society for Bipolar Spectrum Disorders Targeting Cognition Task Force (Miskowiak et al., 2018) stated that cognitive screening allows for the detection of cognitive impairment, identification of patients who present with subjective complaints but whose results are within normative expectations (30%–50%, p. 187), and serial testing to assess changes over time.

COMPUTERIZED COGNITIVE SCREENING

Roebuck-Spencer et al. (2017) provided information about the potential benefits of computerized cognitive screening to assist in the identification of patients who may require more extensive neuropsychological testing. They also described a statement by the Screening and Psychological Assessment, given by the Working Group on Screening and Assessment, as "a collaboration of the American Psychological Association's Board of Professional Affairs and the Committee for the Advancement of Professional Practice" (American Psychological Association Practice Organization, 2014, p. 493). Taken together, these two sources highlight the following potential benefits of computerized cognitive screening measures: (a) early detection for at-risk individuals and contribution to higher detection rates for older adults in primary care settings compared with information provided by collateral sources, (b) good baseline data for further evaluation, (c) limited administration time, (d) focused administration, (e) flexible administration and scoring (e.g., assistants, computers, trained staff), (f) option in some circumstances of self-administration, (g) reduced cost,

(h) increased media attention and public awareness of cognitive health and impairment, (i) legal requirements for assessment of cognitive impairment (i.e., Affordable Care Act; Medical Annual Wellness Visit), (j) reimbursable services, and (k) added information related to decisions about the need for further assessment (Roebuck-Spencer et al., 2017, pp. 492–493).

Limitations of computerized testing were also reported by Roebuck-Spencer et al. (2017), citing the response of Bauer et al. (2012) to the American Academy of Clinical Neuropsychology and the National Academy of Neuropsychology's joint position on computerized neuropsychological assessment devices. In taking a cautionary tone about these guidelines, Bauer et al. (2012) stated, "First, it is important to recognize that even when a traditional examiner-administered test is programmed for computer administration, *it becomes a new and different test*" (p. 179, italics in original). They encouraged user caution in the following areas when considering computerized neuropsychological assessment devices for screening purposes: (a) device marketing and performance claims; (b) end-user issues; (c) technical/hardware/software/firmware issues; (d) privacy, data security, identity verification, and test environment; (e) psychometric development issues; (f) examiner issues like cultural experiential and disability factors; (g) use of computerized testing and reporting services; and (h) checks on validity of responses and results.

COMPREHENSIVE NEUROPSYCHOLOGICAL TESTING

Roebuck-Spencer et al. (2017) recommended a comprehensive neuropsychological evaluation if any one of the following three criteria is positive: "Was screening positive? Is diagnosis needed for treatment planning? Is assessment of functional abilities needed for medical decision-making?" (p. 495). Roebuck-Spencer et al. described how a positive answer to any of these questions is sufficient to trigger an evaluation of neurocognitive disorders. The evaluation can be organized around the following neurocognitive domains (*DSM-5-TR*, American Psychiatric Association, 2022, pp. 669–671): complex attention, executive function, learning and memory, language, perceptual-motor, and social cognition. The evaluator can exercise their clinical judgment when considering evaluating additional domains, such as intellectual functioning, academic achievement, and social–emotional/personality. The American Psychological Association (2020) offered guidance on psychological tele-assessment during the COVID-19 crisis.

CASE STUDY

The following brief case study illustrates the challenge of differentiating bipolar spectrum disorders from other related disorders.[1] The patient, a middle-aged, left-handed man, was referred by his psychiatrist for an assessment of cognitive

---

[1] The identity of the person whose history and test results are cited in this chapter has been disguised to protect their confidentiality.

status and personality. The patient was curious about a possible "mild bipolar disorder," despite having no history of this diagnosis. Anger management when feeling hurt and earning trust were concerns. There was a family history of ADHD. Developmentally, there were no birth or pregnancy complications. Milestones were met within normal limits. There was no history of concussions or seizures. Current medications were for sleep, anxiety-impulse control, and depression.

The patient met Roebuck-Spencer et al.'s (2017) criteria for neuropsychological assessment of functional abilities for purposes of treatment planning. The patient had been diagnosed at different points with speech-language deficits; ADHD, predominantly combined presentation; learning disabilities in mathematics, reading comprehension, and written expression; persistent depression; generalized anxiety; and polysubstance abuse. The patient had varying degrees of short-term success with different types of treatments.

The assessment was conducted in person, with COVID accommodations (masks, partition shield when appropriate, hand sanitizers, ventilation). The patient was cooperative, hard-working, and easy to evaluate. Gait, language, prosody, right–left distinctions, vision, hearing, and fine motor skills were intact. Mood was euthymic. Affect was anxious. A neuropsychological battery was developed to evaluate the domains of effort, intelligence, academic achievement, executive functioning, processing speed, attention, verbal memory, visual memory, constructional skill, fine-motor dexterity, social cognition, and personality. The battery is summarized in Table 11.1.

Results were considered valid and presented as follows. Effort on the Inventory of Problems–29 (Viglione & Giromini, 2020) was credible. Observations and embedded measures supported credible effort. Performance on the Wechsler Adult Intelligence Scale–Fourth Edition (Wechsler, 2008) was average for Verbal Comprehension, Perceptual Reasoning, and Processing Speed. Working memory was low average. Digit span was the only below-average subtest.

Performance on the Wechsler Individual Achievement Test–Fourth Edition (Wechsler, 2020) was average for word reading, spelling, essay composition, pseudoword decoding, oral reading fluency, and multiplication fluency; low average on addition fluency and math fluency; and below average for written fluency. Timed arithmetic on the Wide Range Achievement Test–Fifth Edition (Wilkinson & Robertson, 2017) was low average. Timed reading comprehension on the Nelson Denny Reading Test (NDRT; Fishco, 2019) was average; only 55% of the problems were completed within the standard time limit, but 95% of the items attempted were correct. Reading rate on the NDRT was below average.

Performance on the Halstead–Reitan Speech-Sound Perception Test (Reitan & Wolfson, 1993) was normal. Processing speed on the Symbol Digit Modalities Test (Smith, 2000) was below average. Executive functioning on the Wisconsin Card Sorting Test (Heaton et al., 1993) was above average for concept sorting, normal for sequencing Halstead–Reitan Trails Making Test Forms A and B (Reitan & Wolfson, 1993), average for work fluency on the Controlled Oral

TABLE 11.1. Neuropsychological Domains and Tests Administered

Domain	Tests and measures
Effort	Inventory of Problems–29 (IOP-29); behavioral observations; embedded measures
Intelligence	Wechsler Adult Intelligence Scale–Fourth Edition (WAIS-IV)
Achievement	Wechsler Individual Achievement Test–Fourth Edition (WIAT-4); Nelson Denny Reading Test (NDRT); Wide Range Achievement Test–Fifth Edition (WRAT-5)–Arithmetic subtest
Processing	Halstead–Reitan Speech-sound Perception Test (S-s PT); Symbol Digit Modalities Test (SDMT); WAIS-IV Processing Speed Index (PSI)
Executive functioning	Wisconsin Card Sorting Test (WCST); Halstead–Reitan Trails Making Test Forms A and B (TMT); Controlled Oral Word Association Test (COWAT); Boston Naming Test (BNT); Behavior Rating Inventory of Executive Functions (BRIEF)
Attention	WAIS-IV Digit Span subtest; Conners Auditory Test of Attention (CATA); Conners Continuous Performance Test-3 (CPT-3); Digit's Vigilance Test (DVT); Stroop Color and Word Test (Stroop); Conners Adult Attention Rating Scale (CAARS)
Memory	California Verbal Learning Test–Third Edition (CVLT-3); Rey Complex Figure Design and Recognition Trial-Immediate, Delayed, and Recognition Trial (REY)
Fine-motor dexterity	Grooved Pegboard Test
Visuo-constructional	REY Design Copy
Social cognition	Social Cognition and Object Relations Scale–Global Rating Method (SCORS-G)
Personality	Paulhus Deception Scale (PDS); Rorschach Performance Assessment System (R-PAS); Thematic Apperception Test (TAT); Personality Assessment Inventory (PAI)

Word Association Test (Benton & Hamsher, 1976), and proximal to average for spontaneous object-naming on the Boston Naming Test (Kaplan et al., 2001). Self-reports on the Behavior Rating Inventory of Executive Functions (BRIEF; Roth et al., 2005) suggested significant problems with executive functioning. Parent ratings on the BRIEF were in agreement for no clinically significant problems with behavior regulation and for clinically significant problems with metacognition.

As regards attention, he showed some indication of inattentiveness on measures of auditory attention on the Conners Auditory Test of Attention (Conners, 2014a) and visual attention on the Conners Continuous Performance Test-3 (Conners, 2014b). Performance on the Digit's Vigilance Test (Lewis, 1995), a cancellation measure, was average. Slow reading rate affected performance on a measure of response inhibition on the Stroop Color and Word Test (Golden, 2002). Self-report suggested more problems with attention than parent's report on the Conners Adult Attention Rating Scale (Conners & Ehrardt, 1998) suggested significant problems with attention.

Verbal memory on the California Verbal Learning Test–Third Edition (Delis et al., 2017) was average for five-trial verbal learning, free recall, cued recall, and new list learning, but below average for intrusions, repetitions, and false positives on a recognition task. Immediate and delayed visual recall were below average on the Rey Complex Figure Design and Recognition Trial-Immediate, Delayed, and Recognition Trial (REY; Meyers & Meyers, 1996). In the area of perceptual-motor skill, fine-motor dexterity was average on the Grooved Pegboard Test. (Matthews & Klove, 1964), but below average on the REY design copy, which was marked by omissions and imprecisions (Meyers & Meyers, 1996).

Social cognition on a storytelling measure suggested primarily basic descriptions of object relations using the Social Cognition and Object Relations Scale–Global Rating Method (Stein & Slavin-Mulford, 2018). Personality assessment indicated variable efforts to manage impression on the Personality Assessment Inventory (PAI; Morey, 1991) and Paulhus Deception Scale (Paulhus, 1999). Performance on the Rorschach Performance Assessment System (Meyer et al., 2011) and Thematic Apperception Test (Murray, 1943) suggested difficulty with relationships, struggles against expressing dependency (but wanting contact with others), painful introspection, some pessimism, and self-doubt. The PAI (Morey, 1991) indicated problems in the areas of depression and substances, but not in the area of mania.

Diagnostic impression considered that the patient performed solidly in areas where deficit might be expected (e.g., concept sorting, memory) and showed deficits in other areas (e.g., processing speed; visuoconstructional, visual memory). His history was also considered: childhood diagnosis of a mixed ADHD subtype and learning disabilities, along with generalized anxiety, persistent depression (and possible major depression), polysubstance use/dependence, and multiple learning disabilities by history; no family history of bipolar disorder; and no prior diagnosis of bipolar disorder. This information, combined with relatively low ratings on a mania subscale, favored the more conservative diagnoses of ADHD, combined presentation; generalized anxiety disorder; persistent depressive disorder (with a possible history of major depressive disorder); and a specific learning disability in reading rate or fluency. Other diagnoses related to substance and alcohol use were present in history.

Recommendations addressed the need to continue in psychotherapy at a weekly minimum to support personal growth and sobriety, including review of current substance and alcohol status by a drug and alcohol specialist; medication review and management with consideration for neuroimaging given potential for long-term impact on cognitive functioning of persistent substance use; and educational accommodations. Educational recommendations were 100% extended time for all tests, assignments, and standardized examinations with breaks not counting against extended time; private room for testing to minimize distractions; reduced course-load option; audio access to support needs in the area of reading; and study skills support. Feedback was well-received by the patient and his parents. I provided the patient with a report draft, asked for his input, and considered all points raised in his review of the material before finalizing the report.

CONCLUSION

Neuropsychological assessment of cognitive problems in people diagnosed with bipolar spectrum disorders is complex, time-consuming, and never clear-cut. The seriousness and long-term implications of the diagnosis pose challenges to the skill and knowledge of the assessor. Outcomes vary across patients, clinicians, and type of test utilized. Diagnostic criteria are overlapping. Approaching the evaluation with a framework guided by the literature can organize clinical data into a domain-based, patient-centered assessment that provides a sensible narrative to support the patient's psychosocial adjustment and treatment.

REFERENCES

Akiskal, H. S. (1983). The bipolar spectrum: New concepts in classification and diagnosis. In L. Grinspoon (Ed.), *Psychiatry update: The American Psychiatric Association annual review* (Vol. 2, pp. 271–292). American Psychiatric Association.

Akiskal, H. S. (2002). The bipolar spectrum—The shaping of a new paradigm in psychiatry. *Current Psychiatry Reports, 4*(1), 1–3. https://doi.org/10.1007/s11920-002-0001-1

American Psychiatric Association. (2022). *Diagnostic and statistical manual of mental disorders* (5th ed.; text rev.).

American Psychological Association. (2020). *Guidance on psychological tele-assessment during the COVID-19 crises.* https://www.apaservices.org/practice/reimbursement/health-codes/testing/tele-assessment-covid-19

American Psychological Association Practice Organization. (2014, December). *Distinguishing between screening and assessment for mental and behavioral health problems: A statement from an American Psychological Association Practice Organization work group on screening and psychological assessment.* http://www.apapracticecentral.org/reimbursement/billing/assessment-screening.aspx

Bauer, R. M., Iverson, G. L., Cernich, A. N., Binder, L. M., Ruff, R. M., & Naugle, R. I. (2012). Computerized neuropsychological assessment devices: Joint position paper of the American Academy of Clinical Neuropsychology and the National Academy of Neuropsychology. *The Clinical Neuropsychologist, 26*(2), 177–196. https://doi.org/10.1080/13854046.2012.663001

Benton, A. L., & Hamsher, K. (1976). *Multilingual aphasia examination.* University of Iowa.

Conners, C. K. (2014a). *Conners Continuous Auditory Attention Test of Attention.* MHS Assessments.

Conners, C. K. (2014b). *Conners Continuous Performance Test* (3rd ed.). MHS Assessments.

Conners, C. K., & Ehrardt, D. (1998). *(CAARS) Conners Adult ADHD Rating Scale.* Multi-Health Systems.

de Sá Sarmento, S. M., Bittencourt, L., de Mendonca Filho, E. J., Abreu, N., de Lacerda, A. L. T., & Miranda-Scippa, Á. (2020). Neurocognitive impairment in bipolar disorder and associated factors: Using population-based norms and a strict criterion for impairment definition. *Cognitive Behavioral Neurology, 33*(2), 103–112. https://doi.org/10.1097/wnn.0000000000000231

Delis, D. C., Karmer, J. H., Kaplan, E., & Ober, B. A. (2017). *California Verbal Learning Test* (3rd ed.). Harcourt.

Fishco, V. V. (2019). *Nelson-Denny Reading Test Forms I & J.: Examiner's manual.* PRO-ED.

Ghaemi, S. N. (2013). Bipolar spectrum: A review of the concept and a vision for the future. *Psychiatry Investigation, 10*(3), 218–224. https://doi.org/10.4306/pi.2013.10.3.218

Golden, C. (2002). *Stroop Color and Word Test*. Stoelting.

Heaton, R. K., Chelune, G. J., Talley, J. L., Kay, G. G., & Curtiss, G. (1993). *Wisconsin Card Sorting Test manual: Revised and expanded*. Psychological Assessment Resources.

Kaplan, E., Goodglass, H., & Weintraub, S. (2001). *Boston Naming Test* (2nd ed.). PRO-ED.

Kraepelin, E. (1904). *Lectures on clinical psychiatry*. Cornell University Library. https://doi.org/10.1037/10789-000

Lewis, R. F. (1995). *Digit Vigilance Test*. Psychological Assessment Resources.

Lin, K., Xu, G., Lu, W., Ouyang, H., Dang, Y., Guo, Y., So, K. F., & Lee, T. M. (2015). Neuropsychological performance of patients with soft bipolar spectrum disorders. *Bipolar Disorders, 17*(2), 194–204. https://doi.org/10.1111/bdi.12236

Matthews, C. G., & Klove, K. (1964). *Instruction manual for the Adult Neuropsychology Test Battery*. University of Wisconsin Medical School.

Meyer, G. J., Viglione, D. J., Mihura, J. L., Erard, R. E., & Erdberg, P. (2011). *Rorschach Performance Assessment System: Administration, coding, interpretation, and technical manual*. Rorschach Performance Assessment System.

Meyers, J., & Meyers, K. (1996). *Rey Complex Figure Design and the Recognition Trial: Professional manual*. Psychological Assessment Resources.

Miskowiak, K. W., Burdick, K. E., Martinez-Aran, A., Bonnin, C. M., Bowie, C. R., Carvalho, A. F., Gallagher, P., Lafer, B., López-Jaramillo, C., Sumiyoshi, T., McIntyre, R. S., Schaffer, A., Porter, R. J., Purdon, S., Torres, I. J., Yatham, L. N., Young, A. H., Kessing, L. V., & Vieta, E. (2018). Assessing and addressing cognitive impairment in bipolar disorder: The International Society for Bipolar Disorders Targeting Cognition Task Force recommendations for clinicians. *Bipolar Disorders, 20*(3), 184–194. https://doi.org/10.1111/bdi.12595

Morey, L. C. (1991). *Personality Assessment Inventory professional manual*. Psychological Assessment Resources.

Murray, H. A. (1943). *Thematic Apperception Test*. Harvard University Press.

O'Connell, K. S., & Coombes, B. J. (2021). Genetic contributions to bipolar disorder: Current status and future directions. *Psychological Medicine, 51*(13), 2156–2167. https://doi.org/10.1017/S0033291721001252

Paris, J. (2012). *The bipolar spectrum: Diagnosis or fad?* Routledge. https://doi.org/10.4324/9780203121061

Paulhus, D. L. (1999). *Paulhaus Deception Scales*. Multi-Health Systems.

Perugi, G., & Akiskal, H. S. (2002). The soft bipolar spectrum redefined: Focus on the cyclothymic, anxious-sensitive, impulse-dyscontrol, and binge-eating connection in bipolar II and related conditions. *The Psychiatric Clinics of North America, 25*(4), 713–737. https://doi.org/10.1016/S0193-953X(02)00023-0

Reitan, R. M., & Wolfson, D. (1993). *The Halstead–Reitan Neuropsychological Test Battery: Theory and clinical interpretation* (2nd ed.). Neuropsychology Press.

Roebuck-Spencer, T. M., Glen, T., Puente, A. E., Denney, R. L., Ruff, R. M., Hostetter, G., & Bianchini, K. J. (2017). Cognitive screening tests versus comprehensive neuropsychological test batteries: A National Academy of Neuropsychology Education Paper. *Archives of Clinical Neuropsychology, 32*(4), 491–498. https://doi.org/10.1093/arclin/acx021

Roth, R. M., Isquith, P. K., & Gioia, G. A. (2005). *Behavior Rating Inventory of Executive Function–Adult version: Professional manual*. Psychological Assessment Resources.

Smith, A. (2000). *Symbol-Digit Modalities Test*. Western Psychological Associates.

Sole, B., Bonnin, C. M., Torrent, C., Martinez-Aran, A., Popovic, D., Tabarés-Seisdedos, R., & Vieta, E. (2012). Neurocognitive impairment across the bipolar spectrum. *CNS Neuroscience & Therapeutics, 18*(3), 194–200. https://doi.org/10.1111/j.1755-5949.2011.00262.x

Stein, M. B., & Slavin-Mulford, J. (2018). *The Social Cognition and Object Relations Scale-Global Rating Method (SCORS-G): A comprehensive guide for clinicians*. Routledge.

Varo, C., Jiménez, E., Solé, B., Bonnín, C. M., Torrent, C., Lahera, G., Benabarre, A., Saiz, P. A., de la Fuente, L., Martnez-Aéan, A., Vieta, E., & Reinares, M. (2019). Social cognition in bipolar disorder: The role of sociodemographic, clinical, and neurocognitive variables in emotional intelligence. *Acta Psychiatrica Scandinavica, 139*(4), 369–380. https://doi.org/10.1111/acps.13014

Viglione, D. J., & Giromini, L. (2020). *Inventory of Problems–29.* IOP-Test.

Wechsler, D. (2008). *Wechsler Adult Intelligence Scale* (4th ed.). Harcourt.

Wechsler, D. (2020). *Wechsler Individual Achievement Test* (4th ed.). Harcourt.

Wilkinson, G. S., & Robertson, G. J. (2017). *Wide Range Achievement Test: Manual.* Pearson.

IV

CONSIDERATIONS IN
DIFFERENTIAL DIAGNOSIS

12

Assessment of Bipolar Spectrum Disorders, Disruptive Mood Dysregulation Disorder, and ADHD in Children and Adolescents

Anthony D. Bram and Kate G. Edwards

When a child or adolescent is referred for formal psychological assessment, it is almost axiomatic that they are in some way and to some extent struggling with emotional regulation, necessitating the need to further understand this disruptive and distressing symptom presentation. Conceptually and clinically, we think of emotional regulation as a core ego function or psychological capacity central to adaptive functioning and crucial to treatment planning (Bram, 2013; Bram & Peebles, 2014).[1] When our young patient's emotional dysregulation manifests in intense or frequent oscillations of mood, temper outbursts, aggression, or other dangerous or disruptive behavior, the referral inevitably involves the following question: Do they "have bipolar"? That is, does our young patient's pattern of emotional dysregulation meet criteria for a bipolar spectrum disorder (encompassing bipolar I, bipolar II, or cyclothymia)

---

[1] *Ego functions* refer to processes through which a person tries to adapt their internal experience and needs to the reality of their environment (Marcus, 2017).

https://doi.org/10.1037/0000356-013
Psychological Assessment of Bipolar Spectrum Disorders, J. H. Kleiger and I. B. Weiner (Editors)

as defined in the *Diagnostic and Statistical Manual of Mental Disorders* (5th ed., text rev.; *DSM-5-TR*; American Psychiatric Association, 2022)?

Historically, this has not been—and still is not—an easy diagnostic question to answer. In part, this difficulty stems from long-standing controversies about whether bipolar disorders can be diagnosed in children and, if so, the extent to which and ways in which it looks similar to or different from the adult form of the condition. Part of the controversy relates to the idea that bipolar conditions are considered biologically driven afflictions that need to be managed over a lifetime, often involving treatment with potent medications. Therefore, there is much at stake in arriving at this diagnosis for a young person for whom there remains much yet to unfold developmentally.

There have been primarily two opposing schools of thought about bipolar conditions in children and adolescents. The first is narrower, predicated on the definition of mania associated with the diagnosis of bipolar illness in adults, the hallmarks being episodes of elevated mood, heightened energy, expansive/grandiose thinking, and psychomotor acceleration. The second broadens the definition of mania for children beyond the adult criteria mentioned previously, encompassing dispositions to irritability, and proneness to frequent and prolonged rages and tantrums. With this expanded definition, more children fall under the umbrella of the bipolar spectrum and are considered to have a "juvenile phenotype" of the disorder. A problem with this expanded definition of mania for children has been that there is not much evidence that children displaying primary symptoms of irritability and explosive anger meet criteria for bipolar illness as adults. Prospective studies do not show the expected continuity between this purported juvenile phenotype and adult forms of mania (Duffy et al., 2020).

The controversy has attenuated somewhat over the past decade, since the authors of the *DSM-5* introduced the disruptive mood dysregulation disorder (DMDD; American Psychiatric Association, 2013, 2022) category to describe children and adolescents whose behavioral struggles primarily revolve around irritability, tantrums, and angry outbursts and who do not also exhibit episodes of elevated mood, expansive thinking, grandiosity, and psychomotor acceleration (Goldstein et al., 2017). As such, children whose condition was previously conceptualized as "bipolar disorder not otherwise specified" based on the *DSM-IV* criteria (American Psychiatric Association, 1994) could now be viewed as meeting the criteria for DMDD. Our current perspective on diagnosing bipolar conditions in children is consistent with the first, more limited view of what constitutes mania, the view also articulated in the guidelines of the American Academy of Child and Adolescent Psychiatry (AACAP; McClellan et al., 2007), and is in line with the *DSM-5-TR* criteria (American Psychiatric Association, 2022).

But even with the clarity added by the DMDD category, the process of differential diagnosis involving the bipolar spectrum in pediatric populations remains challenging. For example, with children prone to emotional dysregulation, ruling out and/or assessing for possible co-occurring conditions remains necessary. Considerations to keep in mind include but are not limited to the role of anxiety, trauma, emerging personality problems, and/or the role an underlying neurodevelopmental disorder (e.g., an autism spectrum disorder) could be playing in the symptom presentation. However, perhaps the most common question of differential diagnosis we encounter in the practice of clinical assessment involves disentangling symptoms of bipolar spectrum disorders from those consistent with DMDD and attention-deficit/hyperactivity disorder (ADHD). Thus, this chapter focuses on assessment considerations of differential diagnoses among the bipolar spectrum, DMDD, and ADHD.

GENERAL CONSIDERATIONS FOR ASSESSMENT OF EMOTIONAL DYSREGULATION

Although this chapter emphasizes *DSM-5-TR* differential diagnostics with ADHD and DMDD, we acknowledge that this is only one aspect of assessing a child or adolescent's emotional dysregulation. In practice, we are equally interested in, and encourage using, a multimethod approach (see Bram, 2010, 2018; Bram & Peebles, 2014) to learn more about the *psychological processes* involved in a young person's emotional dysregulation. This includes addressing questions such as: In what way and under what conditions is the child prone to dysregulation? What feelings are most problematic and difficult to contain? What is the child's self-protective style? What are the psychological costs of their dysregulation, and what functions might the symptoms serve? What are the child's psychological strengths, and what helps them recover from dysregulation? These dynamic considerations are addressed in more depth by Bram (2010, 2018) and Bram and Peebles (2014).

Considering the complicated nature of diagnosing psychopathology in children, our approach to assessing their emotional regulation in general—and bipolar spectrum conditions in particular—stays close to the data. We may feel pressure from our referring colleagues and the families of our patients (and our own ideals of what an assessor should be able to do) to pin down, yea or nay, whether a dysregulated child or adolescent is suffering a bipolar illness. We also do not want to miss a diagnosis of bipolar disorder because we recognize that doing so has costs in terms of trials of possibly contraindicated medications or delayed initiation of mood-stabilizing medication, heightening the risk of various disruptions in functioning and well-being (Singh & Rajput, 2006). But in real-world practice, even with a multimethod approach, this differential diagnosis is often far from crystal clear. Not uncommonly, the assessment findings are mixed with some data sources supporting a diagnosis and other sources less so. When the data are equivocal, we describe how the picture is consistent with the bipolar spectrum and how it is not. This is no different from our overall approach to inference making (see Bram & Peebles, 2014), but we highlight it here because of the profound, lifelong implications of concluding that a child has this severe and persistent mental illness (McClellan et al., 2007). Humbly, when assessing children, we recognize that there is still much to unfold developmentally that we cannot predict; the younger the child, the more this is the case.

CONSIDERATION OF BASE RATES FOR BIPOLAR DISORDER IN CHILDREN AND ADOLESCENTS AND SOME CAVEATS

As with any other condition, an accurate diagnosis of a bipolar spectrum illness involves considering base rates of that condition in the setting in which the assessor practices (Youngstrom, Choukas-Bradley et al., 2015; Youngstrom et al., 2012). Youngstrom et al. (2012) reported estimated base rates for pediatric bipolar disorder to be 2% (4% for all bipolar spectrum conditions) in the general population, 5% to 10% in patients receiving outpatient/community mental health care, 11% in youth in a state foster-care system, 2% to 22% in incarcerated adolescents, and 25% to 40% in psychiatrically hospitalized children and adolescents (see p. 18, Table 2 in Youngstrom et al., 2012, for references). Essentially, the more intensive or acute the clinical setting, the higher the base rate for bipolar diagnoses. The base rate can also be expected to be higher the more specialized the setting is for the evaluation and treatment of mood disorders. Youngstrom, Choukas-Bradley, et al. (2015) reminded us that the lower the base rate, the greater the "burden of proof" required to support the diagnosis.

It makes sense that in more intensive and specialized settings with a higher frequency of bipolar spectrum diagnoses, it is likelier that the patient currently being assessed will also be found to have that diagnosis. We encourage assessors working in such settings to hold this in mind simultaneously with an awareness of some familiar diagnostic pitfalls such as confirmation bias, false dichotomy (or black-and-white thinking), and reduction fallacies (e.g., Kahneman & Tversky, 1972; Klayman, 1995). Our impression is that some highly specialized clinics and programs (e.g., for bipolar disorder, ADHD, autism, borderline personality) are vulnerable to viewing complex patients through their narrow diagnostic lens such that they (a) overlook, minimize, or otherwise fail to integrate data inconsistent with their diagnostic specialty and thus (b) do not adequately consider alternate or complementary conceptualizations and treatment modalities.

ACCOUNTING FOR DEVELOPMENTAL AND FAMILIAL FACTORS BEARING ON A POSSIBLE BIPOLAR SPECTRUM DIAGNOSIS

Assessment begins before the child or adolescent enters our office for one-to-one evaluation sessions. To clarify the context to address the referral questions, we want to have a handle on the child's family and developmental history, elicited through some combination of questionnaires and/or interviews with parents or caregivers. Although what to ask in a thorough developmental history is beyond the scope of this chapter (e.g., see Cepeda & Gotanco, 2017), five crucial points to probe when there are questions about a possible bipolar spectrum condition include whether (a) there is a family history of bipolar illness; (b) the child has had adverse reactions to selective serotonin reuptake inhibitor (SSRI) antidepressants; (c) the child has had a recent physical exam with laboratory work, ruling out other medical explanations; (d) there are concerns about alcohol or substance use; and (e) the course of symptoms is consistent with patterns more typically observed in children with bipolar illness. Most of these considerations involve the identification of risk factors that can be integrated with what we know about base rates in our setting to inform the probability of a bipolar spectrum diagnosis (Youngstrom, Choukas-Bradley, et al., 2015; Youngstrom et al., 2012).

Family History of Bipolar Illness

As there is a strong genetic component to bipolar conditions (McGuffin et al., 2003), with a confirmed diagnosis of bipolar disorder in at least one biological relative, there is an increased likelihood that a child or adolescent will eventually meet the criteria for the condition. Although the risk is lower when a second-degree or more distant biological relative has had this diagnosis, it is still much higher than in the general population (McGuffin et al., 2003). The critical point here is that a familial diagnosis of bipolar disorder ought to be weighted and integrated with base rates and data from self-report, collateral-report, and performance-based data.

Adverse Reactions to SSRI Antidepressant Medication

There is evidence from both observational studies and clinical trials that in some child and adult patients, the use of SSRI medications (especially in "mono-therapy," i.e., prescribed in the absence of other psychotropics) is associated with triggering manic symptoms (a "manic switch"; e.g., Allain et al., 2017). Though Joseph et al. (2009) cautioned that the empirical jury may still be out on this explanation, from an assessment standpoint, it is meaningful to know that a child or adolescent has had such an adverse reaction, as this can lend some weight to other evidence pointing in the direction of a bipolar diagnosis.

Recent Medical Evaluation

As numerous physical conditions can mimic bipolar/manic symptoms, we want to ensure that our physician colleagues have carefully ruled them out. Among such conditions are hyperthyroidism, lupus, encephalitis, temporal lobe epilepsy, or head injuries (Kowatch et al., 2005).

Concerns About Alcohol and Substance Abuse

Manic-like symptoms such as overconfidence/grandiosity, euphoric mood, racing thoughts, and risk-taking behaviors can be secondary to alcohol and recreational drug use. Especially with adolescents, it is valuable to tease out to what extent such symptoms are circumscribed or exacerbated around alcohol or substance use (e.g., cannabis, amphetamines, hallucinogens). If manic symptoms are circumscribed around drug use, there is more reason to conceptualize the symptoms as substance-induced rather than a primary bipolar condition (American Psychiatric Association, 2022).

Course of Illness

Although there is variation in the course of a developing bipolar spectrum condition, the more the child's or adolescent's trajectory resembles a typical course, the more confident we can be that their condition is consistent with the diagnosis. Duffy et al. (2020) noted that for children who eventually meet criteria for a bipolar illness as adults, the trend is for an early childhood marked by anxiety and disrupted sleep and an adolescence marked by episodic alternation between depressive and manic/hypomanic states. By contrast, children who show early neurodevelopmental challenges, including symptoms of ADHD, and whose adolescence involves more chronic mood dysregulation, trend toward meeting criteria for DMDD or depressive disorders as adults.

MULTIMETHOD ASSESSMENT OF BIPOLAR SPECTRUM CONDITIONS

Typically, when a dysregulated child or adolescent is referred to us for a formal psychological evaluation, they have already been assessed by another clinician—such as a therapist, psychiatrist, or other physician—who has made use of clinical interview and observational methods. But something essential remains puzzling about their young patient and how to help them, leading to their referral to us for a more specialized assessment. Central to what sets our evaluations apart from such more routine clinical assessments (Youngstrom, Choukas-Bradley, et al., 2015; Youngstrom et al., 2012) is our multimethod approach, that is, the integration of self-report, collateral-report, and performance-based methods (e.g., Chapter 1 of this volume; Bram & Peebles, 2014; Hopwood & Bornstein, 2014; Yalof & Bram, 2021). In this section, we review an array of collateral-report, self-report, and performance-based measures to consider for assessing the possibility of a bipolar spectrum condition. The greater convergence of findings across the various methods, the more confidence we have in them, and when there is divergence across methods, we aim to make sense of it in a way that illuminates a more nuanced understanding of the patient (Bram & Peebles, 2014). Based on Weiner's (2000) invaluable suggestion to convey test findings with a level of confidence commensurate with the evidence in the data, it is acceptable to conclude that findings are mixed or equivocal, specifying in what ways.

Collateral-Report Measures to Assess Emotional Regulation in General

Typically, collateral-report measures to assess emotional regulation in general, and bipolar spectrum conditions in particular, are completed by parents or caregivers because as compared with self- and teacher-report, parent/caregiver ratings correlate most strongly with diagnoses based on structured interviews (Youngstrom, Genzlinger, et al., 2015), such as the Kiddie Schedule for Affective Disorders and Schizophrenia for School-Aged Children, Present and Lifetime Version, for the *DSM-5* (K-SADS-PL *DSM-5*; Kaufman et al., 2016; see also Chapter 2 in this volume). However, Duffy et al. (2020) and Youngstrom et al. (2012) reminded us of the value of using data from multiple informants, which illuminates conditions under which a patient's functioning varies. As is the case for the self-report measures discussed later, collateral-report measures of emotional dysregulation can be classified according to whether they are broadband or bipolar-specific.

Broadband Collateral-Report Measures of Emotional Regulation

Collateral-report broadband measures include parent/caregiver- and teacher-report forms of multiscale measures such as the Behavioral Assessment Scale for Children, Third Edition (BASC-3; Reynolds & Kamphaus, 2015) or the Child Behavior Checklist (Achenbach & Rescorla, 2001). These types of broadband scales are discussed in Chapter 7 of this volume, so we will not go into great detail here. Youngstrom et al. (2012) alerted us to the value of attending to such measures' subscales that capture externalizing behaviors (e.g., oppositionality, aggression, hyperactivity, risk-taking). Low externalizing scores are weighted heavily in helping to rule out bipolar, whereas high scores must be further investigated with bipolar-specific measures to mitigate high rates of false positives.

Collateral-Report Measures Specific to Bipolar Conditions

Any evaluation where there is a question of bipolar illness ought to include a caregiver/parent-report scale that assesses for symptoms of mania. Three such bipolar-specific collateral scales for assessors to consider include the Child Mania Rating Scale, Parent Version (Pavuluri et al., 2006), the Parent Version of the Young Mania Rating Scale (P-YMRS; Gracious et al., 2002), and the parent report of the Mood Disorder Questionnaire, Adolescent Version (Wagner et al., 2006). Such measures are reviewed in Chapter 7 of this volume. We add that with any of these bipolar-specific collateral-report measures, assessors can consider augmenting the instructions as Marchand et al. (2005) did with the P-YMRS: If the patient is effectively medicated or otherwise stabilized at the time of evaluation, instruct the parent to complete ratings based on the child/adolescent's functioning before stabilization. Additionally, when a parent has endorsed multiple symptoms on any of the resulting in a score at or above the research-based threshold for differential diagnosis and the endorsed items are more specific to mania or hypomania (e.g., uncharacteristically expansive/elevated mood, grandiosity, increased energy, decreased need for sleep, hypersexuality) as opposed to primarily irritability and aggression, which are transdiagnostic in nature, the assessor can follow up a focused interview to determine the extent to which these symptoms cluster into discrete episodes.

The assessor strives to clarify with the parent the frequency, onset, duration, and offset of such episodes.

Self-Report Measures to Assess Emotional Regulation in General

Self-Report by Interview

If our principal objective is a hard-and-fast ruling in or ruling out of a bipolar spectrum condition, ideally, the cornerstone assessment method would be a structured or semistructured interview anchored to *DSM-5-TR* (or the latest psychiatric taxonomic system) criteria. The caveat is that such measures have primarily been developed in and for research settings, making application to clinical assessment more cumbersome and less practical (Kleiger & Khadivi, 2015). The K-SADS-PL *DSM-5* mentioned previously (Kaufman et al., 2016) is the semistructured interview that, though covering a wide range of neurodevelopmental and psychiatric conditions, has been used most extensively in research into pediatric bipolar disorder. This interview is reviewed, among others, in Chapter 2 of this volume.

Self-Report by Questionnaire

Self-report questionnaires are relatively time- and cost-effective methods that allow us to appreciate the child or adolescent's own perspective on their emotional functioning. These measures include both (a) symptom- and disorder-specific scales (reviewed in Chapter 7 of this volume) and (b) broadband personality measures. The latter include adolescent measures such as the Minnesota Multiphasic Personality Inventory–Adolescent version (MMPI-A; Butcher et al., 1992), the Minnesota Multiphasic Personality Inventory–Adolescent–Restructured Form (MMPI-A-RF; Archer et al., 2016), the Personality Assessment Inventory–Adolescent version (PAI-A; Morey, 2007), and the Millon Adolescent Clinical Inventory–Second Edition (MACI-II; Millon et al., 2020). These measures' respective bipolar-relevant scales are as follows: MMPI-A Scale 9 plus subscales that include Psychomotor Acceleration and Ego Inflation; MMPI-A-RF Scale RC9 Hypomanic Activation; PAI-A Mania scale and subscales of Activity Level, Grandiosity, and Irritability; and BASC-3 Mania scale. The MACI-II has a scale specific to Disruptive Mood Dysregulation. Endorsed items that elevate the bipolar-related scales can be clarified with subsequent inquiry.

Performance-Based Measures and Methods to Assess for Bipolar Spectrum Conditions

Including performance-based methods in our battery enables us to sample a child/adolescent's *implicit processes* of emotional (dys)regulation in real time (see Chapter 5 in Bram & Peebles, 2014). Performance-based data complement what the child/adolescent and collaterals tell us explicitly about their feelings, mood, and behavior. Compared with collateral and self-report measures, performance-based measures are less central in determining *DSM-5-TR* diagnoses, but they can provide converging or refuting evidence. Most notably, cognitive scores from the Rorschach test (Exner, 2003; Meyer et al., 2011) can inform us about our patient's vulnerability to lapse into certain kinds of hypomanic thinking that research has associated with bipolar conditions (summarized in Kleiger, 1999, 2017; see also Chapters 8 and 9 in this volume). In particular, we look for patterns of (a) combinative thinking (Fabulized Combinations and Incongruous Combinations) that are associated with enlivened, playful, jocular content and/or delivery and (b) tangential, often excitable or flippant, responses (coded as Deviant Responses [DRs]).[2] Here is an example of each, offered by an emotionally dysregulated 9-year-old:

> Card III. Ooooh! Two monkeys dancing the jig. With music notes whirling and swirling around them! (FAB1)

> Card II. Clowns celebratin' at birthday party! When's your birthday? Mine is in June! I told my mom I want an Xbox. [laughing and singing] Happy birthday to me! Happy birthday to me! (DR1)

We emphasize, though, that having such responses in a Rorschach protocol is not sufficient in and of itself to conclude a bipolar spectrum diagnosis. We need additional, critical evidence from collateral and self-report symptom measures. Also, it is important to keep in mind that some combinative thinking is not unusual in the protocols of young children (Leichtman, 1995), so we need to compare our patient's scores against age-based norms (Exner, 2003; Meyer et al., 2007, 2011). When these scores are elevated, and responses have the kind of hypomanic flavor illustrated previously, we have some evidence in the direction of a bipolar condition.

CONSIDERATIONS FOR *DSM-5-TR* DIFFERENTIAL DIAGNOSES: BIPOLAR SPECTRUM, DMDD, AND ADHD

Having presented self-report, collateral-report, and performance-based measures to consider in a multimethod evaluation, we now turn to specific considerations about (a) where on the bipolar spectrum a patient lies and (b) differential diagnosis of bipolar disorders relative to DMDD and ADHD.

Locating the Patient on the Bipolar Spectrum

To determine where the child or adolescent is located along the bipolar spectrum, we rely most heavily on caregivers' reports of manic/hypomanic and depressive symptoms and their clustering, onset/offset, and frequency of recurrence. According to the American Psychiatric Association (2022), for bipolar I disorder, there needs to be at least a week of three symptoms of mania

---

[2] Note that the research on which this is based (summarized by Kleiger, 1999, 2017) has predominantly been conducted with adults. Because we are operating on the premise of continuity between childhood and adulthood versions of mania, we extrapolate from this literature to our assessment of children and adolescents.

(or four, if the primary symptom is irritability as opposed to elevated mood). For bipolar II, the duration of the same criteria must be met for at least 4 consecutive days (but fewer than 7). In this case, it is termed hypomania as opposed to mania. Often overlooked by clinicians and understudied by researchers, cyclothymic disorder (sometimes informally referred to as bipolar III) is more challenging to diagnose (Van Meter & Youngstrom, 2012). For a child or adolescent to be diagnosed with cyclothymia, they must experience over the course of a year or longer multiple periods of (a) hypomanic symptoms that fall short of a hypomanic episode and (b) depressive symptoms that fall short of a depressive episode. Further, during that period of a year or more, a patient must experience the aforementioned symptoms at least 50% of the time and be free of these symptoms for no more than 2 months (American Psychiatric Association, 2022). One can appreciate how challenging it could be for caregivers to retrospectively report these kinds of complex and nuanced patterns in a way conducive to an accurate diagnosis of cyclothymia, so it requires effort on the assessor's part to try to parse this out by interview.

The Bipolar Spectrum and Differential Diagnosis

Problems with emotional regulation in children can manifest in symptoms of various *DSM-5-TR* conditions, among them bipolar spectrum disorders, DMDD, and ADHD. The synopses offered next are not intended as substitutes for a careful review of all *DSM-5-TR* criteria in the service of a final diagnosis. Instead, they are provided to give a framework for assessors' conceptualization.

Bipolar Spectrum Versus DMDD

As described earlier, DMDD is the *DSM-5-TR* authors' attempt to resolve the controversy surrounding pediatric bipolar disorder, specifically cases previously considered by many clinicians to be ultradian (less than a day but longer than an hour) rapid cycling subtype of the disorder (American Psychiatric Association, 2022). Irritable and volatile moods could indicate either DMDD or a bipolar spectrum disorder. Thus, the primary distinguishing features are the intertwined (a) *chronicity* of symptoms in DMDD versus the *episodic* course in pediatric bipolar disorder and (b) the specificity of elevated mood, grandiosity, and other features of mania or hypomania to bipolar conditions. In the instance where the child or adolescent exhibits an episode of primarily irritable—as opposed to elevated or expansive—mood, they must also show heightened energy and goal-directed activity most of the day for at least 4 days (hypomania/bipolar II) to at least a week (mania/bipolar I) to meet the criteria for a bipolar diagnosis (American Psychiatric Association, 2013).[3] Irritability in the absence of energized and goal-directed activity is more in the realm of DMDD. The differential diagnosis

---

[3] When mood is elevated or expansive, the same additional requirement for heightened energy and goal-directed behavior applies to meet criteria for a bipolar disorder. We emphasize irritability because when it is primary, it is more challenging to differentiate between bipolar and DMDD.

between DMDD and bipolar is either/or, but not both. Also, it is worth reiterating that children meeting DMDD criteria are rarely diagnosed with a bipolar spectrum illness later in life (Althoff et al., 2010; Copeland et al., 2013), further establishing the two disorders as having distinct symptom profiles. If the multi-method measures described earlier do not illuminate discrete episodic clusters of manic or hypomanic symptoms, DMDD becomes a more likely diagnostic conclusion.

Bipolar Spectrum and ADHD

When evaluating a child or adolescent who is prone to emotional dysregulation, a common but challenging differential diagnosis involves distinguishing between the bipolar spectrum and ADHD. Further complicating this differential is that bipolar spectrum and ADHD diagnoses can co-occur, and, in actuality, co-occurrence is quite common. A recent meta-analysis examining the prevalence of ADHD in children with bipolar spectrum disorders estimated such co-occurrence to be as high as 73% in childhood and 43% in adolescence (Sandstrom et al., 2021). The psychiatrist and researcher Gabrielle Carlson offered a conceptualization that can assist assessment clinicians to tease apart the confusingly overlapping characteristics of the two conditions: (a) Both involve distractibility and sleep problems, (b) manic activity of bipolar conditions and the hyperactivity of ADHD can mimic each other, (c) manic lapses in judgment can be confused with the impulsivity of ADHD, and (d) bipolar irritability and the poor frustration tolerance of ADHD resemble each other (Miller, n.d.). Again, the episodic nature of bipolar manic symptoms in contrast to the chronicity of those of ADHD (American Psychiatric Association, 2022) is a crucial distinguisher. For example, Miller (n.d.; based on her interview with Carlson) explained that "the low frustration tolerance of ADHD does not go away, while a child with bipolar disorder could be severely irritable for six months and then not have another episode for years." Related to this is the episodic grandiosity that is a hallmark of manic states in bipolar spectrum disorders but is not part of an ADHD picture (American Psychiatric Association, 2022). Along similar lines, impulsivity centered on excessive spending, sexual disinhibition, and substance use points more toward the bipolar spectrum than ADHD (Jensen et al., 2001).

In considering the chronicity of ADHD symptoms, however, it is also essential to consider that there can be a situational exacerbation of irritability, impulsivity, restlessness, and fidgeting (Marangoni et al., 2015). For instance, hyperactivity may increase relative to task demand, such as in the classroom or when asked to engage in activities that require focus and prolonged effort. Also note that in ADHD, mood lability may be observed within the same day and not over the 4- to 7-plus-day day requirement for a hypomanic/manic episode (American Psychiatric Association, 2022). If that same-day pattern of mood lability involves persistent irritability and frequent severe verbally and/or physically aggressive outbursts for at least a year, the possibility of DMDD (see the previous section) ought to be considered instead of or in addition to ADHD.

Some research shows that children diagnosed with bipolar spectrum disorders, ADHD, or both show weaknesses on a performance-based test of executive functioning (Passarotti et al., 2016). Interestingly, although the three groups (bipolar, ADHD, and bipolar plus ADHD) did not differ from each other on this performance-based measure, differences in the severity and nature of their executive functioning were evident based on the Parent Form of the Behavior Rating Inventory of Executive Functioning (Gioia et al., 2015):

> While all three groups were impaired in General Executive Functioning and Metacognition only the two [pediatric bipolar] groups revealed more extensive [executive functioning] dysfunction, in both, only the two [pediatric bipolar] groups revealed more extensive [executive functioning] dysfunction in cognitive and emotional control domains, relative to the ADHD group. Conversely, the ADHD group exhibited selective deficits in cognitive domains such as working memory, planning/organization, monitoring, and metacognition. The two [pediatric bipolar] groups showed greater impairment than the ADHD group in the domains of Inhibition, Shifting, Monitoring and Emotional Control. (p. 185)

These findings have implications for considering a parent-report measure of executive functioning such as the Behavior Rating Inventory of Executive Function, Second Edition (Gioia et al., 2015) for inclusion in the test battery when this differential is salient. Elevated indicators of emotional dyscontrol point toward the bipolar spectrum (or in the absence of indicators of mania on other measures, perhaps toward DMDD).

When there is a question of ADHD—whether or not a bipolar spectrum condition is also suspected—it is routine for assessors to query a thorough history of the onset, nature, severity, and duration of symptoms as well as to administer disorder-specific, norm-based self-, parent-, and teacher-report measures such as the Conners, Third Edition (Conners, 2008); Vanderbilt Assessment Scales, Third Edition (Zurhellen et al., 2019); or Attention Deficit Disorders Evaluation Scale, Fifth Edition (ADDES-5; McCarney & House, 2019). In more comprehensive evaluations, assessors also make use of attention-specific computerized performance tests (e.g., Conners Continuous Performance Test–3 [CPT-3]; Conners, 2014b; Conners Kiddie Continuous Performance Test [K-CPT]; Conners, 2015; Conners Continuous Auditory Test of Attention [CATA]; Conners, 2014a) alongside other neuropsychological and psychoeducational performance-based tests aimed at discerning the degree and type of executive dysfunction and other potential learning disabilities.

SUMMARY AND CONCLUDING THOUGHTS

In this chapter, we have offered assessment considerations for the diagnosis of bipolar spectrum disorders in children and adolescents. We have highlighted the importance of attending to base rates to determine the degree of "burden of proof" (Youngstrom, Choukas-Bradley, et al., 2015) required to conclude that a young person meets the criteria for a bipolar spectrum condition. We have also emphasized the need to weigh family psychiatric history, the developmental course of illness, and previous adverse medication reactions to gauge the likelihood of a bipolar condition. In addition, we have noted the need to rule out medical conditions as well as the role of alcohol and substance use in accounting for bipolar-like symptoms. We have then reviewed collateral-report, self-report, and performance-based methods specific to clarifying whether an emotionally dysregulated child or adolescent is best understood on the bipolar spectrum. Subsequently, we have discussed factors determining where on the bipolar spectrum a patient might fall. Finally, we have offered consideration for differentiating dysregulation on the bipolar spectrum from DMDD and ADHD.

As we have suggested previously, applying and integrating all of these considerations in a multimethod evaluation of a dysregulated young person is challenging. In Chapter 19 of this volume, Kleiger offers a detailed case illustration that provides a sense of how the measures and mindset that we have presented can be implemented to clarify the presence or absence of a bipolar spectrum disorder and other aspects of differential diagnosis in a complex adolescent.

To conclude, we reiterate four key points. First, a limitation of this chapter is that although we have addressed differential diagnoses among bipolar spectrum disorders, DMDD, and ADHD, space limitations precluded the consideration of other important differentials and potential co-occurring conditions with which assessors often grapple. These include trauma/PTSD, various anxiety disorders, disruptive behavior disorders, the autism spectrum, emerging personality psychopathology, and learning disabilities, among others.

Second, the determination of *DSM-5-TR* diagnoses—including differentials related to the bipolar spectrum—is just one way that assessors contribute to a meaningful understanding of a patient's emotional dysregulation. Although not the focus of the present chapter, it is arguably the strength of multimethod psychological assessment to clarify the patient's processes of emotional dysregulation (e.g., self-protective style, variability under different conditions, function and cost of symptoms, strengths) and associated psychotherapeutic implications (Bram, 2010, 2018; Bram & Peebles, 2014). Third, it is sometimes the case—perhaps more often than we would like to admit—that our multimethod data are equivocal about a bipolar diagnosis. Despite internal and external pressures to fit complicated people neatly into diagnostic boxes, there is no shame in acknowledging and embracing the ambiguity and messiness inherent in efforts to understand a real person. Our task is to report what we find—that is, ways in which our young patient matches and does not match a bipolar prototype. In part, this is what it means to practice evidence-based assessment. In such instances, we describe for the patient's caregivers and treaters what kinds of symptoms and behavior to look for that would increase certainty about a bipolar diagnosis or help rule it out more definitively. Fourth, given that a bipolar spectrum diagnosis is associated with lifelong implications as an often severe and persistent mental illness, we must be extraordinarily thoughtful—particularly around whether criteria for manic/hypomanic episode are met—before assigning this diagnosis to a young person whose developmental trajectory is uncertain and unfolding.

REFERENCES

Achenbach, T. M., & Rescorla, L. A. (2001). *Manual for the ASEBA School-Age Forms & Profiles*. University of Vermont, Research Center for Children, Youth, & Families.

Allain, N., Leven, C., Falissard, B., Allain, J.-S., Batail, J.-M., Polard, E., Montastruc, F., Drapier, D., & Naudet, F. (2017). Manic switches induced by antidepressants: An umbrella review comparing randomized controlled trials and observational studies. *Acta Psychiatrica Scandinavica, 135*(2), 106–116. https://doi.org/10.1111/acps.12672

Althoff, R. R., Verhulst, F. C., Rettew, D. C., Hudziak, J. J., & van der Ende, J. (2010). Adult outcomes of childhood dysregulation: A 14-year follow-up study. *Journal of the American Academy of Child & Adolescent Psychiatry, 49*(11), 1105–1116. https://doi.org/10.1097/00004583-201011000-00004

American Psychiatric Association. (1994). *Diagnostic and statistical manual of mental disorders* (4th ed.).

American Psychiatric Association. (2013). *Diagnostic and statistical manual of mental disorders* (5th ed.).

American Psychiatric Association. (2022). *Diagnostic and statistical manual of mental disorders: DSM-5-TR* (5th ed., text rev.).

Archer, R. P., Handel, R. W., Ben-Porath, Y. S., & Tellegen, A. (2016). *Minnesota Multiphasic Personality Inventory–Adolescent–Restructured Form (MMPI-A-RF): Manual for administration, scoring, interpretation, and technical manual*. University of Minnesota Press.

Bram, A. (2018). Understanding a therapeutic impasse: Use of R-PAS in a multi-method assessment of alliance dynamics and underlying developmental disruption. In J. Mihura & G. Meyer (Eds.), *Applications of the Rorschach performance assessment system* (pp. 119–137). Guilford Press.

Bram, A. D. (2010). The relevance of the Rorschach and patient–examiner relationship in treatment planning and outcome assessment. *Journal of Personality Assessment, 92*(2), 91–115. https://doi.org/10.1080/00223890903508112

Bram, A. D. (2013). Psychological testing and treatment implications: We can say more. *Journal of Personality Assessment, 95*(4), 319–331. https://doi.org/10.1080/00223891.2012.736907

Bram, A. D., & Peebles, M. J. (2014). *Psychological testing that matters: Creating a road map for effective treatment*. American Psychological Association. https://doi.org/10.1037/14340-000

Butcher, J. N., Williams, C., Graham, J. R., Archer, R. P., Tellegen, A., & Ben-Porath, Y. S. (1992). *Minnesota Multiphasic Personality Inventory–Adolescent (MMPI-A): Manual for administration, scoring, and interpretation*. University of Minnesota Press.

Cepeda, C., & Gotanco, L. (2017). *Psychiatric interview of children and adolescents*. American Psychiatric Association.

Conners, C. K. (2008). *Conners* (3rd ed.). Multi-Health Systems.

Conners, C. K. (2014a). *Conners Continuous Auditory Test of Attention*. Multi-Health Systems.

Conners, C. K. (2014b). *Conners Continuous Performance Test* (3rd ed.). Multi-Health Systems.

Conners, C. K. (2015). *Conners Kiddie Continuous Performance Test* (2nd ed.). Multi-Health Systems.

Copeland, W. E., Angold, A., Costello, E. J., & Egger, H. (2013). Prevalence, comorbidity, and correlates of *DSM-5* proposed disruptive mood dysregulation disorder. *The American Journal of Psychiatry, 170*(2), 173–179. https://doi.org/10.1176/appi.ajp.2012.12010132

Duffy, A., Carlson, G., Dubicka, B., & Hillegers, M. H. J. (2020). Pre-pubertal bipolar disorder: Origins and current status of the controversy. *International Journal of Bipolar Disorders, 8*(1), Article 18. https://doi.org/10.1186/s40345-020-00185-2

Exner, J. E. (2003). *The Rorschach: A comprehensive system: Vol. 1. Basic foundations and principles of interpretation* (4th ed.). Wiley.

Gioia, G. A., Isquith, P. K., Guy, S. C., & Kenworthy, L. (2015). *Brief Rating Inventory of Executive Function* (2nd ed.). Psychological Assessment Resources.

Goldstein, B. I., Birmaher, B., Carlson, G. A., DelBello, M. P., Findling, R. L., Fristad, M., Kowatch, R. A., Miklowitz, D. J., Nery, F. G., Perez-Algorta, G., Van Meter, A., Zeni, C. P., Correll, C. U., Kim, H. W., Wozniak, J., Chang, K. D., Hillegers, M., & Youngstrom, E. A. (2017). The International Society for Bipolar Disorders Task Force report on pediatric bipolar disorder: Knowledge to date and directions for future research. *Bipolar Disorders, 19*(7), 524–543. https://doi.org/10.1111/bdi.12556

Gracious, B. L., Youngstrom, E. A., Findling, R. L., & Calabrese, J. R. (2002). Discriminative validity of a parent version of the Young Mania Rating Scale. *Journal of the American Academy of Child & Adolescent Psychiatry, 41*(11), 1350–1359. https://doi.org/10.1097/00004583-200211000-00017

Hopwood, C. J., & Bornstein, R. F. (Eds.). (2014). *Multimethod clinical assessment*. Guilford Press.

Jensen, P. S., Hinshaw, S. P., Swanson, J. M., Greenhill, L. L., Conners, C. K., Arnold, L. E., Abikoff, H. B., Elliott, G., Hechtman, L., Hoza, B., March, J. S., Newcorn, J. H., Severe, J. B., Vitiello, B., Wells, K., & Wigal, T. (2001). Findings from the NIMH Multimodal Treatment Study of ADHD (MTA): Implications and applications for primary care providers. *Journal of Developmental and Behavioral Pediatrics, 22*(1), 60–73. https://doi.org/10.1097/00004703-200102000-00008

Joseph, M. F., Youngstrom, E. A., & Soares, J. C. (2009). Antidepressant-coincident mania in children and adolescents treated with selective serotonin reuptake inhibitors. *Future Neurology, 4*(1), 87–102. https://doi.org/10.2217/14796708.4.1.87

Kahneman, D., & Tversky, A. (1972). Subjective probability: A judgment of representativeness. *Cognitive Psychology, 3*(3), 430–454. https://doi.org/10.1016/0010-0285(72)90016-3

Kaufman, J., Birmaher, B., Axelson, D., Perepletchikova, F., Brent, D., & Ryan, N. (2016). *K-SADS-PL DSM-5*. Western Psychiatric Institute & Clinic.

Klayman, J. (1995). Varieties of confirmation bias. *Psychology of Learning and Motivation, 32*, 385–418. https://doi.org/10.1016/S0079-7421(08)60315-1

Kleiger, J. H. (1999). *Disordered thinking and the Rorschach: Theory, research, and differential diagnosis*. The Analytic Press.

Kleiger, J. H. (2017). *Rorschach assessment of psychotic phenomena: Clinical, conceptual, and empirical developments*. Routledge. https://doi.org/10.4324/9781315271385

Kleiger, J. H., & Khadivi, A. (2015). *Assessing psychosis: A clinician's guide*. Routledge. https://doi.org/10.4324/9781315882086

Kowatch, R. A., Fristad, M., Birmaher, B., Wagner, K. D., Findling, R. L., Hellander, M., & the Child Psychiatric Workgroup on Bipolar Disorder. (2005). Treatment guidelines for children and adolescents with bipolar disorder. *Journal of the American Academy of Child & Adolescent Psychiatry, 44*(3), 213–235. https://doi.org/10.1097/00004583-200503000-00006

Leichtman, M. (1995). *The Rorschach: A developmental perspective*. The Analytic Press.

Marangoni, C., De Chiara, L., & Faedda, G. L. (2015). Bipolar disorder and ADHD: Comorbidity and diagnostic distinctions. *Current Psychiatry Reports, 17*(8), Article 604. https://doi.org/10.1007/s11920-015-0604-y

Marchand, W. R., Clark, S. C., Wirth, L., & Simon, C. (2005). Validity of the Parent Young Mania Rating Scale in a community mental health setting. *Psychiatry, 2*(3), 31–35.

Marcus, E. R. (2017). *Psychosis and near psychosis: Ego function, symbol structure, treatment* (3rd ed.). Routledge. https://doi.org/10.4324/9781315675855

McCarney, S. B., & House, S. N. (2019). *Attention Deficit Disorder Evaluation Scale* (5th ed.). Hawthorne Educational Services.

McClellan, J., Kowatch, R., Findling, R. L., & the Work Group on Quality Issues. (2007). Practice parameter for the assessment and treatment of children and adolescents with bipolar disorder. *Journal of the American Academy of Child & Adolescent Psychiatry, 46*(1), 107–125. https://doi.org/10.1097/01.chi.0000242240.69678.c4

McGuffin, P., Rijsdijk, F., Andrew, M., Sham, P., Katz, R., & Cardno, A. (2003). The heritability of bipolar affective disorder and the genetic relationship to unipolar depression. *Archives of General Psychiatry, 60*(5), 497–502. https://doi.org/10.1001/archpsyc.60.5.497

Meyer, G. J., Erdberg, P., & Shaffer, T. W. (2007). Toward international normative reference data for the comprehensive system. *Journal of Personality Assessment, 89*(Suppl. 1), S201–S216. https://doi.org/10.1080/00223890701629342

Meyer, G. J., Viglione, D. J., Mihura, J. L., Erard, R. E., & Erdberg, P. (2011). *Rorschach Performance Assessment System: Administration, coding, interpretation, and technical manual.* Rorschach Performance Assessment System.

Miller, C. (n.d.). *Is it ADHD or bipolar disorder?* https://childmind.org/article/is-it-adhd-or-bipolar-disorder/

Millon, T., Tringone, R., Grossman, S., & Millon, C. (2020). *Millon Adolescent Clinical Inventory–II (MACI-II).* Pearson.

Morey, L. C. (2007). *Personality Assessment Inventory–Adolescent (PAI-A).* Psychological Assessment Resources.

Passarotti, A. M., Trivedi, N., Dominguez-Colman, L., Patel, M., & Langenecker, S. A. (2016). Differences in real world executive function between children with pediatric bipolar disorder and children with ADHD. *Journal of the Canadian Academy of Child and Adolescent Psychiatry, 25*(3), 185–195.

Pavuluri, M. N., Henry, D. B., Devineni, B., Carbray, J. A., & Birmaher, B. (2006). Child mania rating scale: Development, reliability, and validity. *Journal of the American Academy of Child & Adolescent Psychiatry, 45*(5), 550–560. https://doi.org/10.1097/01.chi.0000205700.40700.50

Reynolds, C. R., & Kamphaus, R. W. (2015). *Behavior Assessment System for Children* (3rd ed.). Pearson.

Sandstrom, A., Perroud, N., Alda, M., Uher, R., & Pavlova, B. (2021). Prevalence of attention-deficit/hyperactivity disorder in people with mood disorders: A systematic review and meta-analysis. *Acta Psychiatrica Scandinavica, 143*(5), 380–391. https://doi.org/10.1111/acps.13283

Singh, T., & Rajput, M. (2006). Misdiagnosis of bipolar disorder. *Psychiatry, 3*(10), 57–63.

Van Meter, A. R., & Youngstrom, E. A. (2012). Cyclothymic disorder in youth: Why is it overlooked, what do we know and where is the field headed? *Neuropsychiatry, 2*(6), 509–519. https://doi.org/10.2217/npy.12.64

Wagner, K. D., Hirschfeld, R. M., Emslie, G. J., Findling, R. L., Gracious, B. L., & Reed, M. L. (2006). Validation of the Mood Disorder Questionnaire for bipolar disorders in adolescents. *The Journal of Clinical Psychiatry, 67*(5), 827–830. https://doi.org/10.4088/JCP.v67n0518

Weiner, I. B. (2000). Making Rorschach interpretation as good as it can be. *Journal of Personality Assessment, 74*(2), 164–174. https://doi.org/10.1207/S15327752JPA7402_2

Yalof, J., & Bram, A. D. (Eds.). (2021). *Psychoanalytic assessment applications for different settings.* Routledge.

Youngstrom, E. A., Choukas-Bradley, S., Calhoun, C. D., & Jensen-Doss, A. (2015). Clinical guide to the evidence-based assessment approach to diagnosis and treatment.

Cognitive and Behavioral Practice, 22(1), 20–35. https://doi.org/10.1016/j.cbpra. 2013.12.005

Youngstrom, E. A., Genzlinger, J. E., Egerton, G. A., & Van Meter, A. R. (2015). Multivariate meta-analysis of the discriminative validity of caregiver, youth, and teacher rating scales for pediatric bipolar disorder: Mother knows best about mania. *Archives of Scientific Psychology, 3*(1), 112–137. https://doi.org/10.1037/arc0000024

Youngstrom, E. A., Jenkins, M. M., Jensen-Doss, A., & Youngstrom, J. K. (2012). Evidence-based assessment strategies for pediatric bipolar disorder. *The Israel Journal of Psychiatry and Related Sciences, 49*(1), 15–27.

Zurhellen, W., Lessin, H. R., Chan, E., Allan, C. C., Wolraich, M., Sprecher, E., & Evans, S. W. (2019). *Caring for children with ADHD: A practical resource toolkit for clinicians* (3rd ed.). American Academy of Pediatrics.

13

Assessment of Bipolar Spectrum and Medical Conditions

Khai Tran and Panagiota Korenis

Bipolar spectrum disorders have many similarities in clinical presentation with medical conditions. Once a person is suspected to be experiencing any of the bipolar spectrum disorders, it is important to clearly distinguish whether it is primary or secondary mania. Primary mania is brought on due to decompensation of either bipolar disorder or schizoaffective disorder; secondary mania is induced by organic causes such as drugs or other medical conditions. In this chapter, we focus on a better understanding of some of the causes of medical conditions that may present similar to bipolar spectrum disorders.

As a clinician, it is critical to understand the etiology of disease—in particular, if there is a primary organic cause. This is relevant especially if the person experiencing the symptoms is not responding well to classical treatments of bipolar spectrum disorders and might respond better to a different clinical approach or referral to a different medical specialist to manage the underlying medical condition. In a number of these instances, there can be an amelioration of the bipolar spectrum-like symptoms if the underlying medical condition is managed or in control. In other instances, however, the inability to manage the patient's symptoms may further shed light on the complicated nature of the medical condition and help the clinician further educate the patient and their family about potential residual symptoms that may exist.

https://doi.org/10.1037/0000356-014
Psychological Assessment of Bipolar Spectrum Disorders, J. H. Kleiger and I. B. Weiner (Editors)

THE ROLE OF THE NEUROTRANSMITTER

When discussing the abnormal affect, it is imperative to understand the significant regulatory components of neurophysiological aspects, the neurotransmitters. Neurotransmitters are essential signaling chemical molecules that control all neural activities in the body. For mood regulation, there are several important neurotransmitters that are involved in complex networks and pathways to maintain neural homeostasis (see Exhibit 13.1). Any aberrant fluctuation in these levels will result in changes in mood and mental status.

Dopamine

One of the most important regulatory neurotransmitters in the neural network. There are four critical neural pathways that involve dopamine:

- *Mesocortical*: Originating from the ventral tegmental area (VTA) and projected to the cortex, this pathway is responsible for cognition, memory and learning, and motivation.

- *Mesolimbic*: Originating from the VTA and projected into the limbic system, this pathway regulates emotion, external perception of stimuli, and reward.

- *Nigrostriatal*: Originating from the VTA, continuing to the substantia nigra, and ultimately ending at the dorsal striatum, this is the motor control center of the brain.

- *Tuberoinfundibular*: Unlike the other pathways, this one originates at the arcuate nucleus and the paraventricular nucleus of the hypothalamus, and projects to the pituitary gland where it controls sensory processing and hormonal regulation, most significantly the hormone prolactin.

When the level of dopamine increases, the excess dopamine results in the overstimulation as well as upregulation of dopaminergic receptors. These pathways explain manic symptoms observed in patients. It is also important to note

---

EXHIBIT 13.1

Neurotransmitters and the Mood-Regulating Functions

Neurotransmitter	Essential function in mood regulation
Adrenaline	Fight or flight
Noradrenaline	Concentration
Dopamine	Pleasure
Serotonin	Mood regulation
GABA	Calming
Acetylcholine	Learning
Glutamate	Memory
Endorphins	Euphoria

Note. GABA = gamma-aminobutyric acid.

that dopamine is responsible for the reward system in the brain. The reward system is the modulator for pleasure, learning, and behavioral conditioning. When treating manic symptoms, one of the most important aspects to consider is high impulsivity. The current proposed neuropsychological model for under-standing rewards and behaviors is the concept of motivational salience. In this model, there are two factors that drive behaviors. The "want" or "seeking" factor is responsible for the motivation and behaviors to obtain a reward, whereas the "like" factor leads to consumption-type behaviors.

Gamma-Aminobutyric Acid

Gamma-aminobutyric acid (GABA) is an inhibitory neuromodulator that helps to coordinate cortical functions. A decreasing level of GABA relative to dopamine results in the loss of inhibition of dopamine, leading to the manifestation of manic symptoms. Takato et al. (2020) explored the relation-ship between hyperactive behaviors and GABA in mice: The GABAergic neurons in the ventral midbrain and pons were ablated, and these mice began to display manic behaviors such as hyperactivity, loss of rebound sleep, reduced level of anxiety responses, and increased risk-taking behaviors despite consequences.

Serotonin

This is a neurotransmitter that is associated with biological functioning such as sleep, wakefulness, eating, sexual behavior, impulsivity, learning, and memory; it also helps to regulate anxiety, sense of happiness, and mood. Serotonin is made and distributed from the Raphe nucleus in the brain and spread through-out the central nervous system. While there is extensive research regarding the relationship between low levels of serotonin and depression (Shiah & Yatham, 2000), there is very little research focused on its role in inducing manic symptoms. It is known that in patients with bipolar depression, giving anti-depressants as monotherapy increases the risk of triggering a manic episode, suggesting that elevated levels of serotonin are related to inducing a manic state. Similarly, in patients with serotonin syndrome, some of the symptoms are similar to that of a manic state. However, research shows that low levels of serotonin also contribute to the induction of a manic episode (Lakshmi et al., 2010). It has been shown that in patients with bipolar disorders undergoing a manic episode at the time of study, there was a reduction in 5HT2 receptor activities. In another study involving mice (Maddaloni et al., 2018) there was a correlation between low levels of serotonin and hippocampal neuroplasticity resulting in manic-like behaviors that were reversible by increased stress levels.

Norepinephrine

Norepinephrine in the brain is synthesized in the locus ceruleus, with global projections to all parts of the brain as well as to the adrenal gland via the vagal

FIGURE 13.1. Relationship Between Neurotransmitters in Mood Regulation

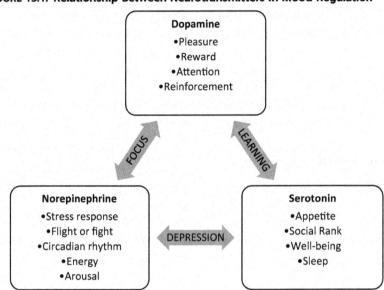

nerve pathway. Increased levels of norepinephrine will trigger the sympathetic nervous system, resulting in the "fight or flight" response. It is also responsible for the hyperactivity, increased spontaneity, and impulsive behaviors that can be seen in a manic episode (see Figure 13.1).

Other Hormones

Other hormones, such as cortisol, thyroid, and parathyroid hormones, seen in specific medical conditions, could result in manic symptoms. In Cushing's syndrome, hypercortisolism can cause manic behaviors. Hyperthyroidism affects the function of serotonin and beta-adrenergic receptors, leading to increased levels of dopamine. Finally, there are studies that showed the efficacy of using calcium-channel blockers in the treatment of bipolar disorders (Cipriani et al., 2016).

MEDICAL, PHYSICAL, AND OTHER CAUSES OF MANIC EPISODES

Bipolar spectrum disorders can be triggered secondarily, as a consequence of a variety of medical conditions. Following are some of the more common conditions that can trigger bipolar disorder spectrum symptoms.

Substance-Induced Mania

These episodes are brought on either by exposure to a substance or soon after the withdrawal of the offending agents. One of the highest risk factors for increased susceptibility is a previous history of psychiatric illnesses. Most substances that can induce mania are prescription medications and illicit substances. Exhibit 13.2 shows medications that may induce mania.

EXHIBIT 13.2

Mania-Inducing Medications

Antidepressants

- Strongest: SSRIs, venlafaxine (SNRI).
- Monotherapy may precipitate mixed/manic episode in patients with bipolar disorder.
- Treatment-emergent mania or hypomania in patients with unipolar major depressive disorder (MDD) reported.
- Mechanism: Non-dose related. Unclear to what extent mood switches represent an uncovering of unrecognized bipolar disorder or a more direct pharmacologic effect, independent of diagnosis.
- Risk factors: Family history of bipolar, depressive episode with psychotic symptoms, young age at depression diagnosis, treatment-resistant depression.

Bromocriptine and cabergoline

- D2 receptor agonist that is used for lactation suppression.
- Associated with increased risk of postpartum psychosis—usually occurs within the first 2 weeks postpartum. Initial symptoms include severe insomnia not related to the care of the newborn.

Levodopa

- Dopamine agonist.
- Proposed mechanism through hypersensitivity of limbic dopamine receptors.
- Psychiatric symptoms are usually reversible with dose reduction.
- Risk factors: Higher doses, older adults with history of dementia.

Glucocorticoids

- Increased risk of manic symptoms in older adults, especially in case of higher dosage or long treatment duration.

Anabolic-adrenergic steroids

- Activate androgen receptors.
- Women are at higher risk.

Metoclopramide

- Dopamine antagonist that is used as an antiemetic for gastroparesis.
- A few case reports showed patients became manic while on medication and, when rechallenged with medication, became manic again. Can be treated with amitriptyline during manic episode.
- Mechanism is likely through mesolimbic dopamine receptor supersensitivity.

Chloroquine and hydroxychloroquine

- Antimalarial drugs.
- Manic episode can develop within a few hours up to 11 weeks after medication initiation; symptoms resolve after 1 week of medication cessation.

Levetiracetam

- Antiepileptic medication.
- Only a few case reports on manic episodes, mostly psychotic symptoms.

(continues)

EXHIBIT 13.2

Mania-Inducing Medications (*Continued*)

Baclofen

- GABA-B agonist.
- >50% of reported cases have pre-existing bipolar diagnosis.
- Risk of mania increased significantly when combined with ropeginterferon alfa-2b.

Alprazolam, triazolam

- Benzodiazepines, enhancers at GABA-A receptor.
- Higher risk in patients with depression.

Other medications to consider

1. Procarbazine: MAO inhibitor
2. Cyclobenazprine: Amitryptyline analog
3. Clonidine:
   - Noradrenergic agonist used in hypertension, ADHD, and to treat vasomotor symptoms in menopausal women
   - Withdrawal can potentiate symptoms in manic patient
4. Isoniazid:
   - Antituberculosis medication, should be used together with pyridoxine
   - Monotherapy increases risk of psychosis, mania, and obsessive–compulsive neurosis
   - Proposed mechanism is due to accumulation of S-adenosylmethionine and pyridoxine deficiency
5. Cyproheptadine: H1 receptor antagonist
6. Disulfram: Aldehyde dehydrogenase inhibitor, increased risk at high doses
7. Felbamate: Anticonvulsant
8. L-glutamate: Over-the-counter supplement
9. Procainamide: Class Ia antiarrhythmic agent
10. Propafenone: Class Ic antiarrhythmic agent
11. Zidovudine: Antiretroviral medication
12. Cimetidine: H2 receptor antagonist, increased risk in depressed patients
13. Yohimbine: Alpha 2 adrenergic antagonist
14. Procyclidine: Anticholinergic agents
15. Pseudoephedrine: Alpha and beta agonist, uses as decongestant
16. Captopril: ACE inhibitor
17. Phencyclidine (PCP, angel dust):
    - Noncompetitive antagonist of NMDA receptors resulting in excess release of glycine, glutamate, and aspartate
    - Inhibits reuptake of dopamine, norepinephrine, and serotonin
18. Cocaine: Inhibits the dopamine transporters
19. Amphetamine: Increases release of dopamine, norepinephrine, and serotonin
20. Other medications that can induce mania upon withdrawal: diltiazem, isocarboxazid, atenolol, and propranolol.

Note. SSRI = selective serotonin reuptake inhibitor; SNRI = serotonin–norepinephrine reuptake inhibitor; GABA = gamma-aminobutyric acid; MAO = monoamine oxidase; ADHD = attention-deficit/hyperactivity disorder; PCP = phenylcyclohexyl piperidine.

Specific Medical Conditions

Stroke

Stroke results in a reduction of blood flow, leading to brain damage due to oxygen and nutrient deprivation. Poststroke mania is commonly seen in older male patients with high cardiovascular risks, such as obesity, a sedentary lifestyle, smoking, and hypercholesterolemia. The affected areas in patients with poststroke mania are commonly noted to be in the orbitofrontal and basotemporal cortices of the right hemisphere. Functional magnetic resonance imaging (fMRI) in manic patients shows an increased blood flow to the orbitofrontal cortex (see Figure 13.2). The timeline of developing mania can range between immediately after vascular insult or up to 2 years after the onset of the stroke.

Systemic Lupus Erythematosus

Systemic lupus erythematosus (SLE) is an autoimmune disease that affects multiple systems in the body. The most commonly affected systems are the skin, joints, kidneys, heart, and brain. Approximately 15% to 80% of SLE patients will develop either mania or psychosis during their lifetime. The proposed model is a combination of immune dysfunction, dopamine imbalance, and vascular inflammation resulting in neuronal damage. Patients with SLE are often taking immunosuppressants and/or corticosteroids as their primary treatment, which also increases the risk of developing mania, not only from the disease itself but also from steroid use.

Frontotemporal Dementia

This is the second most common type of dementia. In frontotemporal dementia, there is significant atrophy of the frontal and temporal lobes. Patients with prominent right-sided atrophy will have a higher risk of developing manic

FIGURE 13.2. MRI of a Poststroke Patient With Manic Symptoms Showing Affected Right Frontal Area

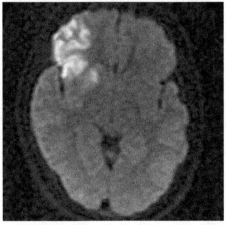

symptoms (see Figure 13.3). In patients with frontotemporal dementia, the prognosis is poor; once diagnosed, the patient has a life expectancy of between 2 and 10 years. There is no treatment or way to slow down the progression of the illness.

Kleine–Levin Syndrome

Kleine–Levin syndrome is a rare and complex neurological condition in which patients experience cyclical episodes of hypersomnia and hypersexuality. Episodes may last from days to months. During the episodes, patients can exhibit manic behaviors. Currently, there are no known causes for this illness; the onset often follows a viral infection. The currently proposed mechanism for this condition is hypoperfusion to the thalamic and frontotemporal areas, there are also suggestions of abnormal metabolism of serotonin and dopamine in the brain.

Anti-NMDA Receptor Encephalitis

This autoimmune condition is mediated by antibodies targeting *N*-methyl-D-aspartate receptors in the brain. Cross-reactivity is often followed by a viral illness with a prodromal phase of flu-like symptoms. Neurological symptom onset often happens weeks to months later.

COVID-19-Induced Mania

Severe acute respiratory syndrome coronavirus-2 is a respiratory virus that led to a global pandemic killing millions of individuals. People who suffered from

FIGURE 13.3. MRI of a Patient With Frontotemporal Dementia Showing Atrophied Areas

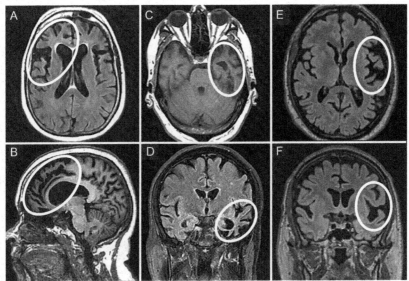

COVID-19 pneumonia experienced severe and debilitating multisystemic symptoms, with lasting sequelae. Currently, there are few theories as to how COVID infections might result in neuropsychiatric symptoms. Evans et al. (2021) reported that there are multiple case reports demonstrating psychotic and manic symptoms in patients with no psychiatric history who contracted the virus.

Infectious Illnesses

Neurological symptoms are brought on by chronic illnesses. The most common infectious causes of mania are HIV encephalitis, syphilis, Lyme disease, viral encephalitis, and cryptococcal meningitis.

Insomnia

There are a number of conditions that can lead to insomnia or the inability to sleep. Insomnia may present with an inability to initiate sleep or maintain a sleep state, with periods of wakefulness. People with insomnia may present with symptoms of affective dysregulation, irritability, pressured speech, distractibility, and poor focus. It is imperative to understand the etiology of the insomnia, as there are a number of medical conditions, including sleep apnea, irregular sleep habits, increased stress, neurological conditions, and medications that can trigger episodes of insomnia.

Direct Physical Causes

Direct physical trauma to the brain can lead to neuropsychiatric symptoms. While the brain is the best-protected organ in the body from everything from physical insults to microscopic dangers, it is still very vulnerable when there are injuries. Any injury to the head can result in concussive damage to the brain. These physical injuries are called traumatic brain injuries, and depending on the severity and location of the injuries, different symptoms can manifest.

Similarly, from within, the blood–brain barrier protects the brain from microscopic invaders that can pose a threat to the neural network, but not so much from the body's own cells. Brain tumors or metastatic spread from the body can lead to mass effect on the brain, leading to psychiatric symptoms. As mentioned previously, manic and similar mood symptoms are often manifested when the right hemispheric frontotemporal regions are affected. The following case reports demonstrate how trauma and tumors can lead to the development of manic symptoms in patients.

Primary Brain Tumor (Glioblastoma Multiforme)

The patient is a 76-year-old man who was admitted to the psychiatric unit with a euphoric mood, hypersexuality, excessive money spending, and grandiose

FIGURE 13.4. MRI Progression of a Patient With Glioblastoma

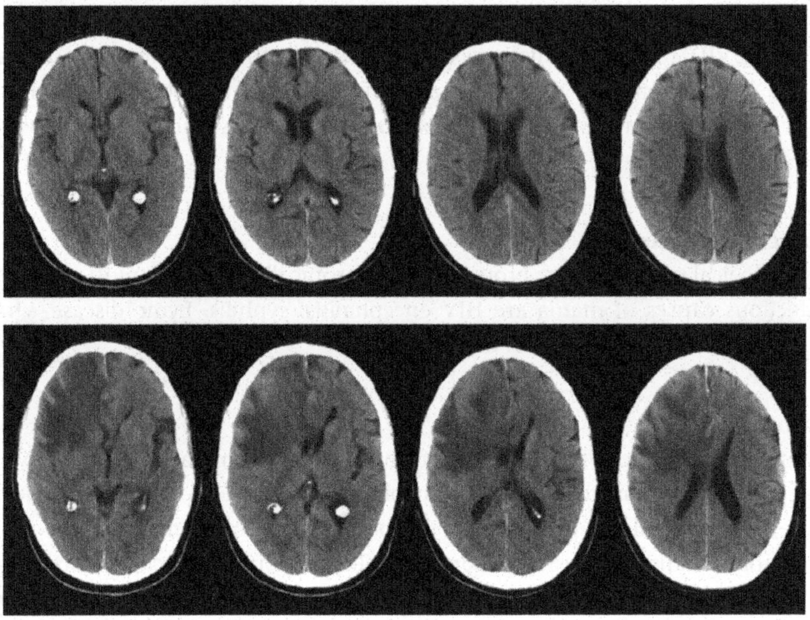

Note. The top figure is at presentation and the bottom figure is at 5 months following demonstrating a mass effect.

capacity for the past 2 months.[1] Physical, neurological, and psychiatric evaluations were normal; blood work and urinalysis only showed mild leukocytosis; brain computerized tomography scan (CT), electrocardiogram, and chest X-ray demonstrated no abnormality. The patient was started on valproic acid and risperidone, leading to full remission of his affective symptoms. After discharge, the patient started to show some cognitive decline. Five months after discharge, a follow-up CT showed a large right-sided frontal mass (see Figure 13.4).

Metastatic Tumor (Non-Small Cell Lung Carcinoma)
This 65-year-old man with metastatic Stage III non-small cell carcinoma was brought to the hospital after a sudden, acute change in mental status and manic-like symptoms. The patient was initially diagnosed with adenocarcinoma of the lung and began chemotherapy. After 2 years, the patient completed chemotherapy and stopped taking monoclonal antibody medication. Six months after the cessation of medication, he reported headaches to his oncologist; later on, he presented to the hospital. A head CT scan at the time showed a right-sided temporal brain metastatic lesion (see Figure 13.5).

Direct Traumatic Brain Injuries
A 60-year-old man with no previous psychiatric history presented to the emergency department accompanied by his wife for newly developed aggression and legal problems. He had been in a normal state of health until 5 months ago,

---

[1] Identities of the individuals in case examples have been disguised to protect privacy.

FIGURE 13.5. MRI Showing a Metastatic Mass in a Patient With a Non-Small Cell Carcinoma

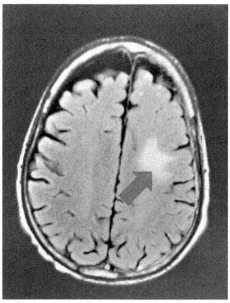

when he started developing syncopal episodes. During one of his episodes, he fell and hit his head, resulting in surgical staples for a scalp laceration. Head CT at the time did not show any acute brain injuries. The patient's spouse reported that shortly after his injury, the patient experienced a short period of depression and then developed behavioral and personality changes. The patient became irritable, euphoric in mood, and grandiose, sleeping only 2 to 3 hours a night. He also began watching pornography (which he never had an interest in before) and went on shopping sprees costing $10,000 to 20,000 a month. He also got arrested multiple times for aggravated assault. The patient was admitted to an inpatient unit and was resistant to treatment; when discharged, he was noncompliant with medication. The patient did not have any history of mood or familial history of mental illness, and these psychiatric symptoms emerged after his head injuries.

Depression

When assessing individuals for bipolar disorder, it is critical to ensure that both manic and depressed symptoms are considered. Failure to properly differentiate bipolar depression from unipolar depression can result in iatrogenically inducing a manic episode by prescribing an antidepressant. Therefore, it is important to screen for a history of manic symptoms in depressive patients (see Chapter 7 in this volume). In bipolar spectrum disorders, maintaining a euthymic state is a delicate balancing act between the levels of neurotransmitters. As described previously, neurotransmitter levels are the key to maintaining homeostasis. Therefore, with any fluctuating level that produces mania, its opposite level will lead to the development of depressive symptoms. It is easy to draw a correlation when comparing manic and depressive symptoms (see Table 13.1).

Like with manic presentation, when patients are presenting with depressive symptoms, it is important to differentiate if it is primary or secondary depression so that the appropriate treatment plan can be formulated. It is essential to rule out organic causes for secondary depression before considering primary psychiatric causes.

Medication/Substance-Induced Depressions

With substance-induced depressive symptoms, patients often present with prominent and persistent depressed mood and marked anhedonia. These can be through either taking or withdrawing from any of the specific substances listed in the following subsections.

Medications. Much like mania-induced medication, the following extensive list of medications is known to trigger depressive symptoms. The most likely include (a) anabolic steroids, (b) angiotensin converting enzyme inhibitors, (c) beta-blockers, (d) corticosteroids, (e) inteferon alpha, (f) isotretinoin, and (g) reserpine. Other medications that may induce depression include acyclovir, anticonvulsives, baclofen, benzodiazepines, bromocriptine, calcium-channel blockers, ciprofloxacin, clonidine, digitalis, disulfiram, estrogen, guanethidine, H2-receptor blockers, interleukin-2, levodopa, methyldopa, metoclopramide, metrizamide, metronidazole, nonsteroidal anti-inflamatory drugs most commonly seen with

TABLE 13.1. Correlating Neurotransmitters With Manic and Depressed Symptoms

Neurotransmitter	Elevated level	Depressed level
Dopamine	Mania, increased reward anticipation	Depression, loss of interest in activities (decreased reward pathway)
GABA	Highly inhibitory, depression, stupor, anhedonia	Mania, loss of inhibition, promotion of risk-taking behaviors
Serotonin	Decreased sleep, enhanced wakefulness, increased impulsivity, elevation of mood	Increased sleep, decreased appetite, lack of interest
Norepinephrine	Hyperactivity, increased spontaneity	Slowed body activity, stupor, psychomotor retardation
Cortisol	Irritability, heightened stress response	Increased stress, depressive symptoms
Thyroid	Anxiety, irritability, insomnia, impaired attention, overactivity	Anhedonia, lack of interest, decreased appetite, attention, and cognitive deficits
Parathyroid hormone	Increased anxiety, excitatory	Depressive symptoms

Note. GABA = gamma-aminobutyric acid.

EXHIBIT 13.3

Medical Conditions Triggering Depressive Symptoms

Neoplasm

- Pancreatic cancer
- Brain tumors
- Paraneoplastic syndromes
- Immune disorder: AIDS
- Systemic lupus erythematosus
- Infectious diseases: neurosyphilis

Infections

- AIDS
- COVID-19

Cardiac[a]

- Poststroke
- Post MI
- Coronary heart disease

Endocrine

- Hypothyroidism
- Cushing's disease
- Diabetes

Neurological diseases

- Multiple sclerosis
- Epilepsy
- TBI
- Parkinson's disease
- Huntington's disease
- Alzheimer's disease
- Stroke

Obstructive sleep apnea

Note. TBI = traumatic brain injury; AIDS = acquired immunodeficiency syndrome; COVID = coronavirus disease; MI = myocardial infarction.
[a] It is well-reported that patients who experience a cardiac event will develop depressive symptoms that are likely to persist for an extended period of time.

---

indomethacin, opioids, pergolide, sulfonamides, thiazide diuretics, topiramate, vinblastine, and vincristine.

Illicit Substances. The majority of illicit substances are classified as either stimulants or depressants. Depressive symptoms can be brought on through withdrawal of stimulants or intoxication with depressants. The most common stimulants include cocaine, phencyclidine, inhalants, and amphetamines. Depressants include alcohol and drugs from the sedative/hypnotic/anxiolytic class such as benzodiazepine, anticonvulsants, opioids, and heroin. Finally, the most common hallucinogens are D-lysergic acid diethylamide, psilocybin, mescaline, *NN*-trimethyltryptamine, ketamine, dextromethorphan (cough syrup), and salvia.

Medical Illness–Induced Depression. Exhibit 13.3 shows many of the medical conditions that directly trigger depressive symptoms as their pathophysiological consequences.

IMPORTANT LAB TESTS

When patients present with either manic or depressive symptoms, especially with a history of comorbid medical conditions, foundational and explorative laboratory tests are a useful tool to either rule out or determine the likelihood of causes (see Exhibit 13.4).

EXHIBIT 13.4

Essential Laboratory Tests

Test	Rule out
Complete blood count	Anemias, infections
Complete metabolic panel	Electrolyte abnormalities, SIADH, DI
Glucose	Diabetes, hypoglycemia
BUN, creatinine	Renal disease
TSH	Thyroid disease
Vitamin B12, folate	Vitamin deficiencies
Urine toxicology	Substance use
Brain MRI	Organic brain causes
Urinalysis	To rule out UTI, especially in elderly patients
Pregnancy test	Hormonal causes, also as contraindication result to start certain medications
EKG	Cardiac causes, arrhythmias or when planning to use certain medication
Polysomnography	Sleep apnea signs and symptoms
RPR/FTA	Neurosyphilis
CD4 counts, HIV (with patient's consent)	AIDS

Note. SIADH = syndromes of inappropriate antidiuretic hormones secretion; DI = diabetes insipidius; BUN = blood urea nitrogen; TSH = thyroid stimulating hormone; UTI = urinary tract infection; RPR = rapid plasma regain; FTA = fluorescent treponemal antibody absorption test; CD4 = cluster of differentiation 4.

CONCLUSION

When assessing patients with dysregulated mood symptoms, it is of the utmost importance to do a thorough medical screening and medication review. While it is important to address the psychiatric symptoms, providing appropriate medical care to address the secondary causes of mood disorders would be an important first step, especially in patients without a previous history of psychiatric illnesses.

REFERENCES

Cipriani, A., Saunders, K., Attenburrow, M. J., Stefaniak, J., Panchal, P., Stockton, S., Lane, T. A., Tunbridge, E. M., Geddes, J. R., & Harrison, P. J. (2016). A systematic review of calcium channel antagonists in bipolar disorder and some considerations for their future development. *Molecular Psychiatry, 21*(10), 1324–1332. https://doi.org/10.1038/mp.2016.86

Evans, S., Alkan, E., Bhangoo, J. K., Tenenbaum, H., & Ng-Knight, T. (2021). Effects of the COVID-19 lockdown on mental health, wellbeing, sleep, and alcohol use in a UK student sample. *Psychiatry Research, 298*, Article 113819. https://doi.org/10.1016/j.psychres.2021.113819

Lakshmi, N., Yatham, P., Liddle, J., Erez, J., Kauer-Sant'Anna, M., Lam, R. W., Imperial, M., Sossi, V., & Ruth, T. J. (2010). Brain serotonin-2 receptors in acute mania. *The British Journal of Psychiatry, 196*(1), 47–51. https://doi.org/10.1192/bjp.bp.108.057919

Maddaloni, G., Migliarini, S., Napolitano, F., Giorgi, A., Nazzi, S., Biasci, D., De Felice, A., Gritti, M., Cavaccini, A., Galbusera, A., Franceschi, S., Lessi, F., Ferla, M. L., Aretini, P., Mazzanti, C. M., Tonini, R., Gozzi, A., Usiello, A., & Pasqualetti, M. (2018). Serotonin depletion causes valproate-responsive manic-like condition and increased hippo-campal neuroplasticity that are reversed by stress. *Scientific Reports, 8*(1), Article 11847. https://doi.org/10.1038/s41598-018-30291-2

Shiah, I. S., & Yatham, L. N. (2000). Serotonin in mania and in the mechanism of action of mood stabilizers: A review of clinical studies. *Bipolar Disorders, 2*(2), 77–92. https://doi.org/10.1034/j.1399-5618.2000.020201.x

Takato, H., Yohko, T., Yoan, C., Mizuno, S., Sugiyama, F., Takahashi, S., Funato, H., Yanagisawa, M., Lazarus, M., & Oishi, Y. (2020). Ablation of ventral midbrain/pons GABA neurons induces mania-like behaviors with altered sleep homeostasis and dopamine D2R-mediated sleep reduction. *iScience, 23*(6), Article 101240. https://doi.org/10.1016/j.isci.2020.101240

14

Assessment of Bipolar Spectrum and Personality Disorders

Robert F. Bornstein

ipolar spectrum disorders (BSDs) are among the most common forms of serious mental illness, with an overall lifetime prevalence rate of just over 2% worldwide (Merikangas et al., 2011). The most well-known and widely studied BSDs are bipolar I disorder, bipolar II disorder, and cyclothymic disorder. Beyond these major categories, the *Diagnostic and Statistical Manual of Mental Disorders* (5th ed., text rev.; *DSM-5-TR*; American Psychiatric Association, 2022) also includes several less common variants of BSD: substance/medication-induced bipolar and related disorder, bipolar and related disorder due to another medical condition, other specified bipolar and related disorder, unspecified bipolar and related disorder, and unspecified mood disorder. Research confirms that BSDs have significant negative impacts on the individual, and substantial societal costs as well. Individuals diagnosed with BSDs show elevated risk for an array of other psychological difficulties, including anxiety and substance use disorders (Merikangas et al., 2011). BSDs are also associated with an increased risk of suicide, significant medical and psychological treatment costs, and substantial financial costs due to absenteeism and diminished productivity in work (Tondo et al., 2016).

Pharmacological interventions are the treatments of choice for bipolar I disorder and bipolar II disorder, with mood stabilizers considered first-line medications for both syndromes (Hede et al., 2019). For both disorders, medications are often supplemented with cognitive-behavioral interventions to maximize efficacy and treatment compliance. Cyclothymic disorder is sometimes

https://doi.org/10.1037/0000356-015
Psychological Assessment of Bipolar Spectrum Disorders, J. H. Kleiger and I. B. Weiner (Editors)

treated with mood stabilizers as well, especially in more severe cases. In addition, cognitive-behavioral therapies and psychoeducational interventions have demonstrated good efficacy in helping manage cyclothymic symptoms (Van Meter et al., 2012). Research suggests that the presence of comorbid psychological disorders—including personality disorders (PDs)—diminishes treatment effectiveness for all three of the major BSD categories and may require some modification in treatment strategy (Frías et al., 2016). As a result, accurate diagnosis and comorbidity assessment are crucial to maximizing BSD treatment effectiveness.

This chapter examines the association between personality pathology and BSDs, focusing on links between PDs and bipolar I disorder, bipolar II disorder, and cyclothymic disorder. The chapter begins with an overview of measures and methods used to diagnose BSDs and PDs, followed by a discussion of BSD–PD comorbidity and symptom overlap. Key distinguishing features of BSDs and PDs are then reviewed, followed by a discussion of psychological assessment tools that facilitate differential diagnosis and help clinicians disentangle the complex relationship between BSDs and PDs.[1]

DIAGNOSING BSDs AND PERSONALITY DISORDERS: TRADITIONAL APPROACHES AND RECENT INNOVATIONS

Accurate diagnosis is a crucial first step in examining BSD–PD comorbidity and symptom overlap, and in elucidating the psychological and behavioral factors that distinguish these two syndromes. In the following sections, widely used methods for diagnosing and assessing BSDs and PDs are described.

Bipolar Spectrum Disorders: Diagnosis and Assessment

The most widely used broadband diagnostic interview used to assess BSDs in clinical settings has been the Structured Clinical Interview for *DSM* Disorders (SCID), which is updated periodically as new editions of the *DSM* appear; the current version is the SCID-5-CV (First, Williams, Karg, & Spitzer, 2016; see also Chapter 7 in this volume). Cerimele et al. (2019) provided a comprehensive review and meta-analysis of the validity and clinical utility of questionnaire and interview measures of BSDs that indicated that the best-validated BSD-specific interview is the Bipolar Inventory of Symptoms Scale (Peluso et al., 2007); patient self-report measures with the greatest clinical utility include the Altman

---

[1] Given the limited evidence bearing on the links between BSDs and traits specified in the alternative model of personality disorders (AMPD; American Psychiatric Association, 2013), and the *International Classifications of Diseases* (11th ed.; *ICD-11*) trait model (World Health Organization, 2019), this chapter focuses on BSD–PD overlap using *DSM-5-TR* PD categories (American Psychiatric Association, 2022). In this context, it is worth noting that borderline PD, the PD diagnosis most strongly comorbid with BSDs, is included as a categorical qualifier in the *ICD-11* trait framework.

Self-Rating Mania Scale (Altman et al., 1997) and the Internal State Scale (Bauer et al., 1991).

Beyond questionnaires and interviews, archival and life history data (e.g., school records, legal documents) are often used as supplementary evidence to help confirm BSD diagnoses (Fowler et al., 2019). Most recently, ambulatory assessment techniques—in particular, Ecological Momentary Assessment (EMA)—have been used to document temporal variations in BSD symptoms that allow clinicians and researchers to (a) gain confidence in conclusions derived from questionnaire and interview BSD measures and (b) aid in determining the nature of a patient's symptoms (e.g., the presence of rapid cycling or seasonal patterns; see Depp et al., 2016).

Personality Disorder Diagnosis and Assessment

Like BSDs, PDs have historically been assessed using questionnaires and interviews, with most PD screening questionnaires designed to be overinclusive and to yield some number of false positive diagnoses. Structured diagnostic interviews are then used to confirm or rule out potential PD diagnoses identified via self-report. Loranger et al.'s (1994) International Personality Disorder Examination screening questionnaire is one of the most widely used self-report PD screening tools, and the gold standard diagnostic interview for *DSM-5-TR* PDs is the SCID-5-PD (First, Williams, Benjamin, & Spitzer, 2016). A number of PD-specific self-report measures are also available, including Tyrer et al.'s (2004) Dependent Personality Questionnaire and Pincus et al.'s (2009) Pathological Narcissism Inventory.

Performance-based test data—particularly those derived from the Rorschach Inkblot Method (RIM)—are frequently used to assess the underlying dynamics associated with different PDs (Bornstein, 2015; Huprich, 2006; see also Chapter 8 in this volume). In addition to providing evidence that enables clinicians and researchers to support a potential PD diagnosis, performance-based test data may also illuminate underlying PD dynamics when these data diverge from findings obtained via questionnaires or interviews. For example, Bornstein (1998) found that college students who qualified for a dependent PD diagnosis obtained elevated scores on both questionnaire and RIM indices of interpersonal dependency, whereas college students who were diagnosed with histrionic PD scored high on RIM-assessed dependency, but low on self-reported dependency. Similar test score divergences have been obtained for other PDs as well (see Bornstein, 2015).

THE COMPLEX RELATIONSHIP BETWEEN BSDs AND PERSONALITY DISORDERS

Three issues are relevant to understanding the BSD–PD relationship: symptom overlap, comorbidity, and differential diagnosis. *Symptom overlap* refers to the degree to which two disorders are characterized by identical or very similar symptoms. For example, dysthymia and major depressive disorder are both characterized by anhedonia and anergia; borderline PD (BPD) and dissociative disorder are both characterized by periods of depersonalization and derealization (i.e., episodes wherein the individual feels as though they are witnessing events as an observer rather than as an active participant, and may also feel disconnected from their surroundings).

Comorbidity refers to the co-occurrence of separate disorders—a situation wherein a patient qualifies for two (or more) diagnoses at the same time. Although high levels of symptom overlap tend to be associated with an increased likelihood of diagnostic comorbidity, it is also possible for two disorders to show significant symptom overlap even when they are not comorbid (e.g., BPD and dissociative disorder show substantial symptom overlap but modest comorbidity). Whereas information regarding symptom overlap is particularly useful in contextualizing diagnosis, information regarding comorbidity is most helpful in determining prognosis, and in treatment planning.

Differential diagnosis refers to the process whereby clinicians attempt to distinguish two or more syndromes that are characterized by similar symptoms. To the extent that two disorders show substantial symptom overlap, differential diagnosis becomes increasingly challenging. Although accurate differential diagnosis can sometimes be made solely on the basis of data derived from diagnostic interviews, in many cases accurate differential diagnosis requires the clinician to look beyond diagnostic criteria and focus on underlying dynamics and expressed behaviors that distinguish ostensibly similar disorders.

Comorbidity and Symptom Overlap: *DSM-5-TR* Guidelines and Empirical Evidence

According to *DSM-5-TR* (American Psychiatric Association, 2022), the only form of personality pathology that shows significant comorbidity with BSDs is BPD. The inclusion of this guideline is not surprising, insofar as BPD is characterized by several symptoms that are also exhibited by individuals with BSDs. These shared symptoms include (a) unstable interpersonal relationships; (b) unstable self-image or sense of self; (c) impulsivity that is potentially self-damaging; (d) suicidal behavior, gestures, or threats; (e) affective instability; and (f) inappropriate, intense anger or difficulty controlling anger.

Two other PDs that would appear to overlap with BSDs based on extant diagnostic criteria are not included in the list of comorbid diagnoses in *DSM-5-TR*, but they are nonetheless worth noting in this context. The first of these is antisocial PD, wherein common symptoms include (a) failure to conform to social norms leading to legal difficulties, (b) impulsivity or failure to plan ahead, and (c) irritability and aggressiveness. Narcissistic PD is also omitted from the list of *DSM-5-TR* BSD comorbid diagnoses, but it is characterized by several symptoms that are also present in BSDs, including (a) a grandiose sense of self; (b) fantasies of unlimited success and power; (c) belief that one is "special" or unique; and (d) arrogant, haughty behaviors or attitudes.

Empirical evidence strongly supports the *DSM-5-TR* assertion regarding BSD–BPD comorbidity. For example, Fornaro et al.'s (2016) meta-analysis of 42 published studies found that the prevalence of BPD among 5,273 individuals diagnosed with bipolar disorder was 21.6%. Consistent with these results, Frías et al.'s (2016) meta-analysis of 28 published investigations reported an overall prevalence rate of BPD in individuals with BSD of just over 20%. Whereas Fornaro et al. and Frias et al. focused exclusively on the comorbidity of BSDs with BPD, Bezerra-Filho et al.'s (2015) meta-analysis examined all 10 *DSM-5* (American Psychiatric Association, 2013) PDs, finding the highest comorbidity rate for BPD (10.1%), followed by histrionic PD (7.7%). BSD comorbidities for narcissistic and antisocial PDs were 4.5% and 0.79%, respectively.

Comorbidity findings aside, evidence also suggests substantial symptom overlap between BSDs and BPD. When Goutaudier et al. (2014) assessed cyclothymic symptoms and symptoms of BPD in a mixed-sex sample of 312 adolescents, they found a large positive correlation ($r = .76$) between scores on self-report measures of these two syndromes. Factor analyses of pooled items from both scales yielded two factors, "anger–impulsivity" and "affective instability," which when combined accounted for the majority of symptom overlap between these cyclothymia and BPD respondents. Other investigations have similarly documented substantial symptom overlap between BPD and bipolar disorders (see Li et al., 2020, for a review).

Differential Diagnosis of Personality Pathology and BSDs

To illuminate the intra- and interpersonal dynamics that distinguish two syndromes with overlapping symptoms, evidence derived from diagnostic interviews must be supplemented with data gathered via psychological assessment. Bornstein (2016) contrasted the processes involved in these two clinical tasks as follows:

> Diagnosis involves identifying and documenting a patient's symptoms, with the goal of classifying that patient into one or more categories whose labels represent shorthand descriptors of complex psychological syndromes (e.g., social anxiety disorder, bulimia nervosa, avoidant personality disorder). Assessment, in contrast, involves collecting broad information, usually with psychological tests, to disentangle the array of dispositional and situational factors that interact to determine a patient's subjective experiences, core beliefs, coping strategies, and behavior patterns. Put another way, diagnosis is key to understanding a patient's pathology; assessment is key to understanding the person with this pathology. (p. 83)

Information regarding the psychological and behavioral factors that may be useful in distinguishing BSDs and BPD comes from two sources: clinical writings and empirical evidence. Regarding the former, Bassett et al.'s (2017) review of the clinical literature on BSDs and BPD identified three dynamics that appear to distinguish these overlapping syndromes. First, patients with BPD are more likely to manifest a "noxious sense of self" (i.e., a pervasive negative evaluation of themselves). Second, BPD patients often rely on the defense mechanism of projective identification, a process wherein the individual projects unacceptable

TABLE 14.1. Distinguishing Features of BSDs and BPD: Empirical Evidence

Study	Distinguishing features
Balling et al. (2019)	Patients with BSD higher on elevated mood, increased goal-directed activity, and episodicity of mood symptoms
Bayes and Parker (2019)	Patients with BPD higher on identity disturbance
Carvalho and Pianowski (2019)	Patients with BPD higher on emotional dependency and aggressivity
Fowler et al. (2019)	Patients with BPD higher on emotional lability, anxiousness, separation insecurity, hostility, depressivity, and risk-taking
Mneimne et al. (2018)	Participants with BPD showed greater event-related reactivity of guilt and shame, and greater persistence of shame
Saunders et al. (2016)	Patients with BPD higher on hostility and impulsivity
Vöhringer et al. (2016)	Patients with BSD higher on elevated mood, increased goal-directed activity, and episodicity of mood symptoms
Wilson et al. (2007)	Patients with BPD higher on hostility and impulsivity

Note. BSD = bipolar spectrum disorder; BPD = borderline personality disorder. All studies used self-report methods to assess distinguishing features except for Mneimne et al. (2018), who used ecological momentary assessment (EMA; i.e., experience sampling in vivo), and Saunders et al. (2016), who assessed behavior in a laboratory negotiation task.

aspects of the self onto another person, causing that person to internalize these projected qualities. Third, BPD patients experience more frequent and more intense interpersonal conflicts than BSD patients (which may be due in part to their reliance on projective identification, which often causes the patent's internalized conflicts to be re-enacted in close interpersonal relationships).

Beyond the clinical literature, eight published studies have documented empirically the psychological and behavioral features that differentiate BSDs and BPD; key findings from these investigations are summarized in Table 14.1. As this table shows, relative to patients with BPD, patients with BSDs show (a) more elevated mood, (b) increased goal-directed activity (i.e., task persistence), and (c) greater "episodicity of mood" (i.e., more predictable temporal variations in mood states). Relative to patients with BSDs, patients with BPD show (a) more pronounced identity disturbance, (b) greater impulsivity, (c) higher levels of emotional dependency, (d) higher levels of aggressivity and hostility, and (e) more intense feelings of shame and guilt.

USE OF MULTIMETHOD ASSESSMENT TO DISTINGUISH BSDs FROM BPD

The following sections describe psychological tests and methods that are useful in documenting the distinguishing features listed in Table 14.1. These assessment tools can help clinicians distinguish patients with BSDs from those with BPD in clinical settings, and they may also be useful to researchers examining the underlying dynamics and behavioral correlates of BSDs and BPD. Within each section, tests and measures that employ different formats (e.g., self-report and performance-based) are included wherever possible. As Meyer (2002) and Bornstein (2017) noted, the use of multimethod assessment provides a unique opportunity to illuminate underlying psychological dynamics by scrutinizing cross-method test score convergences and divergences (see also Chapter 1 in the present volume).

Elevation and Episodicity of Mood

Evidence suggests that structured interviews yield the most valid and reliable data regarding temporal and contextual variations in mood state; questionnaire measures tend to yield less reliable data, in part because they are confounded by self-presentation effects but also because people show significant limitations in memory for episodes of mood elevation (Yen et al., 2016). Among the most well-validated measures in this area are the appropriate modules of the Longitudinal Interview Follow-up Evaluation (Keller et al., 1987) for use in adults and the Kiddie Schedule for Affective Disorders and Schizophrenia for School-Age Children (Kaufman et al., 1997) for use with children.

About a dozen studies have examined the utility of EMA in assessing elevation and episodicity of mood (Miguelez-Fernandez et al., 2018). Although evidence supports the validity of these measures with respect to variations in mood states, until recently no researchers had examined BSD patients' compliance with EMA tasks, which is crucial for the use of this method in clinical contexts. Gershon et al. (2019) addressed this issue, using EMA to assess variations in mood in a sample of adolescents with BSDs over 21 days. Results indicated that patients showed adequate but not excellent adherence to the task (i.e., 80% compliance). Additional evidence is needed before EMA may be used in this context, but initial results are promising.

Goal-Directed Activity

Studies indicate that, unlike for variations in mood, questionnaire measures are useful for assessing goal-directed activity in BSD patients. For example, Goldberg et al. (2012) used the Mood Disorder Questionnaire (MDQ) to assess various features of bipolar disorders in a large, mixed-sex sample of adults, and found strong concordance between scores on the MDQ index of goal-directed activity and clinician ratings based on interview and archival data. Additional evidence bearing on the validity and clinical utility of the MDQ goal-directed activity index was provided by Hirschfeld et al. (2003; see also Chapter 7 in this volume).

Approaching this question from a novel perspective, Johnson et al. (2000) hypothesized that increases in goal-directed activity would occur in BSD patients following exposure to cues that signal the possibility of external reward (i.e., being compensated for completing a task). The hypothesized patterns were in fact obtained in a mixed-sex sample of adults with BSD, with scores on Leenstra et al.'s (1995) four-item Goal Attainment Scale (GAS) predicting context-driven variations in goal-directed activity. Because increases in goal-directed activity do not occur specifically in response to the presence of external cues in patients with BPD, the GAS may be a useful measure in helping differentiate these two syndromes.

Identity Disturbance

One of the most useful self-report measures of identity disturbance is the Personality Structure Questionnaire (PSQ; Pollock et al., 2001), which asks participants to rate the extent to which eight items reflect their sense of self (e.g., "My sense of myself is always the same" vs. "How I act or feel is constantly changing"), with each item rated on a 5-point bipolar scale. As Berrios et al. (2016) noted, an advantage of the PSQ in clinical settings is that it is one of the few brief measures of identity disturbance that has been validated cross-culturally. Clarkin et al.'s (2019) Structured Interview of Personality Organization–Revised— which focuses on the assessment of consolidated identity versus identity disturbance, the use of adaptive versus maladaptive defenses, and intact versus loss of reality testing—may also be helpful in this context.

In addition, a number of Rorschach Comprehensive System (RCS; Weiner, 2003) and Rorschach Performance Assessment System (R-PAS; Meyer et al., 2011) variables are associated with identity impairment (see also Chapters 8 and 9 in this volume). Elevated scores on these identity impairment variables might suggest the presence of BPD in lieu of (or in addition to) BSD. These variables include the RCS H:(H) + Hd + (Hd) ratio (the number of human percepts divided by the number of quasihuman and human detail percepts) and the R-PAS PHR/GHR ratio (the number of percepts reflecting poor representation of humans divided by the number of human percepts with good or poor quality).

Interpersonal Dependency

Bornstein and Hopwood (2017) reviewed evidence bearing on the validity and clinical utility of widely used measures of interpersonal dependency. Among the most useful self-report dependency scales are Hirschfeld et al.'s (1977) Interpersonal Dependency Inventory and Bornstein et al.'s (2003) Relationship Profile Test, which yields separate scores for Destructive Overdependence, Dysfunctional Detachment, and Healthy Dependency. In addition, Krueger et al.'s (2013) Personality Inventory for *DSM-5* is useful for assessing the components of dependent personality disorder included in the alternative model of personality disorders (i.e., Submissiveness, Anxiousness, and Separation Insecurity).

The Rorschach Oral Dependency (ROD) scale, now included in R-PAS as the Oral Dependent Language (ODL) scale, is the most widely used and well-validated performance-based measure of interpersonal dependency. Information regarding the construct validity of the ROD/ODL scale was provided by Bornstein and Hopwood (2017); strategies for integrating ROD/ODL scores with scores on self-report measures of dependency were described by

Bornstein (2012). As Bornstein (2012) noted, divergences between scores of self-report and performance-based dependency tests may enable the clinician to determine whether a patient is minimizing or exaggerating the intensity of their underlying dependency needs.

Aggressivity and Hostility

Two self-report measures are useful in this context. Carpiniello et al.'s (2011) Aggression Questionnaire is a 29-item scale that yields separate scores for Physical Aggressiveness, Verbal Aggressiveness, and Anger and Hostility, in addition to an overall/composite aggressivity score. Along somewhat different lines, the Ambiguous Intentions Hostility Questionnaire (AIHQ; Combs et al., 2007) assesses aggression-related cognitions. AIHQ items describe conflict-related events that are ambiguous, intentional, or accidental, and respondents indicate their attributions regarding each event. Higher scores reflect an attributional style characterized by hostility along with negative expectations of other people.

Beyond self-reports, several Rorschach-derived indices are useful in assessing underlying aggression and hostility. These include the RCS AG (aggressive movement) score, the R-PAS AGC (aggressive content) index, and Meloy and Gacono's (1992) AgC (aggressive content) score (Katko et al., 2010). Used in conjunction with self-report tests, these performance-based measures can help clinicians identify divergences between a patient's self-reported and underlying aggression.

Shame and Guilt

Two self-report scales are particularly useful in assessing shame and guilt in clinical settings. Tangney et al.'s (2000) 11-item Test of Self-Conscious Affect–3 assesses an array of negative emotions, including shame and guilt. Elison et al.'s (2006) 48-item Compass of Shame Scale (CoSS) is a scenario-based self-report measure that yields scores reflecting the frequency with which participants use several emotion-focused coping strategies, including shame. A 12-item version of the CoSS is also available and shows good psychometric properties (see Robins et al., 2007).

In addition, Gazzillo et al. (2017) developed a 15-item clinician-rated index of guilt, the Interpersonal Guilt Rating Scale–15 (IGRS-15), which yields scores for four manifestations of guilt (Separation/Disloyalty, Omnipotent Responsibility, Survivor Guilt, and Self-Hate). The IGRS-15 is useful in obtaining a multidimensional index of guilt in clinical settings and examining convergences and divergences between patient-reported and clinician-assessed guilt.

CONCLUSION

BPD and BSDs represent two of the more severe forms of psychopathology, with substantial costs for the individual and society. Accurate assessment of these disorders is crucial for effective treatment planning and intervention.

Maximizing the clinical utility of assessment for these two syndromes requires not only the use of well-validated, psychometrically sound assessment tools but also the implementation of an evidence-based procedure for integrating the results of tests that employ different methods and tap contrasting psychological processes. Where possible, multimethod assessment is the strategy of choice when assessing the underlying features of BPD and BSDs, and in situations where a differential diagnosis is an assessment goal.

This chapter has reviewed evidence bearing on the relationship between BSDs and personality pathology, with a focus on BPD, the PD that shows the greatest comorbidity with BSDs. Evidence bearing on this issue will evolve in the coming years, as diagnostic criteria for BSDs and PDs are revised in future versions of the *DSM* and *International Statistical Classification of Diseases and Related Health Problems* (*ICD*). Although the diagnostic criteria for PDs did not change in *DSM-5-TR*, personality pathology is conceptualized very differently in *ICD-11*, with the categorical framework replaced by a dimensional model wherein PDs are represented by (a) an overall index of personality impairment, along with (b) specification of "trait qualifiers" that characterize each patient's personality functioning and interpersonal behavior. This reconceptualization of personality pathology will require not only the development of new assessment tools but also a wholesale shift in thinking about what it means for a clinical disorder to be comorbid with personality pathology. This shift will bring with it a new set of challenges, and new opportunities as well.

REFERENCES

Altman, E. G., Hedeker, D., Peterson, J. L., & Davis, J. M. (1997). The Altman Self-Rating Mania Scale. *Biological Psychiatry*, *42*(10), 948–955. https://doi.org/10.1016/S0006-3223(96)00548-3

American Psychiatric Association. (2013). *Diagnostic and statistical manual of mental disorders* (5th ed.).

American Psychiatric Association. (2022). *Diagnostic and statistical manual of mental disorders* (5th ed., text rev.).

Balling, C., Chelminski, I., Dalrymple, K., & Zimmerman, M. (2019). Differentiating borderline personality from bipolar disorder with the Mood Disorder Questionnaire (MDQ). *Comprehensive Psychiatry*, *88*(1), 49–51. https://doi.org/10.1016/j.comppsych.2018.11.009

Bassett, D., Mulder, R., Outhred, T., Hamilton, A., Morris, G., Das, P., Berk, M., Baune, B. T., Boyce, P., Lyndon, B., Parker, G., Singh, A. B., & Malhi, G. S. (2017). Defining disorders with permeable borders: You say bipolar, I say borderline! *Bipolar Disorders*, *19*(5), 320–323. https://doi.org/10.1111/bdi.12528

Bauer, M. S., Crits-Christoph, P., Ball, W. A., Dewees, E., McAllister, T., Alahi, P., Cacciola, J., & Whybrow, P. C. (1991). Independent assessment of manic and depressive symptoms by self-rating. Scale characteristics and implications for the study of mania. *Archives of General Psychiatry*, *48*(9), 807–812. https://doi.org/10.1001/archpsyc.1991.01810330031005

Bayes, A. J., & Parker, G. B. (2019). Cognitive and behavioral differentiation of those with borderline personality disorder and bipolar disorder. *Journal of Nervous and Mental Disease*, *207*(8), 620–625. https://doi.org/10.1097/NMD.0000000000001024

Berrios, R., Kellett, S., Fiorani, C., & Poggioli, M. (2016). Assessment of identity distur-bance: Factor structure and validation of the Personality Structure Questionnaire in an Italian sample. *Psychological Assessment, 28*(4), e27–e35. https://doi.org/10.1037/pas0000143

Bezerra-Filho, S., Galvão-de Almeida, A., Studart, P., Rocha, M. V., Lopes, F. L., & Miranda-Scippa, Â. (2015). Personality disorders in euthymic bipolar patients: A systematic review. *Revista Brasileira de Psiquiatria, 37*(2), 162–167. https://doi.org/10.1590/1516-4446-2014-1459

Bornstein, R. F. (1998). Implicit and self-attributed dependency needs in dependent and histrionic personality disorders. *Journal of Personality Assessment, 71*(1), 1–14. https://doi.org/10.1207/s15327752jpa7101_1

Bornstein, R. F. (2012). From dysfunction to adaptation: An interactionist model of dependency. *Annual Review of Clinical Psychology, 8*(1), 291–316. https://doi.org/10.1146/annurev-clinpsy-032511-143058

Bornstein, R. F. (2015). Process focused assessment of personality pathology. In S. K. Huprich (Ed.), *Personality disorders: Toward theoretical and empirical integration in diagnosis and assessment* (pp. 271–290). American Psychological Association. https://doi.org/10.1037/14549-012

Bornstein, R. F. (2016). Personality traits and dynamics. In J. C. Norcross, G. R. VandenBos, & D. K. Freedheim (Eds.), *APA handbook of clinical psychology: Vol. III. Applications and methods* (pp. 81–101). American Psychological Association. https://doi.org/10.1037/14861-005

Bornstein, R. F. (2017). Evidence based psychological assessment. *Journal of Personality Assessment, 99*(4), 435–445. https://doi.org/10.1080/00223891.2016.1236343

Bornstein, R. F., & Hopwood, C. J. (2017). Evidence based assessment of interpersonal dependency. *Professional Psychology: Research and Practice, 48*(4), 251–258. https://doi.org/10.1037/pro0000036

Bornstein, R. F., Languirand, M. A., Geiselman, K. J., Creighton, J. A., West, M. A., Gallagher, H. A., & Eisenhart, E. A. (2003). Construct validity of the relationship profile test: A self-report measure of dependency-detachment. *Journal of Personality Assessment, 80*(1), 67–74. https://doi.org/10.1207/S15327752JPA8001_15

Carpiniello, B., Lai, L., Pirarba, S., Sardu, C., & Pinna, F. (2011). Impulsivity and aggressiveness in bipolar disorder with co-morbid borderline personality disorder. *Psychiatry Research, 188*(1), 40–44. https://doi.org/10.1016/j.psychres.2010.10.026

Carvalho, L. F., & Pianowski, G. (2019). Differentiating borderline personality disorder and bipolar disorder through emotional dependency, emotional instability, impul-siveness and aggressiveness traits. *European Journal of Psychiatry, 33*(2), 91–95. https://doi.org/10.1016/j.ejpsy.2019.03.001

Cerimele, J. M., Goldberg, S. B., Miller, C. J., Gabrielson, S. W., & Fortney, J. C. (2019). Systematic review of symptom assessment measures for use in measurement-based care of bipolar disorders. *Psychiatric Services, 70*(5), 396–408. https://doi.org/10.1176/appi.ps.201800383

Clarkin, J. F., Caligor, E., Stern, B., & Kernberg, O. F. (2019). *Structured Interview for Personality Disorder, revised.* Personality Disorders Institute, Weill Medical College of Cornell University.

Combs, D. R., Penn, D. L., Wicher, M., & Waldheter, E. (2007). The Ambiguous Intentions Hostility Questionnaire (AIHQ): A new measure for evaluating hostile social-cognitive biases in paranoia. *Cognitive Neuropsychiatry, 12*(2), 128–143. https://doi.org/10.1080/13546800600787854

Depp, C. A., Moore, R. C., Dev, S. I., Mausbach, B. T., Eyler, L. T., & Granholm, E. L. (2016). The temporal course and clinical correlates of subjective impulsivity in bipolar disorder as revealed through ecological momentary assessment. *Journal of Affective Disorders, 193*, 145–150. https://doi.org/10.1016/j.jad.2015.12.016

Elison, J., Lennon, R., & Pulos, S. (2006). Investigating the compass of shame: The development of the Compass of Shame Scale. *Social Behavior and Personality, 34*(3), 221–238. https://doi.org/10.2224/sbp.2006.34.3.221

First, M. B., Williams, J. B. W., Benjamin, L. S., & Spitzer, R. L. (2016). *Structured Clinical Interview for* DSM-5 *Personality Disorders.* American Psychiatric Association.

First, M. B., Williams, J. B. W., Karg, R. S., & Spitzer, R. L. (2016). *Structured Clinical Interview for* DSM-5 *Disorders, Clinician Version.* American Psychiatric Association.

Fornaro, M., Orsolini, L., Marini, S., De Berardis, D., Perna, G., Valchera, A., Gananca, L., Solmi, M., Veronese, N., & Stubbs, B. (2016). The prevalence and predictors of bipolar and borderline personality disorders comorbidity: Systematic review and meta-analysis. *Journal of Affective Disorders, 195*(5), 105–118. https://doi.org/10.1016/j.jad.2016.01.040

Fowler, J. C., Madan, A., Allen, J. G., Oldham, J. M., & Frueh, B. C. (2019). Differentiating bipolar disorder from borderline personality disorder: Diagnostic accuracy of the Difficulty in Emotion Regulation Scale and Personality Inventory for *DSM-5. Journal of Affective Disorders, 245*, 856–860. https://doi.org/10.1016/j.jad.2018.11.079

Frías, Á., Baltasar, I., & Birmaher, B. (2016). Comorbidity between bipolar disorder and borderline personality disorder: Prevalence, explanatory theories, and clinical impact. *Journal of Affective Disorders, 202*, 210–219. https://doi.org/10.1016/j.jad.2016.05.048

Gazzillo, F., Gorman, B., Bush, M., Silberschatz, G., Mazza, C., Faccini, F., Crisafulli, V., Alesiani, R., & De Luca, E. (2017). Reliability and validity of the Interpersonal Guilt Rating Scale–15 (IGRS-15): A new clinician-reporting tool for assessing interpersonal guilt according to control-mastery theory. *Psychodynamic Psychiatry, 45*(3), 362–384. https://doi.org/10.1521/pdps.2017.45.3.362

Gershon, A., Kaufmann, C. N., Torous, J., Depp, C., & Ketter, T. A. (2019). Electronic Ecological Momentary Assessment (EMA) in youth with bipolar disorder: Demographic and clinical predictors of electronic EMA adherence. *Journal of Psychiatric Research, 116*(1), 14–18. https://doi.org/10.1016/j.jpsychires.2019.05.026

Goldberg, J. F., Garakani, A., & Ackerman, S. H. (2012). Clinician-rated versus self-rated screening for bipolar disorder among inpatients with mood symptoms and substance misuse. *The Journal of Clinical Psychiatry, 73*(12), 1525–1530. https://doi.org/10.4088/JCP.12m07926

Goutaudier, N., Melioli, T., Valls, M., Bouvet, R., & Chabrol, H. (2014). Relations between cyclothymic temperament and borderline personality disorder traits in non-clinical adolescents. *European Review of Applied Psychology, 64*(6), 345–351. https://doi.org/10.1016/j.erap.2014.08.006

Hede, V., Favre, S., Aubry, J. M., & Richard-Lepouriel, H. (2019). Bipolar spectrum disorder: What evidence for pharmacological treatment? A systematic review. *Psychiatry Research, 282*, Article 112627. https://doi.org/10.1016/j.psychres.2019.112627

Hirschfeld, R. M. A., Holzer, C., Calabrese, J. R., Weissman, M., Reed, M., Davies, M., Frye, M. A., Keck, P., McElroy, S., Lewis, L., Tierce, J., Wagner, K. D., & Hazard, E. (2003). Validity of the Mood Disorder Questionnaire: A general population study. *The American Journal of Psychiatry, 160*(1), 178–180. https://doi.org/10.1176/appi.ajp.160.1.178

Hirschfeld, R. M. A., Klerman, G. L., Gough, H. G., Barrett, J., Korchin, S. J., & Chodoff, P. (1977). A measure of interpersonal dependency. *Journal of Personality Assessment, 41*(6), 610–618. https://doi.org/10.1207/s15327752jpa4106_6

Huprich, S. K. (Ed.). (2006). *Rorschach assessment of the personality disorders.* Lawrence Erlbaum. https://doi.org/10.4324/9781410615640

Johnson, S. L., Sandrow, D., Meyer, B., Winters, R., Miller, I., Solomon, D., & Keitner, G. (2000). Increases in manic symptoms after life events involving goal attainment. *Journal of Abnormal Psychology, 109*(4), 721–727. https://doi.org/10.1037//0021-843x.109.4.721

Katko, N. J., Meyer, G. J., Mihura, J. L., & Bombel, G. (2010). A principal components analysis of Rorschach aggression and hostility variables. *Journal of Personality Assessment, 92*(6), 594–598. https://doi.org/10.1080/00223891.2010.513309

Kaufman, J., Birmaher, B., Brent, D., Rao, U., Flynn, C., Moreci, P., Williamson, D., & Ryan, N. (1997). Schedule for Affective Disorders and Schizophrenia for School-Age Children–Present and Lifetime Version (K-SADS-PL): Initial reliability and validity data. *Journal of the American Academy of Child & Adolescent Psychiatry, 36*(7), 980–988. https://doi.org/10.1097/00004583-199707000-00021

Keller, M. B., Lavori, P. W., Friedman, B., Nielsen, E., Endicott, J., McDonald-Scott, P., & Andreasen, N. C. (1987). The longitudinal interval follow-up evaluation. A comprehensive method for assessing outcome in prospective longitudinal studies. *Archives of General Psychiatry, 44*(6), 540–548. https://doi.org/10.1001/archpsyc.1987.01800180050009

Krueger, R. F., Derringer, J., Markon, K. E., Watson, D., & Skodol, A. E. (2013). *Personality Inventory for* DSM-5. American Psychiatric Association.

Leenstra, A. S., Ormel, J., & Giel, R. (1995). Positive life change and recovery from depression and anxiety. A three-stage longitudinal study of primary care attenders. *The British Journal of Psychiatry, 166*(3), 333–343. https://doi.org/10.1192/bjp.166.3.333

Li, B., Valles, N.-L., Saunders, J., Vyas, A., Naqvi, M., & Shah, A. A. (2020). Can we differentiate borderline personality disorder from bipolar disorder? *Psychiatric Annals, 50*(1), 19–23. https://doi.org/10.3928/00485713-20191126-01

Loranger, A. W., Sartorius, N., Andreoli, A., Berger, P., Buchheim, P., Channabasavanna, S. M., Coid, B., Dahl, A., Diekstra, R. F., Ferguson, B., Jacobsberg, L. B., Mombour, W., Pull, C., Ono, Y., & Regier, D. A. (1994). The international personality disorder examination. The World Health Organization/Alcohol, Drug Abuse, and Mental Health Administration international pilot study of personality disorders. *Archives of General Psychiatry, 51*(3), 215–224. https://doi.org/10.1001/archpsyc.1994.03950030051005

Meloy, J. R., & Gacono, C. B. (1992). The aggression response and the Rorschach. *Journal of Clinical Psychology, 48*(1), 104–114. https://doi.org/10.1002/1097-4679(199201)48:1<104::AID-JCLP2270480115>3.0.CO;2-1

Merikangas, K. R., Jin, R., He, J.-P., Kessler, R. C., Lee, S., Sampson, N. A., Viana, M. C., Andrade, L. H., Hu, C., Karam, E. G., Ladea, M., Medina-Mora, M. E., Ono, Y., Posada-Villa, J., Sagar, R., Wells, J. E., & Zarkov, Z. (2011). Prevalence and correlates of bipolar spectrum disorder in the world mental health survey initiative. *Archives of General Psychiatry, 68*(3), 241–251. https://doi.org/10.1001/archgenpsychiatry.2011.12

Meyer, G. J. (2002). Implications of information-gathering methods for a refined taxonomy of psychopathology. In L. E. Beutler & M. Malik (Eds.), *Rethinking the* DSM*: Psychological perspectives* (pp. 69–105). American Psychological Association. https://doi.org/10.1037/10456-003

Meyer, G. J., Viglione, D. J., Mihura, J. L., Erard, R. E., & Erdberg, P. (2011). *Rorschach Performance Assessment System: Administration, coding, interpretation, and technical manual.* Rorschach Performance Assessment System.

Miguelez-Fernandez, C., de Leon, S. J., Baltasar-Tello, I., Peñuelas-Calvo, I., Barrigon, M. L., Capdevila, A. S., Delgado-Gómez, D., Baca-García, E., & Carballo, J. J. (2018). Evaluating attention-deficit/hyperactivity disorder using ecological momentary assessment: A systematic review. *Attention Deficit and Hyperactivity Disorders, 10*(4), 247–265. https://doi.org/10.1007/s12402-018-0261-1

Mneimne, M., Fleeson, W., Arnold, E. M., & Furr, R. M. (2018). Differentiating the everyday emotion dynamics of borderline personality disorder from major depressive disorder and bipolar disorder. *Personality Disorders, 9*(2), 192–196. https://doi.org/10.1037/per0000255

Peluso, M. A. M., Hatch, J. P., Glahn, D. C., Monkul, E. S., Sanches, M., Najt, P., Bowden, C. L., Barratt, E. S., & Soares, J. C. (2007). Trait impulsivity in patients with mood disorders. *Journal of Affective Disorders, 100*(1–3), 227–231. https://doi.org/10. 1016/j.jad.2006.09.037

Pincus, A. L., Ansell, E. B., Pimentel, C. A., Cain, N. M., Wright, A. G. C., & Levy, K. N. (2009). Initial construction and validation of the Pathological Narcissism Inventory. *Psychological Assessment, 21*(3), 365–379. https://doi.org/10.1037/a0016530

Pollock, P. H., Broadbent, M., Clarke, S., Dorrian, A., & Ryle, A. (2001). The Personality Structure Questionnaire (PSQ): A measure of the multiple self states model of identity disturbance in cognitive analytic therapy. *Clinical Psychology & Psychotherapy, 8*(1), 59–72. https://doi.org/10.1002/cpp.250

Robins, R. W., Noftle, E. E., & Tracy, J. L. (2007). *Assessing self-conscious emotions*. Guilford Press.

Saunders, K. E. A., Goodwin, G. M., & Rogers, R. D. (2016). Borderline personality disorder, but not euthymic bipolar I disorder, is associated with prolonged post-error slowing in sensorimotor performance. *Journal of Affective Disorders, 198*, 163–170. https://doi.org/10.1016/j.jad.2016.03.027

Tangney, J., Dearing, R., Wagner, P., & Gramzow, R. (2000). *The Test of Self-Conscious Affect–short form (TOSCA-S)*. George Mason University.

Tangney, J. P., Stuewig, J., & Hafez, L. (2011). Shame, guilt and remorse: Implications for offender populations. *Journal of Forensic Psychiatry & Psychology, 22*(5), 706–723. https://doi.org/10.1080/14789949.2011.617541

Tondo, L., Pompili, M., Forte, A., & Baldessarini, R. J. (2016). Suicide attempts in bipolar disorders: Comprehensive review of 101 reports. *Acta Psychiatrica Scandinavica, 133*(3), 174–186. https://doi.org/10.1111/acps.12517

Tyrer, P., Morgan, J., & Cicchetti, D. (2004). The Dependent Personality Questionnaire (DPQ): A screening instrument for dependent personality. *The International Journal of Social Psychiatry, 50*(1), 10–17. https://doi.org/10.1177/0020764004038754

Van Meter, A. R., Youngstrom, E. A., & Findling, R. L. (2012). Cyclothymic disorder: A critical review. *Clinical Psychology Review, 32*(4), 229–243. https://doi.org/10.1016/ j.cpr.2012.02.001

Vöhringer, P. A., Barroilhet, S. A., Alvear, K., Medina, S., Espinosa, C., Alexandrovich, K., Riumallo, P., Leiva, F., Hurtado, M. E., Cabrera, J., Sullivan, M., Holtzman, N., & Ghaemi, S. N. (2016). The International Mood Network (IMN) Nosology Project: Differentiating borderline personality from bipolar illness. *Acta Psychiatrica Scandinavica, 134*(6), 504–510. https://doi.org/10.1111/acps.12643

Weiner, I. B. (2003). *Principles of Rorschach interpretation* (2nd ed.). Lawrence Erlbaum. https://doi.org/10.4324/9781410607799

Wilson, S. T., Stanley, B., Oquendo, M. A., Goldberg, P., Zalsman, G., & Mann, J. J. (2007). Comparing impulsiveness, hostility, and depression in borderline personality disorder and bipolar II disorder. *The Journal of Clinical Psychiatry, 68*(10), 1533–1539. https:// doi.org/10.4088/JCP.v68n1010

World Health Organization. (2019). *International statistical classification of diseases and related health problems* (11th ed.).

Yen, S., Stout, R., Hower, H., Killam, M. A., Weinstock, L. M., Topor, D. R., Dickstein, D. P., Hunt, J. I., Gill, M. K., Goldstein, T. R., Goldstein, B. I., Ryan, N. D., Strober, M., Sala, R., Axelson, D. A., Birmaher, B., & Keller, M. B. (2016). The influence of comorbid disorders on the episodicity of bipolar disorder in youth. *Acta Psychiatrica Scandinavica, 133*(4), 324–334. https://doi.org/10.1111/acps.12514

15

Assessment of Bipolar and Psychological Trauma Spectrum Disorders

F. Barton Evans, Bethany L. Brand, and Nancy Kaser-Boyd

This chapter addresses the knotty problem of differentiating bipolar spectrum disorders (BSDs) from what we are terming trauma spectrum disorders (TSpD) and how multimethod psychological assessment can be especially valuable for clinicians. As Phelps (2016) noted, one of three most difficult challenges in differentiating BSDs is the extensive overlap of symptoms and clinical presentation with posttraumatic stress disorder (PTSD). As we further discuss, this overlap becomes even more complex when differentiating BSDs from TSpD includes considering other trauma-based diagnoses of complex posttraumatic stress disorder (CPTSD) and dissociative disorders (DD). Further compounding this complexity is the reality that traumatized individuals may suffer from bipolar disorders and individuals with bipolar disorders may become traumatized by the consequences of their bipolar disorder. In accordance with the diathesis-stress (Monroe & Simons, 1991; Rosenthal, 1970) and kindling (Post et al., 2000) models, psychological trauma (PT), especially PT in childhood, may contribute environmental loading to the causation of expression of bipolar disorders (see Bender & Alloy, 2011; Maguire et al., 2008; Malkoff-Schwartz et al., 1998). The literature abounds with bicausality of these two disorder clusters.

As noted in the Introduction to this book, bipolar disorders are increasingly viewed as existing on a spectrum. Consequences of dimensional, rather than categorical, approach suggests the importance of greater nuance and complexity in assessment, especially in determining the nonmanic or submanic expression

https://doi.org/10.1037/0000356-016
Psychological Assessment of Bipolar Spectrum Disorders, J. H. Kleiger and I. B. Weiner (Editors)

of the disorder such as bipolar II disorder. This determination has real-life consequences; for example, underdiagnosing of the nonmanic or submanic expression of the disorder can lead to treatment of, for example, unipolar depression using antidepressive medication, which can be of little help or even make BSDs symptoms worse (see Merikangas et al., 2007).

Further, consistent with current thinking and research, we use the designation of psychological TSpD to cover disorders ranging from PTSD to CPTSD to DD. Unlike the current nomenclature of the *Diagnostic and Statistical Manual of Mental Disorders* (5th ed., text rev.; *DSM-5-TR*; American Psychiatric Association, 2022), the research literature strongly suggests that these three disorders lie on a continuum of severity of trauma exposure and response to this exposure. For example, as originally proposed by Herman (1992) and validated by extensive research (see Brewin et al., 2017), CPTSD, the result of multiple traumatic events occurring over a period of time, has been accepted as a new diagnostic entity in the *International Statistical Classification of Diseases and Related Health Problems* (11th ed.; *ICD-11*). In addition to the symptoms of PTSD, CPTSD includes symptoms of negative self-concept, interpersonal disturbance, and perhaps most importantly for this chapter, affect dysregulation. Further, it is well established that DD is a disorder resulting from severe trauma in childhood (Dalenberg et al., 2012; Putnam, 1997). Changing of mood states resulting from switching between personality states in DD can easily be mistaken for a bipolar disorder. Even clear differentiation among these trauma disorders is frequently difficult, let alone adding the complexity of differentiating them from BSDs; yet ramifications for treatment and therefore assessment are often critical.

SYMPTOM OVERLAP IN BIPOLAR AND TSpD

A critical dimension of differential assessment of these two spectrum disorders is the problem of symptom overlap. As noted by Phelps (2016), BSD symptoms are increasingly conceptualized as including more than the eight *DSM-5-TR* symptoms of bipolar disorders, especially when including nonmanic markers, let alone symptoms of unipolar depressive disorder. Regeer et al. (2015) found that only 22% of individuals with hypomanic symptoms are accurately diagnosed with BSDs, suggesting extensive underdiagnosis of this disorder.

On the other hand, *DSM-5-TR* PTSD diagnostic criteria include 20 symptoms in four clusters, in addition to the traumatic stressor requirement. As Galatzer-Levy and Bryant (2013) noted, using the various combinations of symptoms within each cluster, there are 636,120 ways to have PTSD. Per Evans (2016), most symptoms of PTSD are nonspecific to the disorder in the absence of a clearly defined traumatic event, making a reliable diagnosis difficult, especially using interviews and symptom counting alone. This can easily lead to an overdiagnosis of PTSD unless care is taken (see McNally, 2012; Robinson & Larson, 2010).

Further, there are many symptoms in BSDs that overlap with PTSD, such as irritability and aggression, risky behavior, sleep difficulties, hypervigilance, problems with concentration, and depressive mood. This combination of under-diagnosis and overdiagnosis, co-occurrence, and symptom overlap makes forming a differential diagnosis between BSDs and PTSD/TSpD a highly knotty clinical problem. This complexity can lead potentially to negative consequences of inaccurate assessment in developing targeted psychotherapy and medication treatment plans. Add to this the current pressure on mental health and medical providers to arrive at quick diagnoses. This confluence of complexity and uncertainty with pressure for rapid decisions increases errors in decision making. Intuitive evaluations of probabilistic data are prone to widespread biases due to the use of short-cut mental strategies that streamline information called heuristics (Kahneman et al., 1982). While heuristics allow for faster processing of information than analytic methods, they can lead to errors, because not all information is considered. Differential diagnosis in BSDs and PTSD/TSpD, especially trends of overdiagnosis of PTSD and underdiagnosis of nonmanic BSDs, are all too vulnerable to inaccurate mental health decision-making heuristics. As such, the value of multimethod psychological assessment in bipolar/trauma spectrum differentiation offers a critical correction to decision-making errors. As Armstrong (1991) stated,

> The strength of psychological assessment has long been its ability to describe the organization of psychological processes to gain a detailed knowledge of the individual. As such, in the hands of well-trained clinicians, psychological assessment has been one of the most powerful tools for predicting long-term treatment outcome.

MULTIMETHOD PSYCHOLOGICAL ASSESSMENT IN DIFFERENTIATING BSDs AND TSpD

The major advantage of comprehensive multimethod psychological assessment is that it is empirically grounded and provides objective information that can debias the heuristics errors in clinical judgment. Comprehensive multimethod assessments ideally include structured interview measures, self-report symptom-specific tests, multiscale personality inventories, and performance-based personality tests.

Clinical interviews are naturally at the heart of all mental health practice, providing a path to understanding the client's history, interpersonal relationships, personal experience, and subjective reactions to these experiences and relationships. Naturally, understanding a history of past and present trauma in the case of TSpD and a family history of affective disorders in BSDs is critical for diagnosis. However, unstructured clinical interviews alone have some important disadvantages, the first of which is that it runs the risk of missing crucial information.

Structured interview-based measures are important psychological methods that can systematically assess sign and symptoms of psychological disorders. With the advent of the Structured Clinical Interview for *DSM-III-R*

(Spitzer et al., 1990), the structured interview has become increasingly a gold standard for the reliable diagnosis of mental disorders for research and clinical purposes. In the assessment of PTSD, an example is the gold standard Clinician-Administered PTSD Scale for *DSM-5* (Weathers et al., 2018), which provides both structured and open-ended question for detailed examination of posttraumatic symptoms and their severity.

Self-report symptom-specific tests are psychological assessment instruments, which include straightforward, face-valid instruments measuring a particular disorder or clinical phenomenon. They range from PTSD-specific scales, such as the PTSD Checklist for *DSM-5* (PCL-5; Weathers, Litz, et al., 2013), to comprehensive assessment measures for psychological sequelae of traumatic experiences, such as Briere's (2011) Trauma Symptom Inventory–2 (TSI-2).

Personality tests are designed to broadly assess psychological symptoms, as well as personality traits, behavioral predispositions and inner experiences (see Chapters 3, 4, 5, and 6 in this volume). Examples of personality tests include multiscale self-report tests, that is, inventory-type, question-and-response tests, such as the Minnesota Multiphasic Personality Inventory–2 (MMPI-2; Butcher et al., 1989), Minnesota Multiphasic Personality Inventory–2–Restructured Form (MMPI-2-RF; Ben-Porath & Tellegen, 2008), and the Personality Assessment Inventory (PAI; Morey & Boggs, 2007).

Additionally, *performance-based tests* such as the Rorschach Inkblot Method, using either the comprehensive system (CS; Exner, 2003; Weiner, 2014) or the Rorschach Performance Assessment System (R-PAS; Meyer et al., 2011), are used to assess more subtle aspects of personality. The value of these comprehensive personality-assessment measures is that they assess a wide variety of psychological states and personality traits, allowing the clinician to better understand comorbid mental disorders and underlying personality issues as well as posttraumatic states.

DIFFERENTIATING PTSD, COMPLEX PTSD, AND BSDs

Following the inclusion of PTSD in *DSM-III* (American Psychiatric Association, 1980), a disorder that has since grown in importance and value, the concept of CPTSD was first described in the professional literature by Herman (1992), who identified the more pervasive and serious symptoms of PTSD that arise from repeated, often inescapable, trauma. She outlined five basic descriptors of CPTSD, capturing the ways repeated trauma results in symptoms different from and more unusually severe and chronic than those of PTSD, including multiplicity of symptoms, somatization, dissociation, affective changes, pathological changes in relationships, and pathological changes in identity.

Though Herman (1992) focused on the profound depression that results in chronic trauma, others noted that the affective changes and the arousal symptoms can result in impaired modulation of affect, mania, or shifts in emotion. This is especially where CPTSD can resemble bipolar disorder. Van der Kolk et al. (2005)

proposed a diagnosis of Disorders of Extreme Stress (DESNOS), which identified symptom clusters as (a) alterations in regulation of affect and impulses, (b) alterations in attention or consciousness, (c) alterations in self-perception, (d) alterations in perceptions of other, (e) somatization, and (f) alterations in systems of meaning.

DSM-5 does not offer a diagnostic category for either CPTSD or DESNOS but outlines two PTSD symptom clusters that involve changes in affect. Cluster D involves negative alterations in cognitions and mood associated with the traumatic event and persistent inability to experience positive emotions. Cluster E involves marked alterations in arousal and reactivity, which can involve emotional dysregulation. While *DSM-5* does not list complex PTSD as a diagnosis, it suggests that those with prolonged exposure to trauma, such as abused children or battered women, could be diagnosed with PTSD with associated features.

Based on substantial research (Brewin et al., 2017), the *ICD-11* includes CPTSD as a diagnosis. In the *ICD-11*, CPTSD may develop following exposure to extremely threatening or horrific nature events that are most commonly prolonged or repetitive events from which escape is difficult or impossible (e.g., torture, slavery, genocide campaigns, prolonged domestic violence, repeated childhood sexual or physical abuse). All diagnostic requirements for PTSD must also be met.

Further, *ICD-11* diagnosis of CPTSD is characterized by three main symptom clusters, which are severe, pervasive, and persistent. The first, and perhaps most immediately relevant to differentiation from BSDs are problems in affect regulation, which include, on the one hand, heightened emotional reactivity, violent outbursts, reckless or self-destructive behavior, and dissociative symptoms when under stress, and on the other hand, depressive-like experiences such as emotional numbing and inability to experience pleasure or positive emotions.

The second CPTSD symptom cluster includes beliefs about oneself as worthless, diminished, or defeated, accompanied by feelings of shame guilt or failure related to the traumatic event. Again, this cluster could be mistaken for depressive experiences, with the added feature of its relationship to a traumatic event or events being an important differentiation factor from the depressive phase of BSDs.

The third CPTSD symptom cluster includes difficulties in sustaining relationships and in feeling close to others. The traumatized person may consistently avoid, devalue, or show little interest in social relationships. Alternatively, they may have intense relationships with difficulty sustaining them. A core feature of CPTSD is the interpersonal damage caused by abuse by trusted others, often referred to as betrayal trauma (Freyd, 1996), and the subsequent mistrust, fear, buried longing, and loneliness in relationships. The potential exists for overlap with this essential CPTSD symptom and BSDs. While interpersonal difficulties are not a formal diagnostic criterion in BSDs, the research shows its potent impact on relationships, especially marriage and family, with high rates of impairment including high rates of divorce and family disturbance (see Azorin et al., 2021). Again, a careful assessment of history is essential in sorting out the cause of interpersonal disturbance.

Distinguishing between BSDs and Complex PTSD is no easy endeavor, though the history collected in the interview will determine whether there has been the type of developmental trauma, such as child abuse, torture or genocide, or domestic violence that is fundamental to CPTSD. For individuals from these populations, there may be symptoms that resemble or meet the criteria for bipolar disorders, as well as the criteria for CPTSD, where treatment interventions will need to acknowledge both disorders.

Many researchers and clinicians have explored the shared symptoms of bipolar disorders and PTSD (e.g., Hernandez et al., 2013). This means that it is often not an either–or diagnostic question. As Cerimele et al. (2017) and Hernandez et al. (2013) noted, bipolar disorders and PTSD frequently occur together, complicating clinical presentations. Trauma symptoms are often left undetected in treatment settings where individuals are diagnosed with a serious mental illness (Mueser et al., 1998). Otto et al. (2004) also found that up to 40% of patients with BSDs also have PTSD. Also, BSD is commonly found in patients with PTSD. For example, veterans with PTSD have higher rates of BSDs than veterans without PTSD (Orsillo et al., 1996). BSDs and PTSD have diagnostic symptoms and features in common, including irritability, increased risk-taking, sleep pattern alterations, concentration difficulties, anhedonia, problems maintaining relationships or employment, anxiety, hopelessness, and mood swings (Goldberg & Fagin-Jones, 2004). The main question is often not about which disorder is present, but how to treat the co-occurring symptoms. Because of the damage to trust, a history of trauma often makes treating BSDs more difficult, with patients with a trauma history having more severe symptoms, such as hallucinations, delusions, dissociation, and hostility (Fawcett, 2008).

The overlap between complex PTSD and bipolar disorders has been less well explored. Presumably, the symptoms of affective instability will be like those in PTSD and the differences with CPTSD will surround the profound changes to self and relationships. Because CPTSD results from prolonged, often inescapable traumatic events and the number of traumatic events in the person's life, the first step in assessment beyond a clinical interview is a valid measure of trauma exposure. The Life Events Checklist for *DSM-5* (Weathers, Blake, et al., 2013) and the more extensive Trauma History Screen (Carlson et al., 2011) are systematic ways to review the types of trauma experienced by the patient, while PTSD-specific instruments such as the PCL-5 (Weathers, Litz, et al., 2013) or the Posttraumatic Diagnostic Scale for *DSM-5* (Foa et al., 2016) can assess symptoms of PTSD.

If CPTSD is suspected, the Complex Trauma Inventory (CTI; Litvin et al., 2017), a self-report measure, can be administered. This 20-item questionnaire incorporates symptoms of PTSD with those of CPTSD. The CTI has two factors, including PTSD (re-experiencing, avoidance, sense of threat) and disturbances in self-organization (affect dysregulation, negative self-concept, and disturbances in relationship). Other trauma-specific assessment measures focusing on impaired affect regulation and impaired self-capacities in CPTSD include the Inventory of Altered Self-Capacities (Briere, 2000; Briere & Runtz, 2002) and portions of the TSI-2 (Briere, 2011). The Inventory of Altered Self-Capacities was created specifically to evaluate the symptoms of CPTSD. This self-report inventory taps the areas of relatedness, identity, and affect regulation, with scales assessing domains of interpersonal conflicts, idealization-disillusionment, abandonment concerns, identity impairment, susceptibility to influence, affect dysregulation, and tension reduction. The TSI-2 (Briere, 2011) is a broad, trauma-specific instrument with scales that are relevant to both PTSD and CPTSD. The TSI-2 has two scales that tap aspects of CPTSD: Impaired Self-Reference and Tension Reduction.

Briere and Spinazzola (2005) suggested that assessment should be with a battery that utilizes a broadband "generic" survey of mental disorders and one or more inventories focused on the unique symptoms of CPTSD. They cautioned that validity measures (e.g., F, Fp on the MMPI-2) for trauma disorders are often elevated beyond cutoff scores for other psychiatric diagnoses. For the broadband measures, they suggested the MMPI, the PAI, the Millon Clinical Multiaxial Inventory–IV (MCMI-IV; Millon et al., 2015) or the Rorschach, each of which, they noted, yield information on personality and self-capacity difficulties frequently associated with complex posttraumatic outcomes.

The PAI (Morey, 1991; see Chapter 4 in this volume) provides directly relevant information with separate scales for Traumatic Stress, Mania, Depression, and Somatization, as well as for Borderline traits that resemble those identified in *ICD-11* criteria for CPTSD surrounding impaired sense of self and problematic relationships. The PAI computer-generated report presents a coefficient of fit including all scales for both bipolar I disorder and PTSD. The PAI subscales also provide information that is closer to the functional impairments in CPTSD, including BOR-A (Affective Instability), BOR-I (Identity Problems), BOR-N (Negative Relationships), and BOR-S (Self-Harm). The PAI has dedicated scales for Alcohol Abuse and Drug Abuse, as well as an actuarial method for evaluating suicide risk. Like all generic broadband self-report inventories we will discuss, the PAI has validity scales that assist the evaluator in determining whether symptoms were denied or exaggerated.

The MCMI-IV (see Chapter 5 in this volume) also has specific scales dedicated to BSDs and PTSD, as well as scales to assess drug or alcohol abuse. It also taps the acting out features of CPTSD often seen in Borderline, Paranoid, and Antisocial disorders, as well as the internalizing features of melancholia and masochism. In short, the MCMI-IV can provide very useful information about the serious impairments in self and other seen in CPTSD. A differential diagnosis (CPTSD vs. BSDs) is likely not a simple determination of which scales are the most elevated, but rather a combination of symptoms measured in conjunction with the client's history, including the onset of the symptoms of each disorder, family history of affective disorder, and trauma history.

The use of the MMPI (see Chapter 3 in this volume) is complicated at present because of the different versions—MMPI-2, MMPI-2-RF, and MMPI-3.

The MMPI-2 had a dedicated trauma scale, PK, although it was criticized for measuring mostly the anxiety aspects of PTSD (see Nichols, 2011). Evaluating CPTSD with the MMPI-2, as well as the MMPI-2-RF and MMPI-3 involves a survey of individual scales to determine the ones that contain symptoms of CPTSD. The research literature on the use of the MMPI-2 to assess child sexual abuse (Griffith et al., 1998; Follette et al., 1997) and battered women (Khan et al., 2010; Morrell & Rubin, 2001) can be useful. Studies with these trauma groups often show elevations on MMPI-2 scales F, 2, 4, 6, and 8. Scale 2 captures depression and feelings of worthlessness. Scale 4 captures alienation and the potential for acting out. Scale 6 captures hypervigilance and impairment of trust. Scale 8 captures reality testing and the likelihood of intrusive recollections.

The research literature from the MMPI-2 cannot be easily applied to the MMPI-2-RF because the structure and some of the content is different. However, Ben-Porath and Tellegen (2020) indicated that the research studies of the MMPI-2-RF can be applied to the MMPI-3. The published research on PTSD and the MMPI-2-RF has primarily involved veterans diagnosed with PTSD rather than CPTSD, likely due to the limitations of *DSM-5-TR*. Wolf et al. (2008) presented data from two groups of soldiers: enlisted veterans and National Guard veterans. They found MMPI-2-RF elevations on RCd, RC1, RC2, RC7, and RC8 in male veterans. They also studied a group of female veterans with multiple types of trauma, including sexual assault, combat, physical abuse, and emotional abuse. While this subgroup likely had symptoms of CPTSD, the authors did not compare them to the data from those with PTSD. Female veterans had the same elevations except for RC8. Similarly, Sellbom et al. (2012) looked at injured workers and found MMPI-2-RF elevations on RCd, RC2, RC7, and RC8. They reported elevations on ANX, ACT, SAY, and SFD. ANX measures the basic symptoms of PTSD—re-experiencing, avoidance, and hyperarousal—while ACT measures the PTSD symptoms of Hyperarousal. Of note is that ACT is also the primary scale reported to be sensitive to bipolar disorders (Watson et al., 2010), which may lead to confusion when distinguishing PTSD from BSDs. Since the Restructured Scales appear on the MMPI-3, this could be a starting point for the study of CPTSD, but additional measures would likely be required. Further, the MMPI-2-RF and MMPI-3 scales SAY and SFD, measuring social alienation and avoidance, may add detail about disrupted relationships.

There has been a substantial amount of research on PTSD and CPTSD with the Rorschach. A recent review of Rorschach findings with trauma survivors (Kaser-Boyd, 2021) identifies Rorschach variables from both the Exner Comprehensive System (CS; Exner, 2003) and the R-PAS (Meyer et al., 2012). Kaser-Boyd (2021) reviewed research on torture victims and victims of child abuse, groups that likely met *ICD-11* criteria for CPTSD. Opaas and Hartmann (2013) studied 51 tortured and raped traumatized refugees from 15 countries. Of these protocols, 33% were too short for interpretation, which likely reflects avoidance of traumatic reminders (see Van der Kolk & Ducey, 1989), while the longer records were significant for the Trauma Content Index (TCI), SevCog, and FQ–%, reflecting trauma content, thought disturbance, and perceptual distortion. Zivney et al. (1988) examined the CS Rorschach records of 80 girls aged 9–16 with histories of severe sexual abuse and found that the most disturbed girls experienced early abuse. Over half of these girls manifested disturbed cognition (M−, DVs, and FABCOMs), scores associated with anxiety and helplessness (m and Y), and a preoccupation with themes of neediness and exposure (food and clothes, X-rays). Leifer et al. (1991) administered the Rorschach to 38 sexually abused girls who showed disturbed thinking and impaired reality testing, as well as high levels of distress and negative affect, primitive, disturbed human relationships, and increased sexual preoccupation.

The Rorschach CS has an important trauma indicator called the TCI (Armstrong & Loewenstein, 1990) measuring aggression, a damaged sense of self, sexual preoccupation, blood, and anatomy responses. The CS TCI (like the R-PAS Critical Contents Index) appears to be particularly useful in evaluating CPTSD. The TCI has been used to help identify victims of sexual abuse (Kamphuis et al., 2000) and individuals with dissociative identity disorder (Brand et al., 2006, 2009). Smith et al. (2020) studied incarcerated women with a history of sexual abuse and found the TCI to be high and correlated with the total number of reported traumatic events. Since there are no studies differentiating TSpD from BSDs, Rorschach PTSD/CPTSD trauma presentations will offer a place to start.

DIFFERENTIATING DDs FROM BSDs

The two most relevant DDs are dissociative identity disorder (DID) and the first type of other specified dissociative disorder (OSDD-1). DID is the most severe of the DDs and is characterized by a disruption of identity with two or more distinct personality states and recurring gaps in recollection of everyday events, important personal information, and/or traumatic events (American Psychiatric Association, 2022). OSDD-1 is diagnosed in the presence of chronic and recurrent mixed dissociative symptoms, such as identity disturbance with discontinuities of self without recurrent memory disturbances. OSDD-1 is similar to DID in that both include the presence of dissociative personality states, although dissociative amnesia is lacking in OSDD-1. DID and OSDD-1 share many characteristics and respond to similar types of psychotherapy, so the disorders are often discussed and studied simultaneously, including here.

Putnam (2016) argued that all humans shift states (e.g., wakeful to sleepy then asleep) and that many psychological disorders are characterized as "state change" disorders with shifts in patterns of emotion, behavior, cognition, and arousal that are accompanied by physiological changes. DID, OSDD-1, and BSDs are all state change disorders. Viewed through the lens of changes in state, it follows that DID/OSDD-1 (DD) show changes among state-dependent patterns of emotion, behavior, consciousness, memory, perception, cognition, and/or sensory-motor functioning, rather than the popular (and impossible) misconception that these individuals are essentially switching to different people.

Recognizing that DID, OSDD-1, and BSDs are characterized by significant state changes, it is understandable that the shifting of mood states in BSDs can be challenging to differentiate from the dissociative state changes in DD.

Contributing to the difficulty with differentiating these disorders is the reality that few clinicians receive systematic, evidence-based training about assessing and treating dissociation (Kumar et al., 2022). This lack of training about dissociation, along with misconceptions and myths about DDs, and the symptom complexity and comorbidity common among these DDs, contribute to clinicians failing to recognize and frequently misdiagnosing DDs (Brand, 2016; Brand, Sar, et al., 2016). As such, many clinicians expect patients with DID to present as they do in the movies (Loewenstein, 2018). In contrast to media portrayals, and misinformation sometimes presented about DDs in psychology textbooks (Brand et al., 2019; Wilgus et al., 2016), individuals with DID rarely present with markedly different, dramatic, "Sybil-like" switches.

In reality, DD is characterized by different states subtly shifting and overlapping, rather than theatrically "switching." Individuals with DID experience intrusions from dissociative self-states, such as hearing voices and passive influence phenomena, including feelings, thoughts and behaviors that may not seem to be "theirs" or that are experienced as beyond their control (Loewenstein, 2018). Although some individuals reporting DD proudly display their dissociated-self states on social media, most of these individuals try to avoid knowing about signs of the disorder to themselves as well as to others. Indeed, disowned, disavowed presentation is consistent with the function of dissociation in DD: It serves to hide, distance, and compartmentalize trauma-based emotions, conflicts, and memories.

Another myth is that DID is rare (Brand, Sar, et al., 2016). The lifetime prevalence of any DD ranges from approximately 9% to 18%, with DID occurring in approximately 1% of the general population, making it approximately as common as bipolar disorders and schizophrenia (Foote, 2018). The median prevalence among five outpatient studies was 2.5% (Foote, 2018).

DDs are considered childhood trauma disorders, while biological, genetic, and attachment-related vulnerabilities contribute to DD development (Loewenstein et al., 2017). People with DD report high levels of exposure to early, severe, and chronic child maltreatment (e.g., 95%–97% frequency), with maltreatment reported to have begun before age six, often with multiple abusers (Foote, 2018). Like nonmanic presentation BSDs, DDs are underdiagnosed. For example, Foote et al. (2006) found 29% of the patients met criteria for a DD, yet only 5% had been diagnosed in their medical record. If a patient's dissociation is not recognized, dissociative symptoms will not be treated. Research indicates that DD does not "go away" if not specifically treated, even with extensive trauma treatment (Jepsen et al., 2014). Individuals receive mental health treatment for 5 to 12 years before their DD is diagnosed, at the cost of prolonged suffering and demoralization (Loewenstein, 2018).

DD is often misdiagnosed as schizophrenia, bipolar disorder, and borderline personality disorder (Loewenstein et al., 2017). If DD is misdiagnosed as a BSD or other psychotic disorder, antipsychotic medications may be prescribed, resulting in potential side effects and lack of efficacy. Similarly, if DD is misdiagnosed when the shifts in mood are actually caused by undiagnosed BSDs, the individual is unlikely to receive the medications that are important for mood stabilization and functioning (American Psychiatric Association, 2022). Accurate differential diagnosis is crucial to successfully treating these particular groups of patients.

Individuals with DD typically struggle with several comorbid disorders, including PTSD, treatment resistant depression, substance use/abuse disorders, conversion disorder, somatic symptom disorder, eating disorders, obsessive compulsive disorder, sleep disorders, and traits of avoidant and borderline personality disorders (American Psychiatric Association, 2022; Foote, 2018). These individuals frequently hear voices; have rapid, perplexing shifts in mood and patterns of interacting with others, thinking, and feeling; high rates of suicide attempts and nonsuicidal self-injury; and frequent extensive dissociative symptoms including depersonalization, derealization, amnesia, identity alteration (outward manifestations of different dissociative self-states), and identity confusion (Foote, 2018; Loewenstein et al., 2017). A review of nine studies found that a median of 92% of the patients with DD reported hearing voices; rather than reflective of a psychotic process, these voices are thought to be the voices of dissociated-self states (Foote, 2018).

Individuals with DD usually present as depressed, obsessional, fearful, avoidant, and suffering from numerous somatic complaints, such as severe headaches (Foote, 2018). It is estimated that less than 5% are dramatic or histrionic in presentation (Loewenstein et al., 2017), although, if flooded with traumatic intrusions and dissociative phenomena, they may initially present like borderline or bipolar instability, including with brief periods of intermittent hypersexuality or hostility. DD is more likely the accurate diagnosis if the mood shifts do not last for more than several hours and if they begin and end abruptly, rather than emerging over a day or more, as is typical of BSDs. Furthermore, individuals with bipolar disorders would be expected to hear voices only during psychotic episodes, and their psychotic symptoms and mood instability typically respond to mood stabilizers and antipsychotics, whereas no medications resolve DD voices or mood shifts related to shifting self-states (Loewenstein et al., 2017).

Individuals with bipolar disorders would not be expected to score high on measures of dissociation unless they have experienced overwhelming trauma. Nor would individuals with BSDs report or show periods of amnesia (except perhaps briefly, if highly disorganized and psychotic), identity alteration (such as suddenly acting and feeling like a young child), or identity confusion (e.g., being confused about who they are because they hold such diverse and sometimes contradictory beliefs, emotions, and behaviors that are not circumscribed to mood episodes). Whereas patients with DD may experience their body as "not mine," patients with bipolar disorder do not feel separate or disconnected from their bodies.

Individuals can have BSDs comorbid with DD (Bakim et al., 2016; Tekin et al., 2013). Patients with comorbid DD and bipolar disorders have more severe pathology, as indicated by longer hospitalizations, earlier onset of illness, and more suicide attempts (Bakim et al., 2016; Tekin et al., 2013). Such individuals are prone to becoming manic when their sleep is disrupted for an extended period, and the mood instability due to bipolar disorders can be stabilized with mood stabilizers and antipsychotics. However, the mood shifts and auditory hallucinations due to DD continue persistently even when the manic states due to bipolar disorders are stabilized. Unfortunately, almost no research has compared the psychological testing performance of individuals with bipolar disorders to those with DD, although it would be fascinating and clinically useful. Even reviews of childhood trauma and bipolar disorders fail to review the role of dissociation (e.g., Duarte et al., 2020).

Interviews for Dissociative Disorders

There are two validated interviews, the Structured Clinical Interview for *DSM-IV* (SCID-D-R; Steinberg, 1994a, 1994b) and the Dissociative Disorders Interview Schedule (Ross et al., 1989). The SCID-D-R is considered the most rigorous of the interviews for making differential diagnoses. A meta-analysis indicated that the SCID-D-R can differentiate between DDs and other disorders (Mychailyszyn et al., 2021). The SCID-D-R's follow up questions would clarify nondissociative psychotic presentations and bipolar presentations from dissociative presentations.

Self-Report Measures of Dissociation

We highlight two of the dozen or more self-report measures that are likely to be most available and useful to practicing clinicians to screen for, rather than diagnose, dissociation. The Dissociative Experiences Scale (DES; Bernstein & Putnam, 1986) is the most widely used screen for dissociation. A meta-analysis found that the average DES score for DD individuals was 48.7 compared with bipolar spectrum individuals' average score of 14.8 (Lyssenko et al., 2018). The bipolar spectrum group had the lowest DES scores of 19 psychiatric disorders, with the trauma- and attachment-related disorders, including DDs, PTSD, and borderline personality disorder, ranking the highest and with DD the highest of all. This is consistent with DD being the most severe of the trauma-related disorders (Lyssenko et al., 2018).

The Multiscale Dissociation Inventory (MDI; Briere, 2002) is one of the few dissociation measures that has been standardized on a population-based sample and yields *T* scores. Ellickson-Larew et al. (2020) used MDI subscales, finding that dissociation was linked to almost all types of pathology they investigated.

Broadband Self-Report Methods

Minnesota Multiphasic Personality Inventory–2

The most common findings on the MMPI-2 (Butcher et al., 2001) for patients with DD are elevations on F and 8 (Schizophrenia) scales, which contain many trauma- and dissociation-related items, as well as Scales 2, 4, 6 and 7

(Brand & Chasson, 2015). Individuals with DD score so high on the F scale that their profiles are often technically invalid (Brand & Chasson, 2015). Few items on Scale 8 are frankly indicative of hallucinations and delusions, and many relate to problems with feeling negative toward oneself, feeling alienated and unloved by others, feeling unreal, and having memory problems. Such experiences are typical for many individuals with more severe DDs. Their item endorsement patterns are consistent with trauma exposure (Brand, Chasson, et al., 2016). DD MMPI-2 profiles would typically have higher elevations on validity as well as on most clinical scales. In contrast to individuals with bipolar disorders, those with DD are unlikely to elevate on 9 (Mania) and the Harris–Lingoes Mania subscales. Further, individuals with DD would likely be more socially introverted than those with bipolar disorders (0, Social Introversion).

Personality Assessment Inventory
Stadnik et al. (2013) found that 62% hospitalized patients with DD scored above the cutoff on the PAI's (Morey, 1991) Negative Impression scale (NIM). Research indicates that the NIM has questionable validity with complex trauma survivors, because of items related to memory problems, having dissociative self-states, and unhappy childhood experiences (Rogers et al., 2012). DD significantly predicted NIM scores above and beyond Depression and Borderline Features. The group with DD scored very high on PTSD, anxiety, depression, borderline symptoms, schizophrenia, and suicidal behavior and ideation (Stadnik et al., 2013). Notably, they were not high on the mania scale or subscales, unlike what would be expected for individuals with bipolar disorders.

The Trauma Symptom Inventory–2
Research indicates that individuals with DDs elevate on almost every clinical scale on the TSI-2 (Briere, 2011) including subscales related to anxiety, hyperarousal, depression, intrusions, avoidance, dissociation, somatic symptoms, suicidal ideation and behavior, relational avoidance and sensitivity, reduced self-awareness, excessive focus on others' needs, and discharging tension behaviorally often in self-destructive ways (Palermo & Brand, 2019). The authors are unaware of any study using the TSI-2 with bipolar spectrum individuals. If they have experienced trauma, they may elevate on many subscales, but if not, it would be unlikely they would elevate on the TSI-2.

Performance-Based/Projective Methods

The Rorschach can be a particularly useful measure for assessing trauma-related dissociation. DD Rorschach responses often illustrate how traumatic intrusions temporarily disrupt thinking and overwhelm accurate perception, and responses are interspersed with shutting down and dissociating. The Rorschach does not require trauma survivors to be aware of flooding and then defensively dissociating, as required on self-report measures. The Rorschach is uniquely helpful when the MMPI-2 or PAI are of questionable validity due to high levels of endorsement (Brand et al., 2006, 2009). If the client's thinking and reality testing appear intact until seeing traumatic images on the Rorschach, after which their thinking becomes distorted, disorganized, and illogical, they may have what Armstrong (2002) called a "traumatic thought disorder" rather than true psychosis.

Patients with DD are consistently found to elevate on the TCI, that is, the sum of Bl, Sx, An, AG, and MOR, divided by the number of responses (Armstrong, 1991; Brand et al., 2006, 2009). The mean TCI scores for 100 psychiatric inpatients diagnosed with DID or DDNOS was 0.50; this high score indicates a preoccupation with bodily integrity and sense of being damaged (Brand et al., 2006, 2009). Traumatic avoidance and traumatic intrusion were observed, along with a tendency to become caught up in complexity, distracted and scattered (low Lambda, high blends), yet with less blatant distortions of reality (X–) compared with patients with depression, acute stress disorder, or chronic PTSD. However, the patients with DD also showed heightened illogical thinking (WSum6). Their Rorschachs have not yet been directly compared with those of individuals with bipolar disorders.

The following clinical observations may inform the differential diagnostic process. Dissociative individuals show fearful reactions on the Rorschach, followed by avoidance, restriction, and/or dissociation when they see potentially traumatic imagery (TCI). In contrast, individuals with bipolar disorders tend to give lengthy, rapidly paced protocols replete with sexual, expansive, exploding, and/or otherwise energetic, chaotic percepts with no sign of fear after seeing potentially traumatic content. Many dissociative clients become so flooded with traumatic imagery that behavioral signs indicate they are overwhelmed. Some may refuse a card or push it away, which are attempts at self-protective avoidance. In individuals with bipolar disorders, evidence of poorly controlled ideation (e.g., INC and FAB) that is typical in mania would not be followed by emotional constriction, fear, or a dissociated reaction, as is more common among individuals with DD.

CONCLUSION

We believe that this chapter is the first comprehensive effort to differentiate BSDs from TSpD using multimethod psychological assessment. Throughout, we show the importance of how this discrimination leads to critical treatment decisions, especially with the overlap in symptoms and clinical presentations of BSDs from TSpD. We especially note that this chapter will hopefully spur future research and assessment practices.

REFERENCES

American Psychiatric Association. (1980). *Diagnostic and statistical manual of mental disorders: DSM III*.
American Psychiatric Association. (2022). *Diagnostic and statistical manual of mental disorders: DSM-5-TR* (5th ed., text rev.).

Armstrong, J. (1991). The psychological organization of multiple personality disordered patients as revealed in psychological testing. *The Psychiatric Clinics of North America, 14*(3), 533–546. https://doi.org/10.1016/S0193-953X(18)30288-0

Armstrong, J. G. (2002). Deciphering the broken narrative of trauma: Signs of traumatic dissociation on the Rorschach. *Rorschachiana, 25*(1), 11–27. https://doi.org/10.1027/1192-5604.25.1.11

Armstrong, J. G., & Loewenstein, R. J. (1990). Characteristics of patients with multiple personality and dissociative disorders on psychological testing. *The Journal of Nervous and Mental Disease, 178*(7), 448–454. https://doi.org/10.1097/00005053-199007000-00006

Azorin, J. M., Lefrere, A., & Belzeaux, R. (2021). The impact of bipolar disorder on couple functioning: Implications for care and treatment. A systematic review. *Medicina, 57*(8), Article 771. https://doi.org/10.3390/medicina57080771

Bakim, B., Baran, E., Güleken, M. D., Tankaya, O., Yayla, S., Akpınar, A., Sengul, H. S., Ertekin, H., Özer, Ö. A., & Karamustafalıoğlu, K. O. (2016). Comparison of the patient groups with and without dissociative disorder comorbidity among the inpatients with bipolar disorder. *Family Practice and Palliative Care, 1*(2), 35–42. https://doi.org/10.22391/920.256690

Bender, R. E., & Alloy, L. B. (2011). Life stress and kindling in bipolar disorder: Review of the evidence and integration with emerging biopsychosocial theories. *Clinical Psychology Review, 31*(3), 383–398. https://doi.org/10.1016/j.cpr.2011.01.004

Ben-Porath, Y. S., & Tellegen, A. (2008). *The Minnesota Multiphasic Personality Inventory–2 Restructured Form: Manual for administration, scoring, and interpretation.* University of Minnesota Press.

Ben-Porath, Y. S., & Tellegen, A. (2020). *MMPI-3 technical manual.* University of Minnesota Press.

Bernstein, E. M., & Putnam, F. W. (1986). Development, reliability, and validity of a dissociation scale. *Journal of Nervous and Mental Disease, 174*(12), 727–735. https://doi.org/10.1097/00005053-198612000-00004

Brand, B. L. (2016). The necessity of clinical training in trauma and dissociation. *Journal of Depression & Anxiety, 5*(4), Article 2167-1044. https://doi.org/10.4172/2167-1044.1000251

Brand, B. L., Armstrong, J. G., & Loewenstein, R. J. (2006). Psychological assessment of patients with dissociative identity disorder. *The Psychiatric Clinics of North America, 29*(1), 145–168. https://doi.org/10.1016/j.psc.2005.10.014

Brand, B. L., Armstrong, J. G., Loewenstein, R. J., & McNary, S. W. (2009). Personality differences on the Rorschach of dissociative identity disorder, borderline personality disorder, and psychotic inpatients. *Psychological Trauma: Theory, Research, Practice, and Policy, 1*(3), 188–205. https://doi.org/10.1037/a0016561

Brand, B. L., & Chasson, G. S. (2015). Distinguishing simulated from genuine dissociative identity disorder on the MMPI-2. *Psychological Trauma: Theory, Research, Practice, and Policy, 7*(1), 93–101. https://doi.org/10.1037/a0035181

Brand, B. L., Chasson, G. S., Palermo, C. A., Donato, F. M., Rhodes, K. P., & Voorhees, E. F. (2016). MMPI-2 item endorsements in dissociative identity disorder vs. simulators. *The Journal of the American Academy of Psychiatry and the Law, 44*(1), 63–72.

Brand, B. L., Kumar, S. A., & McEwen, L. E. (2019). Coverage of child maltreatment and adult trauma in graduate psychopathology textbooks. *Psychological Trauma: Theory, Research, Practice, and Policy, 11*(8), 919–926. https://doi.org/10.1037/tra0000454

Brand, B. L., Sar, V., Stavropoulos, P., Krüger, C., Korzekwa, M., Martínez-Taboas, A., & Middleton, W. (2016). Separating fact from fiction: An empirical examination of six myths about dissociative identity disorder. *Harvard Review of Psychiatry, 24*(4), 257–270. https://doi.org/10.1097/HRP.0000000000000100

Brewin, C. R., Cloitre, M., Hyland, P., Shevlin, M., Maercker, A., Bryant, R. A., Humayun, A., Jones, L. M., Kagee, A., Rousseau, C., Somasundaram, D., Suzuki, Y.,

Wessely, S., van Ommeren, M., & Reed, G. M. (2017). A review of current evidence regarding the *ICD-11* proposals for diagnosing PTSD and complex PTSD. *Clinical Psychology Review, 58*, 1–15. https://doi.org/10.1016/j.cpr.2017.09.001

Briere, J. (2000). *Inventory of Altered Self Capacities (IASC)*. Psychological Assessment Resources.

Briere, J. (2002). *The Multiscale Dissociation Inventory: Professional manual*. Psychological Assessment Resources.

Briere, J. (2011). *Trauma Symptom Inventory–2 professional manual*. Psychological Assessment Resources.

Briere, J., & Runtz, M. D. (2002). The Inventory of Altered Self-Capacities (IASC): A standardized measure of identity, affect regulation, and relationship disturbance. *Assessment, 9*(3), 230–239. https://doi.org/10.1177/1073191102009003002

Briere, J., & Spinazzola, J. (2005). Phenomenology and psychological assessment of complex posttraumatic states. *Journal of Traumatic Stress, 18*(5), 401–412. https://doi.org/10.1002/jts.20048

Butcher, J. N., Dahlstrom, W. G., Graham, J. R., Tellegen, A., & Kaemmer, B. (1989). *Manual for the Restandardized Minnesota Multiphasic Personality Inventory: MMPI-2*. University of Minnesota.

Butcher, J. N., Graham, J. R., Ben-Porath, Y. S., Tellegen, A., & Dahlstrom, W. G. (2001). *Manual for the administration and scoring of the MMPI-2*. University of Minnesota Press.

Carlson, E. B., Smith, S. R., Palmieri, P. A., Dalenberg, C., Ruzek, J. I., Kimerling, R., Burling, T. A., & Spain, D. A. (2011). Development and validation of a brief self-report measure of trauma exposure: The Trauma History Screen. *Psychological Assessment, 23*(2), 463–477. https://doi.org/10.1037/a0022294

Cerimele, J. M., Bauer, A. M., Fortney, J. C., & Bauer, M. S. (2017). Patients with co-occurring bipolar disorder and posttraumatic stress disorder. *The Journal of Clinical Psychiatry, 78*(5), e506–e514. https://doi.org/10.4088/JCP.16r10897

Dalenberg, C. J., Brand, B. L., Gleaves, D. H., Dorahy, M. J., Loewenstein, R. J., Cardeña, E., Frewen, P. A., Carlson, E. B., & Spiegel, D. (2012). Evaluation of the evidence for the trauma and fantasy models of dissociation. *Psychological Bulletin, 138*(3), 550–588. https://doi.org/10.1037/a0027447

Duarte, D., Belzeaux, R., Etain, B., Greenway, K. T., Rancourt, E., Correa, H., Turecki, G., & Richard-Devantoy, S. (2020). Childhood-maltreatment subtypes in bipolar patients with suicidal behavior: Systematic review and meta-analysis. *Revista Brasileira de Psiquiatria, 42*(5), 558–567. https://doi.org/10.1590/1516-4446-2019-0592

Ellickson-Larew, S., Stasik-O'Brien, S. M., Stanton, K., & Watson, D. (2020). Dissociation as a multidimensional transdiagnostic symptom. *Psychology of Consciousness, 7*(2), 126–150. https://doi.org/10.1037/cns0000218

Evans, F. B., II. (2016) *Posttraumatic stress disorder diagnosis and assessment: A forensic overview* [Conference session]. Continuing Education Workshop at the American Psychological Association Annual Convention, Denver, CO, United States.

Exner, J. E. (2003). *The Rorschach: A comprehensive system: Vol. 1. Basic foundations and principles of interpretation* (4th ed.). Wiley.

Fawcett, J. (2008). What we have learned from the systematic enhancement program for bipolar disorder (STEP-BD) study. *Psychiatric Annals, 38*(7), 450–456. https://doi.org/10.3928/00485713-20080701-02

Foa, E. B., McLean, C. P., Zang, Y., Zhong, J., Powers, M. B., Kauffman, B. Y., Rauch, S., Porter, K., & Knowles, K. (2016). Psychometric properties of the Posttraumatic Diagnostic Scale for *DSM-5* (PDS-5). *Psychological Assessment, 28*(10), 1166–1171. https://doi.org/10.1037/pas0000258

Follette, W. C., Naugle, A. E., & Follette, V. M. (1997). MMPI-2 profiles of adult women with child sexual abuse histories: Cluster-analytic findings. *Journal of Consulting and Clinical Psychology, 65*(5), 858–866. https://doi.org/10.1037/0022-006X.65.5.858

Foote, B. (2018, June 19). *Dissociative identity disorder: Epidemiology, pathogenesis, clinical manifestations, course, assessment, and diagnosis.* https://www.uptodate.com/contents/dissociative-identity-disorder-epidemiology-pathogenesis-clinical-manifestations-course-assessment-and-diagnosis

Foote, B., Smolin, Y., Kaplan, M., Legatt, M. E., & Lipschitz, D. (2006). Prevalence of dissociative disorders in psychiatric outpatients. *The American Journal of Psychiatry, 163*(4), 623–629. https://doi.org/10.1176/ajp.2006.163.4.623

Freyd, J. J. (1996). *Betrayal trauma: The logic of forgetting childhood abuse.* Harvard University Press.

Galatzer-Levy, I. R., & Bryant, R. A. (2013). 636,120 ways to have posttraumatic stress disorder. *Perspectives on Psychological Science, 8*(6), 651–662. https://doi.org/10.1177/1745691613504115

Goldberg, J. F., & Fagin-Jones, S. (2004). Diagnosing and treating anxiety comorbidity in bipolar disorders. *Psychiatric Annals, 34*(11), 874–884. https://doi.org/10.3928/0048-5713-20041101-16

Griffith, P. L., Myers, R. W., Cusick, G. M., & Tankersley, M. J. (1998). MMPI-2 profiles of women differing in sexual abuse history and sexual orientation. *Journal of Clinical Psychology, 53*(8), 791–800. https://doi.org/10.1002/(SICI)1097-4679(199712)53:8<791::AID-JCLP2>3.0.CO;2-J

Herman, J. L. (1992). Complex PTSD: A syndrome in survivors of prolonged and repeated trauma. *Journal of Traumatic Stress, 5*(3), 377–391. https://doi.org/10.1002/jts.2490050305

Hernandez, J. M., Cordova, M. J., Ruzek, J., Reiser, R., Gwizdowski, I. S., Suppes, T., & Ostacher, M. J. (2013). Presentation and prevalence of PTSD in a bipolar disorder population: A STEP-BD examination. *Journal of Affective Disorders, 150*(2), 450–455. https://doi.org/10.1016/j.jad.2013.04.038

Jepsen, E. K. K., Langeland, W., Sexton, H., & Heir, T. (2014). Inpatient treatment for early sexually abused adults: A naturalistic 12-month follow-up study. *Psychological Trauma: Theory, Research, Practice, and Policy, 6*(2), 142–151. https://doi.org/10.1037/a0031646

Kahneman, D., Slovic, P., & Tversky, A. (Eds.). (1982). *Judgment under uncertainty: Heuristics and biases.* Cambridge University Press. https://doi.org/10.1017/CBO9780511809477

Kamphuis, J. H., Kugeares, S. L., & Finn, S. E. (2000). Rorschach correlates of sexual abuse: Trauma content and aggression indexes. *Journal of Personality Assessment, 75*(2), 212–224. https://doi.org/10.1207/S15327752JPA7502_3

Kaser-Boyd, N. (2021). The Rorschach and trauma: An update. *Rorschachiana, 42*(2), 118–138. https://doi.org/10.1027/1192-5604/a000133

Khan, F. I., Welch, T. L., & Zillmer, E. A. (2010). MMPI-2 profiles of battered women in transition. *Journal of Personality Assessment, 60*(1), 100–111. https://doi.org/10.1207/s15327752jpa6001_7

Kumar, S. A., Brand, B. L., & Courtois, C. A. (2022). The need for trauma training: Clinicians' reactions to training on complex trauma. *Psychological Trauma: Theory, Research, Practice, and Policy, 14*(8), 1387–1394. https://doi.org/10.1037/tra0000515

Leifer, M., Shapiro, J. P., Martone, M. W., & Kassem, L. (1991). Rorschach assessment of psychological functioning in sexually abused girls. *Journal of Personality Assessment, 56*(1), 14–28. https://doi.org/10.1207/s15327752jpa5601_2

Litvin, J. M., Kaminski, P. L., & Riggs, S. A. (2017). The Complex Trauma Inventory: A self-report measure of posttraumatic stress disorder and complex posttraumatic stress disorder. *Journal of Traumatic Stress, 30*(6), 602–613. https://doi.org/10.1002/jts.22231

Loewenstein, R. J. (2018). Dissociation debates: Everything you know is wrong. *Dialogues in Clinical Neuroscience, 20*(3), 229–242. https://doi.org/10.31887/DCNS.2018.20.3/rloewenstein

Loewenstein, R. J., Frewen, P. A., & Lewis-Fernández, R. (2017). Dissociative disorders. In B. J. Sadock, V. A. Sadock, & P. Ruiz (Eds.), *Kaplan & Sadock's comprehensive textbook of psychiatry* (10th ed., Vol. 1, pp. 1866–1952). Wolters Kluwer; Lippincott Williams & Wilkins.

Lyssenko, L., Schmahl, C., Bockhacker, L., Vonderlin, R., Bohus, M., & Kleindienst, N. (2018). Dissociation in psychiatric disorders: A meta-analysis of studies using the Dissociative Experiences Scale. *The American Journal of Psychiatry, 175*(1), 37–46. https://doi.org/10.1176/appi.ajp.2017.17010025

Maguire, C., McCusker, C. G., Meenagh, C., Mulholland, C., & Shannon, C. (2008). Effects of trauma on bipolar disorder: The mediational role of interpersonal difficulties and alcohol dependence. *Bipolar Disorders, 10*(2), 293–302. https://doi.org/10.1111/j.1399-5618.2007.00504.x

Malkoff-Schwartz, S., Frank, E., Anderson, B., Sherrill, J. T., Siegel, L., Patterson, D., & Kupfer, D. J. (1998). Stressful life events and social rhythm disruption in the onset of manic and depressive bipolar episodes: A preliminary investigation. *Archives of General Psychiatry, 55*(8), 702–707. https://doi.org/10.1001/archpsyc.55.8.702

McNally, R. J. (2012). Are we winning the war against posttraumatic stress disorder? *Science, 336*(6083), 872–874. https://doi.org/10.1126/science.1222069

Merikangas, K. R., Akiskal, H. S., Angst, J., Greenberg, P. E., Hirschfeld, R. M., Petukhova, M., & Kessler, R. C. (2007). Lifetime and 12-month prevalence of bipolar spectrum disorder in the National Comorbidity Survey replication. *Archives of General Psychiatry, 64*(5), 543–552. https://doi.org/10.1001/archpsyc.64.5.543

Meyer, G. J., Viglione, D. J., Mihura, J. L., Erard, R. E., & Erdberg, P. (2011). *Rorschach Performance Assessment System: Administration, coding, interpretation and technical manual.* Rorschach Performance Assessment System.

Meyer, G. J., Viglione, D. J., Mihura, J. L., Erard, R. E., & Erdberg, P. (2012). *A manual for the Rorschach Performance Assessment System.* Rorschach Performance Assessment System.

Millon, T., Grossman, S., & Millon, C. (2015). *Millon Clinical Multiaxial Inventory–IV (MCMI-IV).* Pearson Assessments.

Monroe, S. M., & Simons, A. D. (1991). Diathesis-stress theories in the context of life stress research: Implications for the depressive disorders. *Psychological Bulletin, 110*(3), 406–425. https://doi.org/10.1037/0033-2909.110.3.406

Morey, L. C. (1991). *Personality Assessment Inventory.* Psychological Assessment Resources.

Morey, L. C., & Boggs, C. (2007). *Personality Assessment Inventory (PAI).* Psychological Assessment Resources.

Morrell, J. B., & Rubin, L. J. (2001). The Minnesota Multiphasic Personality Inventory–2, posttraumatic stress disorder, and women domestic violence survivors. *Professional Psychology: Research and Practice, 32*(2), 151–156. https://doi.org/10.1037/0735-7028.32.2.151

Mueser, K. T., Goodman, L. B., Trumbetta, S. L., Rosenberg, S. D., Osher, C., Vidaver, R., Auciello, P., & Foy, D. W. (1998). Trauma and posttraumatic stress disorder in severe mental illness. *Journal of Consulting and Clinical Psychology, 66*(3), 493–499. https://doi.org/10.1037/0022-006X.66.3.493

Mychailyszyn, M. P., Brand, B. L., Webermann, A. R., Şar, V., & Draijer, N. (2021). Differentiating dissociative from non-dissociative disorders: A meta-analysis of the Structured Clinical Interview for *DSM* Dissociative Disorders (SCID-D). *Journal of Trauma & Dissociation, 22*(1), 19–34. https://doi.org/10.1080/15299732.2020.1760169

Nichols, D. S. (2011). *Essentials of MMPI-2 assessment* (2nd ed.). Wiley.

Opaas, M., & Hartmann, E. (2013). Rorschach assessment of traumatized refugees: An exploratory factor analysis. *Journal of Personality Assessment, 95*(5), 457–470. https://doi.org/10.1080/00223891.2013.781030

Orsillo, S. M., Weathers, F. W., Litz, B. T., Steinberg, H. R., Huska, J. A., & Keane, T. M. (1996). Current and lifetime psychiatric disorders among veterans with war zone-related posttraumatic stress disorder. *Journal of Nervous and Mental Disease, 184*(5), 307–313. https://doi.org/10.1097/00005053-199605000-00007

Otto, M. W., Perlman, C. A., Wernicke, R., Reese, H. E., Bauer, M. S., & Pollack, M. H. (2004). Posttraumatic stress disorder in patients with bipolar disorder: A review of prevalence, correlates, and treatment strategies. *Bipolar Disorders, 6*(6), 470–479. https://doi.org/10.1111/j.1399-5618.2004. 00151.x

Palermo, C. A., & Brand, B. L. (2019). Can the Trauma Symptom Inventory–2 distinguish coached simulators from dissociative disorder patients? *Psychological Trauma: Theory, Research, Practice, and Policy, 11*(5), 477–485. https://doi.org/10. 1037/tra0000382

Phelps, J. (2016). *A spectrum approach to mood disorders: Not fully bipolar but not unipolar— Practical management.* W. W. Norton.

Post, R. M., Ketter, T. A., Speer, A. M., Leverich, G. S., & Weiss, S. R. B. (2000). Predictive validity of the sensitization and kindling hypotheses. In J. C. Soares & S. Gershon (Eds.), *Bipolar disorders: Basic mechanisms and therapeutic implications* (pp. 387–432). Marcel Dekker.

Putnam, F. W. (1997). *Dissociation in children and adolescents: A developmental perspective.* Guilford Press.

Putnam, F. W. (2016). *The way we are: How states of mind influence our identities, personality, and potential for change.* International Psychoanalytic Books.

Regeer, E. J., Kupka, R. W., Have, M. T., Vollebergh, W., & Nolen, W. A. (2015). Low self-recognition and awareness of past hypomanic and manic episodes in the general population. *International Journal of Bipolar Disorders, 3*(1), Article 22. https://doi.org/10. 1186/s40345-015-0039-8

Robinson, J. S., & Larson, C. (2010). Are traumatic events necessary to elicit symptoms of posttraumatic stress? *Psychological Trauma: Theory, Research, Practice, and Policy, 2*(2), 71–76. https://doi.org/10.1037/a0018954

Rogers, R., Gillard, N. D., Wooley, C. N., & Ross, C. A. (2012). The detection of feigned disabilities: The effectiveness of the Personality Assessment Inventory in a traumatized inpatient sample. *Assessment, 19*(1), 77–88. https://doi.org/10.1177/ 1073191111422031

Rosenthal, D. (1970). *Genetic theory and abnormal behavior.* McGraw-Hill.

Ross, C. A., Heber, S., Norton, G. R., & Anderson, D. (1989). The Dissociative Disorders Interview Schedule: A structured interview. *Dissociation: Progress in the Dissociative Disorders, 2*(3), 169–189.

Sellbom, M., Lee, T. T., Ben-Porath, Y. S., Arbisi, P. A., & Gervais, R. O. (2012). Differentiating PTSD symptomatology with the MMPI-2-RF (restructured form) in a forensic disability sample. *Psychiatry Research, 197*(1–2), 172–179. https://doi.org/10. 1016/j.psychres.2012.02.003

Smith, J. M., Gacono, C. B., & Cunliffe, T. B. (2020). Using the Rorschach Trauma Content Index (TCI) with incarcerated women. *Journal of Projective Psychology & Mental Health, 27*(1), 12–20.

Spitzer, R. L., First, M. B., Gibbon, M., & Williams, J. B. (1990). *Structured Clinical Interview for* DSM-III-R. American Psychiatric Association.

Stadnik, R. D., Brand, B., & Savoca, A. (2013). Personality Assessment Inventory profile and predictors of elevations among dissociative disorder patients. *Journal of Trauma & Dissociation, 14*(5), 546–561. https://doi.org/10.1080/15299732.2013. 792310

Steinberg, M. (1994a). *Interviewer's guide to the Structured Clinical Interview for* DSM-IV *Dissociative Disorders (SCID-D)* (rev. ed.). American Psychiatric Association.

Steinberg, M. (1994b). *The Structured Clinical Interview for* DSM-IV *Dissociative Disorders Revised (SCID-D-R).* American Psychiatric Association.

Tekin, A., Ozdil, E., Guleken, M. D., Bakim, B., Ozer, O. A., & Karamustafalioglu, O. (2013). Dissociation and childhood trauma in patients with bipolar disorder. *Klinik Psikofarmakoloji Bulteni, 23,* Article S178.

Van der Kolk, B. A., & Ducey, C. P. (1989). The psychological processing of traumatic experience: Rorschach patterns in PTSD. *Journal of Traumatic Stress, 2*(3), 259–274. https://doi.org/10.1002/jts.2490020303

van der Kolk, B. A., Roth, S., Pelcovitz, D., Sunday, S., & Spinazzola, J. (2005). Disorders of extreme stress: The empirical foundation of a complex adaptation to trauma. *Journal of Traumatic Stress, 18*(5), 389–399. https://doi.org/10.1002/jts.20047

Watson, C., Quilty, L. C., & Bagby, M. (2010). Differentiating bipolar disorder from major depressive disorder using the MMPI-2-RF. *Journal of Psychopathology and Behavioral Assessment, 33*(3), 368–374. https://doi.org/10.1007/s10862-010-9212-7

Weathers, F. W., Blake, D. D., Schnurr, P. P., Kaloupek, D. G., Marx, B. P., & Keane, T. M. (2013). *The Life Events Checklist for DSM-5 (LEC-5).* National Center for PTSD. https://www.ptsd.va.gov/professional/assessment/te-measures/life_events_checklist.asp

Weathers, F. W., Bovin, M. J., Lee, D. J., Sloan, D. M., Schnurr, P. P., Kaloupek, D. G., Keane, T. M., & Marx, B. P. (2018). The Clinician-Administered PTSD Scale for *DSM-5* (CAPS-5): Development and initial psychometric evaluation in military veterans. *Psychological Assessment, 30*(3), 383–395. https://doi.org/10.1037/pas0000486

Weathers, F. W., Litz, B. T., Keane, T. M., Palmieri, P. A., Marx, B. P., & Schnurr, P. P. (2013). *The PTSD Checklist for DSM-5 (PCL-5).* National Center for PTSD. https://www.ptsd.va.gov/professional/assessment/adult-sr/ptsd-checklist.asp

Weiner, I. B. (2014). *Principles of Rorschach interpretation* (2nd ed.). Routledge.

Wilgus, S. J., Packer, M. M., Lile-King, R., Miller-Perrin, C. L., & Brand, B. L. (2016). Coverage of child maltreatment in abnormal psychology textbooks: Reviewing the adequacy of the content. *Psychological Trauma: Theory, Research, Practice, and Policy, 8*(2), 188–197. https://doi.org/10.1037/tra0000049

Wolf, E. J., Miller, M. W., Orazem, R. J., Weierich, M. R., Castillo, D. T., Milford, J., Kaloupek, D. G., & Keane, T. M. (2008). The MMPI-2 restructured clinical scales in the assessment of posttraumatic stress disorder and comorbid disorders. *Psychological Assessment, 20*(4), 327–340. https://doi.org/10.1037/a0012948

World Health Organization. (2019). *International statistical classification of diseases and related health problems* (11th ed.).

Zivney, O. A., Nash, M. R., & Hulsey, T. L. (1988). Sexual abuse in early versus late childhood: Differing patterns of pathology as revealed on the Rorschach. *Psychotherapy: Theory, Research, Practice, Training, 25*(1), 99–106. https://doi.org/10.1037/h0085328

16

Assessment of Bipolar Spectrum Disorders and Schizophrenia

James H. Kleiger and Ali Khadivi

Distinguishing individuals with bipolar and schizophrenia spectrum disorders can be a challenging diagnostic task for assessment psychologists. Some may ask why this is the case. After all, for more than a century, diagnosticians have separated the disorders into distinct categories of severe psychopathology. Beginning with Kraepelin's distinction between dementia praecox and manic depressive insanity (Kraepelin, 1896/1921a, 1921b), and through multiple iterations in the *Diagnostic and Statistical Manual of Mental Disorders* (*DSM*) and *International Statistical Classification of Diseases and Related Health Problems* (*ICD*), schizophrenia and bipolar disorders have been categorized as different families of mental disorders. However, despite this traditional categorical approach, the boundary between the disorders is not clearly delineated, making differential diagnosis a practical challenge for assessment psychologists.

In this chapter, we examine conceptual and diagnostic issues that make the distinction between bipolar and schizophrenia spectrum disorders a challenge and then look at the distinguishing features of these disorders. In discussing the role of assessment, we will not duplicate instrument-specific findings presented in Parts I and II of this volume, which highlight the role of self-report and performance-based methods in diagnosing bipolar spectrum disorders. Instead, our task is to review contemporary issues and controversies and to identify areas in which schizophrenia and bipolar disorders overlap and diverge, in order to aid in differential diagnostic decision making.

https://doi.org/10.1037/0000356-017
Psychological Assessment of Bipolar Spectrum Disorders, J. H. Kleiger and I. B. Weiner (Editors)

DIAGNOSTIC CRITERIA, CONTROVERSIES, AND SYMPTOM DIMENSIONS

Skill in differential diagnosis requires an understanding of the diagnostic criteria and familiarity with key concepts, symptoms, and controversies. In this section, we review (a) core diagnostic criteria for the spectrum of schizophrenia and bipolar disorders, (b) the diversity of conditions within each spectrum, (c) the lack of clear boundaries separating schizophrenia and bipolar disorders, (d) psychosis as the key area of symptom overlap, and finally, (e) the differences in nature and degrees of cognitive impairment and other characteristics of schizophrenia and bipolar disorders.

Diagnostic Criteria

In the *Diagnostic and Statistical Manual of Mental Disorders* (5th ed., text rev.; *DSM-5-TR*; American Psychiatric Association, 2022), schizophrenia and related conditions are defined by abnormalities in at least one of the several symptom dimensions: delusions, hallucinations, disorganized thinking/speech, negative symptom, and severely disorganized or catatonic behavior, which constitute Criterion A. For all major schizophrenia spectrum disorders (with the exception of schizotypal personality disorder), at least of one of the symptoms must be hallucinations, delusions, or disorganized speech.

As a part of the schizophrenia spectrum, schizoaffective disorder requires Criterion A of schizophrenia together with concurrent major mood episodes. In addition, either delusions or hallucinations need to be present for at least 2 weeks in the absence of depression or mania, and major mood episodes must be present for the majority of the total lifetime duration of the illness. Schizoaffective disorders are specified as either bipolar or depressive type.

Diagnosis of bipolar and related disorders (Types I and II, cyclothymia, substance/medication-induced, and other specified) requires a manic (for bipolar Type I) or hypomanic (for bipolar Type II) episode, along with a major depressive episode. For Type I bipolar disorder, Criterion A specifies that a distinctly elevated, expansive, or irritable mood and increased goal-directed behavior or heightened energy level must be present for a week (Type I) or 4 days (Type II). Criterion B requires at least three behavioral or psychological features that mark a significant change from baseline functioning. These symptoms include (a) inflated self-esteem or grandiosity; (b) decreased need for sleep; (c) more talkative or increased pressure to continue talking; (d) flight of ideas or subjective experience of racing thoughts; (e) distractibility; (f) increase in goal-directed activity socially, at work, or in school; (g) pursuit of sexual activity, or psychomotor agitation; and (h) excessive participation in risky activities that could have negative consequences (e.g., spending, investing, or sexual activities). A major depressive episode is defined by five or more standard symptoms of depression, which must be concurrent over a 2-week period (see *DSM-5-TR* criteria for a major depressive episode; American Psychiatric Association, 2022).

ICD-11 (World Health Organization [WHO], 2019) diagnosis of schizophrenia symptoms mirrors those in *ICD-10* (WHO, 1992). As in *DSM-5* (American Psychiatric Association, 2013), subtypes of schizophrenia were removed because their validity could not be established. However, like *DSM-5* and *DSM-5-TR*, *ICD-11* introduced a set of symptom dimensions, including positive and negative symptoms, cognitive impairment, and mood-related symptoms (depression and mania).

Immediately noticeable is the fact that, unlike the schizophrenia spectrum, psychosis is not a defining characteristic of bipolar-related disorders. Psychotic features may or may not accompany bipolar disorders. Furthermore, when present, psychotic features are tagged by a specifier noting whether the psychotic features are either congruent or incongruent with the predominant mood. Thus, on the bases of *DSM-5* diagnostic criteria, schizophrenia and bipolar spectrum disorders differ in terms of whether the primary symptoms include psychosis, mood disturbance, or a blend of both. Similarly, core symptoms of mania or hypomania characterized by persistently irritable, elevated, and expansive mood, combined with increased energy or goal-directed activities, are not a defining feature of schizophrenia spectrum disorders.

Categories, Spectrums, and Continuums

Whether disorders are best viewed as distinct categories, spectrums of related disorders within each category, or disturbances along a broader continuum of transdiagnostic symptoms, with overlapping boundaries and varying degrees of severity, are controversial issues in how psychopathology is classified and understood.

Separate and Distinct Disorders

Kraepelin (1896/1921a) proposed a simple categorical framework for classifying dementia praecox (schizophrenia) and manic-depression as separate disorders, each with a distinct course. Increasingly, categorical schemas have given way to diagnostic frameworks that view both disorders as more diverse and continuous in nature. For example, recent versions of the *DSM* no longer classify schizophrenia as a single disorder but as a spectrum of schizophrenia and related psychotic disorders (American Psychiatric Association, 1994, 2013, 2022). Thus, the boundaries were expanded to include associated conditions. As discussed in the Introduction to this volume, the classification of bipolar disorders is complex. Authors of the *DSM-5* rejected a unitary Kraepelinian concept of manic-depression and split bipolar and depressive disorders into separate categories that included related conditions varying in form and severity. Thus, one could argue that there are spectrums of depressive and bipolar disorders. However, some urged a return to Kraepelin's unitary manic-depression concept and advocated for a broader spectrum approach to mood disorders including depressive and bipolar disorders (Cassano et al., 2004; Phelps, 2016).

Regardless of whether there should be a return to a unitary concept of a mood or manic depressive spectrum, both schizophrenia and bipolar disorders are now viewed as two fairly heterogeneous categories of severe mental disorders. Thus, *DSM*-5 introduced a spectrum model within each category, while, at the same time, retaining set boundaries between the two. The key point is that, even if the boundaries were firm (which they are not), variability within each category increases the complexity of differential diagnosis.

Overlapping Disorders as a Continuum

To make matters more interesting and challenging, the spectrum concept has also been considered from a broader, transdiagnostic perspective. Despite Kraepelin's categorical distinction between dementia praecox and manic-depression, which influenced the direction of modern diagnostic classification systems, the boundaries between schizophrenia and manic-depression have long been questioned. Luminaries like Karl Jaspers addressed these imprecise boundaries, raising questions about whether the two disorders were best understood as a continuum as opposed to discrete categories (Jaspers, 1946/1963).

Contemporary researchers have questioned the traditional distinction (Allardyce et al., 2007; van Os, 2015) and wondered whether their symptoms actually distinguish between the two disorders (Kendell & Jablensky, 2003; M. A. Taylor, 1992; van Os et al., 2009). Based on shared symptoms and similarities in neurobiological, cognitive, and genetic factors, others view the categorical separation as a reified vestige of Kraepelinian classification and argue, instead, for a broader continuum of severe psychopathology (Buckley et al., 2004; Demily et al., 2009; Ketter et al., 2004; Lapierre, 1994; Möller, 2003). These authors proposed a psychosis continuum from mood disorders to schizophrenia, with bipolar and schizoaffective disorders falling in the intermediate range between depression and schizophrenia (Crow, 1986; Rosen et al., 2012).

Despite the interest in a schizophrenia–bipolar continuum, other experts pointed to differing degrees of brain abnormalities, premorbid cognitive impairment, and developmental risk factors that support the categorical separation of schizophrenia and bipolar disorders (Lawrie et al., 2010; Murray et al., 2004). These critics argued that the continuum model was too simplistic and overlooked cognitive and affective differences between the two illness spectrums (Sorella et al., 2019). Instead, they proposed an expanded view of the continuum hypothesis, in which there is a shared psychotic neural core complemented by separate cognitive and affective networks. The neurological substrata of the cognitive core are more impaired in schizophrenia, while the affective neural network may be more compromised in bipolar disorders.

The dialectic between continua versus categorical models remains a diagnostic Scylla and Charybdis that bedevils efforts to identify the similarities and differences between schizophrenia and bipolar disorders. Some patients may appear typical for one of the categories, making differential diagnosis less problematic. However, others appear to straddle the boundaries and are referred for psychological evaluations to help make a differential diagnosis. Although no general consensus exists, assessment psychologists should be familiar with arguments supporting dimensional, categorical, or mixed models, which ultimately form the basis for inferences about differential diagnosis.

Psychosis

Whereas psychosis is a primary diagnostic feature in schizophrenia, it is a secondary marker in bipolar disorders. Up until the 1970s, psychotic features in patients with bipolar disorders were neglected, in part because bipolar disorders were underdiagnosed in the United States, while schizophrenia was overdiagnosed (Pope & Lipinski, 1978). As a result, bipolar psychosis was not well understood. However, another reason for this lack of attention is that, unlike the schizophrenia spectrum, not all individuals with bipolar disorders present with psychosis. Broadening the boundaries of bipolarity may conceivably decrease the likelihood that individuals within the broader spectrum will present with psychotic symptoms. However, studies have not necessarily shown this to be the case. Lifetime prevalence of psychotic features in those suffering from bipolar disorders is more common than many might suspect (van Bergen et al., 2019). Studies have found that between 42% and 74% of patients with bipolar disorders presented with psychotic symptoms (Kennedy et al., 2005; Yildiz & Sachs, 2003). When the subjects are restricted to bipolar I disorder, the incidence of psychoses tends to be even higher. In contrast, research has shown a comparatively lower occurrence of psychotic features in subjects diagnosed with bipolar II disorder (Mazzarini et al., 2010). Overall findings indicate that at least 50% of patients with bipolar disorders experience psychotic symptoms at some point. It seems logical that psychotic features would portend a poorer outcome for those suffering from bipolar disorders. However, counterintuitively, a recent study found this not to be the case (Burton et al., 2017).

Overlapping Psychotic Features in Schizophrenia and Bipolar Psychoses

There is substantial overlap in the phenomenology of psychotic symptoms in schizophrenia and bipolar disorders. Shared symptoms are those that define a psychotic episode. Thus, psychotic episodes in both conditions must include delusions, hallucinations, and/or disorganized speech (formal thought disorder [FTD]), and possibly catatonia. Delusions may be paranoid or grandiose in nature. Thinking and speech may be disorganized to the point of incoherence.

Until the 1970s, certain qualities of psychotic phenomena were thought pathognomonic of schizophrenia. Schneiderian first-rank symptoms (FRS; Schneider, 1959) included delusions of control and influence; thought broadcasting, insertion, and withdrawal, and auditory hallucinations characterized by a running commentary on one's behavior. Schneider thought these symptoms were hallmarks of schizophrenia, whereas other types of hallucinations, delusions, and thought disorders were second-rank symptoms.

Beginning in the 1970s, studies showed considerable overlap in psychotic symptoms between both disorders (Lipkin et al., 1970; Pope & Lipinski, 1978), as well as the lack of diagnostic specificity of FRS. Although they may have utility as a screening tool, they lack sensitivity and specificity in schizophrenia (Carpenter et al., 1973; Soares-Weiser et al., 2015). However, some have found that FRS are actually more frequent in schizophrenia than in bipolar psychosis (Parameshwara et al., 2017). In their study, Parameshwara et al. found FRS in 88% of patients with schizophrenia compared to only 35% of those with bipolar disorder. However, this study was not restricted to bipolar psychosis and, instead, included a larger sample of subjects with bipolar disorders.

Schizophrenia-Specific Features
Initial symptoms of schizophrenia typically include hallucinations, delusions, and disorganized speech or behavior (Goldstein et al., 2007). Disorganized speech may be classified as either positive or negative thought disorder (Andreasen, 1979a, 1979b). The former is characterized by derailment or distractibility. Disorganized speech may also include clanging associations and, at its most extreme level, become incoherent. In contrast, negative thought disorder reflects restricted thought processes with a poverty of speech and thought content. Speech may be halting and contain peculiar word usage, including neologisms, and reasoning may be patently illogical. Andreasen and Grove (1986) found negative thought disorder more characteristic of schizophrenia. Furthermore, negative thought disorder symptoms are more likely to persist in schizophrenia and to be a strong predictor of poorer outcomes.

The onset of schizophrenia typically occurs in the 20s but may occur in adolescence and, more rarely, childhood. Paranoid delusions and auditory hallucinations occur most commonly in later onset (after age 20) while early onset shows greater negative symptoms and disorganization (Kirkpatrick et al., 2000). The course and progression of the condition often include a premorbid phase, in which subtle changes are followed by a prodromal phase, marked by a gradual decline in adaptive functioning. Research has demonstrated a strong association between premorbid social, educational, and occupational characteristics and the long-term clinical course, including response to treatment, frequency of relapse, and psychosocial adjustment (Fenton & McGlashan, 1987; Gittelman-Klein & Klein, 1969).

Manic-Specific Features
Psychotic symptoms are more common in individuals who have an early onset of a bipolar disorder (Kennedy et al., 2005; Schulze et al., 2002; Schürhoff et al., 2000). Bipolar disorders with psychotic features generally present with florid positive symptoms, including delusions, hallucinations, and disorganized speech in form of flight of ideas, which typically appear during an acute manic episode. Delusions and hallucinations may also occur during a depressive phase. Manic psychotic symptoms usually develop more rapidly, with male patients showing a higher lifetime prevalence of delusions and hallucinations than females (Morgan et al., 2005).

A lifetime history of delusions is present in almost 70% of patients with bipolar I, while only roughly 43% have hallucinations (van Bergen et al., 2019). Delusions may be more prevalent than hallucinations. An Australian study of patients with Type I and II bipolar disorders found that 86% had delusions and only 21% had hallucinations (Morgan et al., 2005). Delusional or hallucinatory content may be either mood-congruent or -incongruent. The symptoms occur in the context of declining behavioral, social, occupational, and academic functioning usually leading to hospitalization.

For early-onset patients with manic disorders, grandiose and persecutory delusions were shown to be nearly equal in frequency (62%–60%), followed by delusions of influence (Kennedy et al., 2005). This study also showed mood-congruent psychotic features occurring in half of the patients and positive thought disorder in 41%. Burton et al. (2017) found grandiose delusions in over half of their subjects with bipolar psychosis, but few endorsing first-rank hallucinations, with a running commentary by two or more voices.

Early onset of bipolar disorder is also associated more with mood-congruent psychotic features, delusions of persecution and influence, and auditory hallucinations (Kennedy et al., 2005). Carlson et al. (2000) found higher levels of grandiose delusions in adolescent-onset psychosis. Patients with hallucinations also had significantly higher levels of childhood maltreatment (van Bergen et al., 2019). Although rare in bipolar psychosis, visual, somatic, and olfactory hallucinations may be present in late-onset patients.

The presence of mood-incongruent psychotic features was significantly associated with the persistence of psychotic symptoms, but not with a poorer outcome after 1 year. However, more than mood-incongruent features, the presence of FRS at the baseline was significantly correlated with both earlier onset, negative symptoms, and poorer outcomes after a year (Conus et al., 2004; Tohen et al., 1992).

Cognitive Impairment

Cognitive impairment is regarded as an essential feature of schizophrenia (Bowie et al., 2013; Heinrichs, 2005; Wilk et al., 2005). Studies of cognitive impairment in bipolar disorders have lagged behind; however, over the last 2 decades, publications have increased nearly sixfold. Currently, it is well-established that both disorders have varying degrees of cognitive impairment (see also Chapter 11 in this volume). Over 80% of those with schizophrenia demonstrate impairment on neuropsychological measures compared with 40% to 58% of individuals with remitted and psychotic bipolar disorders (Reichenberg et al., 2009). The scope of impairment is broad, including attentional functioning, speed of information processing, working memory, language production, visual and verbal learning and memory, and executive functioning (Bowie et al., 2013; see also Chapter 11 in this volume). However, in terms of progressive deterioration in cognitive functioning, patients with bipolar disorders may not show long-term impairment (Samamé et al., 2022).

The consensus indicates that, while the extent of impairment is similar, the severity is somewhat different (Bowie et al., 2013). In a multisite inpatient study, patients with schizophrenia showed more severe impairment in verbal and visual memory, attention and executive functioning, and visual processing (Reichenberg et al., 2009). Consistent with other findings, the group with bipolar disorders revealed mild to moderate impairment in the same neurocognitive domains. In another study of hospitalized patients, those diagnosed with schizophrenia performed worse on all neuropsychological tasks when compared to nonclinical controls (Zanelli et al., 2010). Those suffering from depressive psychosis also showed widespread impairment. In contrast, patients with bipolar disorders performed more poorly on selective neurocognitive measures of verbal memory and fluency.

Negative Symptoms

Negative symptoms have a modest correlation with cognitive impairment in schizophrenia, but they represent different domains (Harvey et al., 2006). Both dimensions are related to impoverished thinking and speech, but, according to Harvey and colleagues (2006), cognitive impairment was correlated with the ability to perform everyday living skills, whereas negative symptoms were related to the likelihood of actually performing those skills.

Negative symptoms may appear in bipolar depression, but the challenge has been distinguishing the impact of depression from the primary disturbance giving rise to negative symptoms. Some researchers maintained that negative symptoms are specific to schizophrenia (Reddy et al., 1992), while others argue that they occur in bipolar depression (Toomey et al., 1998).

DIAGNOSTIC IMPLICATIONS FOR CLINICAL PRACTICE

Research identifies several clinical features that may help clinicians distinguish between bipolar spectrum disorders and schizophrenia. These include (a) characteristics of FTD in mania and schizophrenia, (b) qualitative nature of disordered thinking in bipolar mania, (c) social cognition, (d) insight, and (e) subtle phenomenological differences.

Formal Thought Disorder

Recent research has affirmed that among acute inpatients, there is little difference between the amount of FTD in patients with schizophrenia and bipolar mania (Harrow et al., 1986; Yalincetin et al., 2017). However, differences in the quality of FTD among the two patient groups emerge in three ways: (a) a greater degree of inappropriate combinative thinking in the Rorschach responses of bipolar patients (see also Chapter 9 in this volume), (b) more incidence of poverty of thought content and perseverations in patients with schizophrenia versus those with bipolar disorder, and (c) a higher level of residual thought disorder in stable outpatients with schizophrenia compared to those with bipolar spectrum disorders.

The increased presence of illogical combinative thinking in the Rorschach results of bipolar individuals is discussed later. Regarding the higher incidence of poverty of thought content and perseverative thinking in schizophrenia versus mania, a recent small study showed that subjects matched for age, sex, and neuropsychological status found that, compared with patients with active mania, those with acute schizophrenia demonstrated more vague speech that was repetitive and conveyed little information (Kircher et al., 2022).

The finding that stable patients with schizophrenia exhibited higher levels of FTD than those with bipolar mania (Yalincetin et al., 2017) is consistent with an earlier study by Spohn et al. (1986) that showed that residual milder forms of thought disorder, as measured on the Rorschach by the Thought Disorder Index (TDI; Johnston & Holzman, 1979), were present in medicated patients with schizophrenia, whose acute positive symptoms had remitted. Spohn's group wondered whether milder forms of thought disorder were a diagnostically specific marker of schizophrenia.

Nature of Manic Thought Disorder

Manic thought disorder is characterized by flight of ideas (characterized by both derailed and pressured speech), distractibility, and clanging (Andreasen & Powers, 1974; Kleiger, 2017; Kleiger & Khadivi, 2015). Manic thought is also characterized by the tendency to combine ideas or categories of thought to form new and original connections (combinative thinking). Studies of manic disorders and creativity found that both creative and hypomanic thinking is characterized by fluency, rapidity, and flexibility (Jamison, 1995). Greater speed of thinking may produce a greater quantity of thoughts and associations that may produce some unique ideas and associations. However, unlike healthy creative individuals, manic individuals may have difficulty maintaining focus and filtering out distractions that give their associations a bizarre quality (Andreasen & Powers, 1974). Additionally, speech patterns in mania tended to be more playful and combinative (Holzman et al., 1986; Solovay et al., 1987) while those associated with schizophrenia were more idiosyncratic and impoverished (Cuesta & Peralta, 2011).

Verbal fluency or productivity has been studied as a way to distinguish thought disorder in schizophrenia and bipolar psychosis. It has been argued that subjects with manic disorders have an advantage in semantic verbal fluency tasks because of overactivation of the semantic network, which leads to faster retrieval of more remotely associated words (Raucher-Chéné et al., 2017). A process-oriented measure of verbal fluency showed increased and more rapid switching from one subcategory to another in subjects with manic disorders, which appeared consistent with a flight of ideas (Weiner et al., 2019). Additionally, manic, and to some extent mixed-manic, subjects appeared to use more rhyming and phonologically based associations, similar to clanging.

Listener reactions to speech patterns in mania and schizophrenia showed some distinctions. Harrow et al. (1982) observed how the speech of subjects with manic disorders was more interactive and pulled for examiner responses, albeit in odd and inappropriate ways. By contrast, subjects with schizophrenia interacted in ways that tended to be more solitary, private, and inwardly directed. Perhaps it is the contrast between interactivity on the one hand, and withdrawal, idiosyncrasy, and encapsulation on the other that may cause listeners to attribute "craziness" to the speaker who has schizophrenia, while accepting the speaker with mania as more accessible and less bizarre. Supporting this idea, Lipkin et al. (1970) reported that even delusional ideas embedded in the speech of a subject with a manic disorder may sound more coherent to the listener. Although the speaker may sound pressured and loose, and even include clang associations, listeners may find the ideas less puzzling and foreign to the ear than those of the individual with schizophrenia.

Further research supports the fact that manic thought/speech disorder may sound somewhat less incoherent or alienating than that which is heard in schizophrenia (Hoffman et al., 1986). Andreasen and Pfohl (1976) conducted a linguistic analysis of manic speech and found it to be colorful and filled with adjectives and action verbs. Finally, the expansive mood found in hypomania and mania may have an infectious quality that is engaging and amusing (before it becomes exhausting). In contrast, the affective flatness and communicative characteristics associated with the negative symptoms of schizophrenia may increase the sense of distance between speaker and listener.

The most extensive Rorschach analysis of disordered thinking in mania was conducted by Holzman's TDI research group (Johnston & Holzman, 1979; Solovay et al., 1987). The mean TDI score was found to be lower in manic than subjects with manic disorders schizophrenic. The total TDI scores were similar for both groups; however, there were significant differences in the type of thought disorder identified.

In a principal components factor analysis, the factor that correctly identified the group with mania was "Combinatory Thinking," which included playful confabulation, incongruous and fabulized combinations, and flippant responses. An additional factor that distinguished the manic group was termed "Irrelevant Intrusions" (made up of flippant and loose responses). As Mihura and Gorner point out in Chapter 9 of this volume, the Yalincetin et al. (2017) meta-analysis employed an aggregate of three combinatory scores (playful confabulations, incongruous combinations, and fabulized combinations) from the TDI studies that distinguished manic from schizophrenic thought disorder.

Regarding levels of symptom severity, subjects with schizophrenia demonstrated examples of disordered thinking on the TDI across four levels of severity. By contrast, none of the patients with mania demonstrated thought disorder scores at the most severe level of 1.0 (which included categories of incoherence and neologisms). Based on their data, Solovay et al. (1987) concluded that disorganized thinking in mania is characterized by ideas that are loosely connected, excessively elaborated, and inappropriately combined. According to Solovay et al. (1987), loosely connected and incongruously combined ideas may lead to "irrelevant intrusions into social discourse that at times may appear inappropriately flippant and playful" (Solovay et al., 1987, p. 19).

Khadivi et al. (1997) cross-validated some of these key findings with subjects with manic disorders. Contrasting six thought disorder factors (combinatory thinking, idiosyncratic verbalization, autistic thinking, fluid thinking, absurdity, and confusion) among subjects with paranoid schizophrenia, manic disorders, and schizoaffective disorders, researchers found significantly more combinatory thinking in those with mania. They viewed combinatory thinking as the tendency to connect things that should normally be kept apart. The subject's effort to integrate disparate elements outstrips their adherence to reason, reality, and intellectual capacity. Khadivi et al. also associated this combinatory thinking with distractibility and problems filtering. They noted that, since individuals with mania are driven to respond to unrelated stimuli, they have difficulty screening out irrelevant stimuli and become overinclusive, which leads to a flight of ideas.

Social Cognition

Deficits in processing emotional cues are present in both schizophrenia and bipolar disorders. As with cognitive impairment, the deficits in bipolar disorders appear to be less severe. Although social perception has not been studied as widely in bipolar disorders, some evidence suggests that patients with manic disorders performed significantly worse than nonclinical controls on tasks of social knowledge and judgment, but not as poorly as patients with schizophrenia (Cutting & Murphy, 1990). Studies of theory of mind showed lesser deficits in bipolar disorders compared with schizophrenia (Bora et al., 2009; Kerr et al., 2003; Mitchell & Young, 2016; Sprong et al., 2007).

Insight

Cognitive impairment, psychosis, and mood states are associated with poorer insight (Látalová, 2012). The *DSM-5* mentions impaired insight as an associated feature of both schizophrenia and bipolar I in schizophrenia (American Psychiatric Association, 2013). However, recent research found awareness of illness (a key component of insight) to be more impaired in patients with schizophrenia than those suffering from bipolar I or methamphetamine-induced psychotic disorder; however, all three groups had similar deficits in understanding the effects of medication and the social consequences of their illness (Asgarabad et al., 2022). Most importantly, poor insight in mania is understood as a *state-dependent* condition in mania, which improves with the resolution of the acute manic episode. By contrast, impaired insight is regarded as more of a *trait-like* condition in schizophrenia (Ghaemi & Rosenquist, 2004). It is not surprising that insight is more impaired during acute mania than in unipolar and bipolar depression episodes; however, some research found more impairment during mixed as opposed to pure manic episodes and among patients with bipolar II disorder versus those with bipolar I disorder (Látalová, 2012).

Prodrome

There is growing interest in defining prodromal symptoms of bipolar disorders for early intervention purposes (Correll et al., 2007; Vieta et al., 2018). In terms of key risk factors, studies have found that affective lability and subsyndromal manic symptoms, along with a positive family history of early-onset bipolar disorder in parents were found to be the most significant risk factors for developing bipolar spectrum disorders (R. H. Taylor et al., 2021; Vieta et al., 2018).

Preonset symptoms in schizophrenia and bipolar mania overlap considerably. Although the prodrome in schizophrenia may be slightly longer, a prodromal phase in bipolar mania may also be relatively long and have insidious onsets. Both prodromes consist of a mixture of subthreshold symptoms of mania, depression, and nonspecific psychopathology. Correll et al. (2007) found the following symptoms most prevalent in the mania prodrome: decreased school and work performance (65.4%), followed by decreased concentration and memory (51.9%), increased energy and goal-directed activity (48.3%), depressed mood (46.7%), social isolation (44.2%), and angry outbursts (43.8%). Despite symptom overlap, the schizophrenia prodrome was character-ized primarily by social isolation (55.7%) and strange or unusual ideas (53.3% compared with 18.0% in bipolar prodrome). Additionally, prodromal features in bipolar disorders may include more suicidality, psychomotor agitation, and difficulties thinking and communicating clearly. Subthreshold delusions and hallucinations occurred later in the mania prodrome. In contrast, attenuated psychotic symptoms are seen as initial symptoms in nonaffective psychoses.

Subtle Phenomenological Factors

Phenomenologically oriented researchers suggest that subtle distinctions in aspects of self-experience may be detected in those suffering from bipolar and schizophrenia spectrum disorders (Sass & Pienkos, 2013). The authors maintain that in bipolar psychosis, the individual may experience a oneness with God or the universe. In contrast, schizophrenia may involve a more fundamental collapse of boundaries, in which the individual feels themselves to be God. Finally, this phenomenological perspective suggests that, in schizo-phrenia, the core sense of self is fragmented, whereas in a manic state, the individual may maintain a basic sense of self.

FINAL THOUGHTS

Establishing a lifetime presence of manic or hypomanic episodes is a core diagnostic feature of bipolar spectrum disorders. Similarly, the presence of at least one lifetime positive symptom is an essential diagnostic criterion for schizophrenic spectrum disorders. As described previously, differential diagnosis of bipolar and schizophrenia spectrum is complicated by the fact that psychotic symptoms and manic and depressive episodes can occur in both disorders.

Regarding key differences and similarities in symptom dimensions, focusing on the nature of hallucinations and delusions is not going to aid in the differential diagnosis of bipolar from schizophrenia spectrum disorders. Although there are some subtle differences in phenomenological experiences and in the frequency and nature of psychotic symptoms, patients with bipolar and schizophrenic spectrum disorders can present with similar types of delusions and hallucinations, including bizarre and mood-incongruent psychotic symptoms.

Finally, a key focus for differential diagnosis should be the temporal relationship between manic or depressive episodes and the onset of psychotic symptoms. In bipolar disorder, psychotic symptoms must occur concurrently with a manic or depressive phase of illness (First, 2014; Kleiger & Khadivi, 2015).

REFERENCES

Allardyce, J., Suppes, T., & Van Os, J. (2007). Dimensions and the psychosis phenotype. *International Journal of Methods in Psychiatric Research, 16*(Suppl. 1), S34–S40. https://doi.org/10.1002/mpr.214

American Psychiatric Association. (1994). *Diagnostic and statistical manual of mental disorders* (4th ed.).

American Psychiatric Association. (2013). *Diagnostic and statistical manual of mental disorders* (5th ed.).

American Psychiatric Association. (2022). *Diagnostic and statistical manual of mental disorders: DSM-5-TR* (5th ed., text rev.).

Andreasen, N. C. (1979a). Thought, language, and communication disorders. I. Clinical assessment, definition of terms, and evaluation of their reliability. *Archives of General Psychiatry, 36*(12), 1315–1321. https://doi.org/10.1001/archpsyc.1979.01780120045006

Andreasen, N. C. (1979b). Thought, language, and communication disorders. II. Diagnostic significance. *Archives of General Psychiatry, 36*(12), 1325–1330. https://doi.org/10.1001/archpsyc.1979.01780120055007

Andreasen, N. C., & Grove, W. M. (1986). Evaluation of positive and negative symptoms in schizophrenia. *Psychiatry and Psychobiology, 1*(2), 108–122. https://doi.org/10.1017/S0767399X00003199

Andreasen, N. G., & Pfohl, B. (1976). Linguistic analysis of speech in affective disorders. *Archives of General Psychiatry, 33*(11), 1361–1367. https://doi.org/10.1001/archpsyc.1976.01770110089009

Andreasen, N. J. C., & Powers, P. S. (1974). Overinclusive thinking in mania and schizophrenia. *The British Journal of Psychiatry, 125*(588), 452–456. https://doi.org/10.1192/bjp.125.5.452

Asgarabad, M. H., Hosseini, S. R., Yegaei, P. S., Moradi, S., Lysaker, P. H. (2022). Psychopathology and poor clinical insight in psychotic patients: Does the diagnosis matter? *The Journal of Nervous and Mental Disease, 210*(7), 532–540. https://doi.org/10.1097/NMD.0000000000001475

Bora, E., Yücel, M., & Pantelis, C. (2009). Theory of mind impairment: A distinct trait-marker for schizophrenia spectrum disorders and bipolar disorder? *Acta Psychiatrica Scandinavica, 120*(4), 253–264. https://doi.org/10.1111/j.1600-0447.2009.01414.x

Bowie, C. R., Gupta, M., Holshausen, K., Jokic, R., Best, M., & Milev, R. (2013). Cognitive remediation for treatment-resistant depression: Effects on cognition and functioning and the role of online homework. *Journal of Nervous and Mental Disease, 201*(8), 680–685. https://doi.org/10.1097/NMD.0b013e31829c5030

Buckley, P. F., Gowans, A., Sebastian, C. S., Pathiraja, A., Brimeyer, A., & Stirewalt, E. (2004). The boundaries of schizophrenia: Overlap with bipolar disorders. *Current Psychosis & Therapeutics Reports, 2*(2), 49–56. https://doi.org/10.1007/s11922-004-0031-8

Burton, C. Z., Ryan, K. A., Kamali, M., Marshall, D. F., Harrington, G., McInnis, M. G., & Tso, I. F. (2017). Psychosis in bipolar disorder: Does it represent a more "severe" illness? *Bipolar Disorders, 20*(1), 18–26. https://doi.org/10.1111/bdi.12527

Carlson, G. A., Bromet, E. J., & Sievers, S. (2000). Phenomenology and outcome of subjects with early- and adult-onset psychotic mania. *The American Journal of Psychiatry, 157*(2), 213–219. https://doi.org/10.1176/appi.ajp.157.2.213

Carpenter, W. T., Jr., Strauss, J. S., & Muleh, S. (1973). Are there pathognomonic symptoms in schizophrenia? An empiric investigation of Schneider's first-rank symptoms. *Archives of General Psychiatry, 28*(6), 847–852. https://doi.org/10.1001/archpsyc.1973.01750360069010

Cassano, G. B., Rucci, P., Frank, E., Fagiolini, A., Dell'Osso, L., Shear, M. K., & Kupfer, D. J. (2004). The mood spectrum in unipolar and bipolar disorder: Arguments for a unitary approach. *The American Journal of Psychiatry, 161*(7), 1264–1269. https://doi.org/10.1176/appi.ajp.161.7.1264

Conus, P., Abdel-Baki, A., Harrigan, S., Lambert, M., & McGorry, P. D. (2004). Schneiderian first rank symptoms predict poor outcome within first episode manic psychosis. *Journal of Affective Disorders, 81*(3), 259–268. https://doi.org/10.1016/j.jad.2003.09.003

Correll, C. U., Penzner, J. B., Frederickson, A. M., Richter, J. J., Auther, A. M., Smith, C. W., Kane, J. M., & Cornblatt, B. A. (2007). Differentiation in the preonset phases of schizophrenia and mood disorders: Evidence in support of a bipolar mania prodrome. *Schizophrenia Bulletin, 33*(3), 703–714. https://doi.org/10.1093/schbul/sbm028

Crow, T. J. (1986). The continuum of psychosis and its implication for the structure of the gene. *The British Journal of Psychiatry, 149*(4), 419–429. https://doi.org/10.1192/bjp.149.4.419

Cuesta, M. J., & Peralta, V. (2011). Testing the hypothesis that formal thought disorders are severe mood disorders. *Schizophrenia Bulletin, 37*(6), 1136–1146. https://doi.org/10.1093/schbul/sbr092

Cutting, J., & Murphy, D. (1990). Impaired ability of schizophrenics, relative to manics or depressives, to appreciate social knowledge about their culture. *The British Journal of Psychiatry, 157*(3), 355–358. https://doi.org/10.1192/bjp.157.3.355

Demily, C., Jacquet, P., & Marie-Cardine, M. (2009). L'évaluation cognitive permet-elle de distinguer la schizophrénie du trouble bipolaire? [How to differentiate schizophrenia from bipolar disorder using cognitive assessment?] *L'Encéphale, 35*(2), 139–145. https://doi.org/10.1016/j.encep.2008.03.011

Fenton, W. S., & McGlashan, T. H. (1987). Prognostic scale for chronic schizophrenia. *Schizophrenia Bulletin, 13*(2), 277–286. https://doi.org/10.1093/schbul/13.2.277

First, M. B. (2014). DSM-5 *handbook of differential diagnosis*. American Psychiatric Association.

Ghaemi, S. N., & Rosenquist, K. J. (2004). Is insight in mania state-dependent? A meta-analysis. *Journal of Nervous and Mental Disease, 192*(11), 771–775. https://doi.org/10.1097/01.nmd.0000145036.76435.c3

Gittelman-Klein, R., & Klein, D. F. (1969). Premorbid asocial adjustment and prognosis in schizophrenia. *Journal of Psychiatric Research, 7*(1), 35–53. https://doi.org/10.1016/0022-3956(69)90010-7

Goldstein, G., Allen, A. N., & Haas, G. L. (2007). Schizophrenia. In D. Fujii & I. Ahmed (Eds.), *The spectrum of psychotic disorders* (pp. 15–38). Cambridge University Press. https://doi.org/10.1017/CBO9780511543784.003

Harrow, M., Grossman, L. S., Silverstein, M. L., & Meltzer, H. Y. (1982). Thought pathology in manic and schizophrenic patients. Its occurrence at hospital admission and seven weeks later. *Archives of General Psychiatry, 39*(6), 665–671. https://doi.org/10.1001/archpsyc.1982.04290060027006

Harrow, M., Grossman, L. S., Silverstein, M. L., Meltzer, H. Y., & Kettering, R. L. (1986). A longitudinal study of thought disorder in manic patients. *Archives of General Psychiatry, 43*(8), 781–785. https://doi.org/10.1001/archpsyc.1986.01800080067009

Harvey, P. D., Koren, D., Reichenberg, A., & Bowie, C. R. (2006). Negative symptoms and cognitive deficits: What is the nature of their relationship? *Schizophrenia Bulletin, 32*(2), 250–258. https://doi.org/10.1093/schbul/sbj011

Heinrichs, R. W. (2005). The primacy of cognition in schizophrenia. *American Psychologist, 60*(3), 229–242. https://doi.org/10.1037/0003-066X.60.3.229

Hoffman, R. E., Stopek, S., & Andreasen, N. C. (1986). A comparative study of manic vs schizophrenic speech disorganization. *Archives of General Psychiatry, 43*(9), 831–838. https://doi.org/10.1001/archpsyc.1986.01800090017003

Holzman, P. S., Shenton, M. E., & Solovay, M. R. (1986). Quality of thought disorder in differential diagnosis. *Schizophrenia Bulletin, 12*(3), 360–371. https://doi.org/10.1093/schbul/12.3.360

Jamison, K. R. (1995). Manic-depressive illness and creativity. *Scientific American, 272*(2), 62–67. https://doi.org/10.1038/scientificamerican0295-62

Jaspers, K. (1963). *General psychopathology* (J. Hoenig & M. W. Hamilton, Trans.; 7th ed.). Manchester University Press. (Original work published 1946)

Johnston, M. H., & Holzman, P. S. (1979). *Assessing schizophrenic thinking: A clinical and research instrument for measuring thought disorder* (1st ed.). Jossey-Bass.

Kendell, R., & Jablensky, A. (2003). Distinguishing between the validity and utility of psychiatric diagnoses. *The American Journal of Psychiatry, 160*(1), 4–12. https://doi.org/10.1176/appi.ajp.160.1.4

Kennedy, N., Everitt, B., Boydell, J., Van Os, J., Jones, P. B., & Murray, R. M. (2005). Incidence and distribution of first-episode mania by age: Results from a 35-year study. *Psychological Medicine, 35*(6), 855–863. https://doi.org/10.1017/S0033291704003307

Kerr, N., Dunbar, R. I., & Bentall, R. P. (2003). Theory of mind deficits in bipolar affective disorder. *Journal of Affective Disorders, 73*(3), 253–259. https://doi.org/10.1016/S0165-0327(02)00008-3

Ketter, T. A., Wang, P. W., Becker, O. V., Nowakowska, C., & Yang, Y. (2004). Psychotic bipolar disorders: Dimensionally similar to or categorically different from schizophrenia? *Journal of Psychiatric Research, 38*(1), 47–61. https://doi.org/10.1016/S0022-3956(03)00099-2

Khadivi, A., Wetzler, S., & Wilson, A. (1997). Manic indices on the Rorschach. *Journal of Personality Assessment, 69*(2), 365–375. https://doi.org/10.1207/s15327752jpa6902_8

Kircher, T., Stein, F., & Nagels, A. (2022). Differences in single positive formal thought disorder symptoms between closely matched acute patients with schizophrenia and mania. *European Archives of Psychiatry and Clinical Neuroscience, 272*(3), 395–401. https://doi.org/10.1007/s00406-021-01263-x

Kirkpatrick, B., Castle, D., Murray, R. M., & Carpenter, W. T., Jr. (2000). Risk factors for the deficit syndrome of schizophrenia. *Schizophrenia Bulletin, 26*(1), 233–242. https://doi.org/10.1093/oxfordjournals.schbul.a033443

Kleiger, J. H. (2017). *Rorschach assessment of psychotic phenomena: Clinical, conceptual, and empirical developments.* Taylor & Francis. https://doi.org/10.4324/9781315271385

Kleiger, J. H., & Khadivi, A. (2015). *Assessing psychosis: A clinician's guide.* Routledge. https://doi.org/10.4324/9781315882086

Kraepelin, E. (1921a). *Dementia praecox and paraphrenia* (R. M. Barclay, Trans.). Chicago Medical Books. (Original work published 1896)

Kraepelin, E. (1921b), *Manic-depressive insanity and paranoia*. E&S Livingston. https://doi.org/10.1097/00005053-192104000-00057

Lapierre, Y. D. (1994). Schizophrenia and manic-depression: Separate illnesses or a continuum? *Canadian Journal of Psychiatry, 39*(9, Suppl. 2), S59–S64.

Látalová, K. (2012). Insight in bipolar disorder. *Psychiatric Quarterly, 83*(3), 293–310. https://doi.org/10.1007/s11126-011-9200-4

Lawrie, S. M., Hall, J., McIntosh, A. M., Owens, D. G., & Johnstone, E. C. (2010). The 'continuum of psychosis': Scientifically unproven and clinically impractical. *The British Journal of Psychiatry, 197*(6), 423–425. https://doi.org/10.1192/bjp.bp.109.072827

Lipkin, K. M., Dyrud, J., & Meyer, G. G. (1970). The many faces of mania. Therapeutic trial of lithium carbonate. *Archives of General Psychiatry, 22*(3), 262–267. https://doi.org/10.1001/archpsyc.1970.01740270070009

Mazzarini, L., Colom, F., Pacchiarotti, I., Nivoli, A. M., Murru, A., Bonnin, C. M., Cruz, N., Sanchez-Moreno, J., Kotzalidis, G. D., Girardi, P., Tatarelli, R., & Vieta, E. (2010). Psychotic versus non-psychotic bipolar II disorder. *Journal of Affective Disorders, 126*(1–2), 55–60. https://doi.org/10.1016/j.jad.2010.03.028

Mitchell, R. L., & Young, A. H. (2016). Theory of mind in bipolar disorder, with comparison to the impairments observed in schizophrenia. *Frontiers in Psychiatry, 6*, Article 188. https://doi.org/10.3389/fpsyt.2015.00188

Möller, H. J. (2003). Bipolar disorder and schizophrenia: Distinct illnesses or a continuum? *The Journal of Clinical Psychiatry, 64*(Suppl. 6), 23–27.

Morgan, V. A., Mitchell, P. B., & Jablensky, A. V. (2005). The epidemiology of bipolar disorder: Sociodemographic, disability and service utilization data from the Australian National Study of Low Prevalence (Psychotic) Disorders. *Bipolar Disorders, 7*(4), 326–337. https://doi.org/10.1111/j.1399-5618.2005.00229.x

Murray, R. M., Sham, P., Van Os, J., Zanelli, J., Cannon, M., & McDonald, C. (2004). A developmental model for similarities and dissimilarities between schizophrenia and bipolar disorder. *Schizophrenia Research, 71*(2–3), 405–416. https://doi.org/10.1016/j.schres.2004.03.002

Parameshwara, N. M., Mascascarenhas, J. J., & Mathai, P. (2017). Schneider's first rank symptoms in patients with bipolar affective disorders and schizophrenia—A clinical study. *International Journal of Recent Scientific Research, 8*(2), 15642–15648.

Phelps, J. (2016). *A spectrum approach to mood disorders: Not fully bipolar but not unipolar—Practical management*. W. W. Norton.

Pope, H. G., Jr., & Lipinski, J. F., Jr. (1978). Diagnosis in schizophrenia and manic-depressive illness: A reassessment of the specificity of 'schizophrenic' symptoms in the light of current research. *Archives of General Psychiatry, 35*(7), 811–828. https://doi.org/10.1001/archpsyc.1978.01770310017001

Raucher-Chéné, D., Achim, A. M., Kaladjian, A., & Besche-Richard, C. (2017). Verbal fluency in bipolar disorders: A systematic review and meta-analysis. *Journal of Affective Disorders, 207*, 359–366. https://doi.org/10.1016/j.jad.2016.09.039

Reddy, R., Mukherjee, S., & Schnur, D. B. (1992). Comparison of negative symptoms in schizophrenic and poor outcome bipolar patients. *Psychological Medicine, 22*(2), 361–365. https://doi.org/10.1017/S0033291700030300

Reichenberg, A., Harvey, P. D., Bowie, C. R., Mojtabai, R., Rabinowitz, J., Heaton, R. K., & Bromet, E. (2009). Neuropsychological function and dysfunction in schizophrenia and psychotic affective disorders. *Schizophrenia Bulletin, 35*(5), 1022–1029. https://doi.org/10.1093/schbul/sbn044

Rosen, C., Marvin, R., Reilly, J. L., Deleon, O., Harris, M. S., Keedy, S. K., Solari, H., Weiden, P., & Sweeney, J. A. (2012). Phenomenology of first-episode psychosis in schizophrenia, bipolar disorder, and unipolar depression: A comparative analysis. *Clinical Schizophrenia & Related Psychoses, 6*(3), 145–151. https://doi.org/10.3371/CSRP.6.3.6

Samamé, C., Cattaneo, B. L., Richaud, M. C., Strejilevich, S., & Aprahamian, I. (2022). The long-term course of cognition in bipolar disorder: A systematic review and meta-analysis of patient-control differences in test-score changes. *Psychological Medicine*, *52*(2), 217–228. https://doi.org/10.1017/S0033291721004517

Sass, L., & Pienkos, E. (2013). Varieties of self-experience: A comparative phenomenology of melancholia, mania, and schizophrenia, Part I. *Journal of Consciousness Studies*, *20*(7–8), 103–130.

Schneider, K. (1959). *Clinical psychopathology*. Grune and Stratton.

Schulze, T. G., Müller, D. J., Krauss, H., Gross, M., Fangerau-Lefèvre, H., Illés, F., Ohlraun, S., Cichon, S., Held, T., Propping, P., Nöthen, M. M., Maier, W., & Rietschel, M. (2002). Further evidence for age of onset being an indicator for severity in bipolar disorder. *Journal of Affective Disorders*, *68*(2–3), 343–345. https://doi.org/10.1016/S0165-0327(01)00306-8

Schürhoff, F., Bellivier, F., Jouvent, R., Mouren-Siméoni, M. C., Bouvard, M., Allilaire, J. F., & Leboyer, M. (2000). Early and late onset bipolar disorders: Two different forms of manic-depressive illness? *Journal of Affective Disorders*, *58*(3), 215–221. https://doi.org/10.1016/S0165-0327(99)00111-1

Soares-Weiser, K., Maayan, N., Bergman, H., Davenport, C., Kirkham, A. J., Grabowski, S. , & Adams, C. E. (2015). First rank symptoms for schizophrenia. *The Cochrane Database of Systematic Reviews*, *1*(1), Article CD010653. https://doi.org/10.1002/14651858. CD010653.pub2

Solovay, M. R., Shenton, M. E., & Holzman, P. S. (1987). Comparative studies of thought disorders. I. Mania and schizophrenia. *Archives of General Psychiatry*, *44*(1), 13–20. https://doi.org/10.1001/archpsyc.1987.01800130015003

Sorella, S., Lapomarda, G., Messina, I., Frederickson, J. J., Siugzdaite, R., Job, R., & Grecucci, A. (2019). Testing the expanded continuum hypothesis of schizophrenia and bipolar disorder. Neural and psychological evidence for shared and distinct mechanisms. *NeuroImage: Clinical*, *23*, Article 101854. https://doi.org/10.1016/j.nicl.2019. 101854

Spohn, H. E., Coyne, L., Larson, J., Mittleman, F., Spray, J., & Hayes, K. (1986). Episodic and residual thought pathology in chronic schizophrenics: Effect of neuroleptics. *Schizophrenia Bulletin*, *12*(3), 394–407. https://doi.org/10.1093/schbul/12.3.394

Sprong, M., Schothorst, P., Vos, E., Hox, J., & van Engeland, H. (2007). Theory of mind in schizophrenia: Meta-analysis. *The British Journal of Psychiatry*, *191*(1), 5–13. https:// doi.org/10.1192/bjp.bp.107.035899

Taylor, M. A. (1992). Are schizophrenia and affective disorder related? A selective literature review. *The American Journal of Psychiatry*, *149*(1), 22–32. https://doi.org/10. 1176/ajp.149.1.22

Taylor, R. H., Ulrichsen, A., Young, A. H., & Strawbridge, R. (2021). Affective lability as a prospective predictor of subsequent bipolar disorder diagnosis: A systematic review. *International Journal of Bipolar Disorders*, *9*(1), Article 33. https://doi.org/10.1186/ s40345-021-00237-1

Tohen, M., Tsuang, M. T., & Goodwin, D. C. (1992). Prediction of outcome in mania by mood-congruent or mood-incongruent psychotic features. *The American Journal of Psychiatry*, *149*(11), 1580–1584. https://doi.org/10.1176/ajp.149.11.1580

Toomey, R., Faraone, S. V., Simpson, J. C., & Tsuang, M. T. (1998). Negative, positive, and disorganized symptom dimensions in schizophrenia, major depression, and bipolar disorder. *Journal of Nervous and Mental Disease*, *186*(8), 470–476. https://doi.org/10. 1097/00005053-199808000-00004

van Bergen, A. H., Verkooijen, S., Vreeker, A., Abramovic, L., Hillegers, M. H., Spijker, A. T., Hoencamp, E., Regeer, E. J., Knapen, S. E., Riemersma-van der Lek, R. F., Schoevers, R., Stevens, A. W., Schulte, P. F. J., Vonk, R., Hoekstra, R., van Beveren, N. J., Kupka, R. W., Sommer, I. E. C., Ophoff, R. A., . . . Boks, M. P. M. (2019).

The characteristics of psychotic features in bipolar disorder. *Psychological Medicine,* *49*(12), 2036–2048. https://doi.org/10.1017/S0033291718002854

van Os, J. (2015). The transdiagnostic dimension of psychosis: Implications for psychiatric nosology and research. *Shanghai Archives of Psychiatry, 27*(2), 82–86. https://doi.org/10. 11919/j.issn.1002-0829.215041

van Os, J., Linscott, R. J., Myin-Germeys, I., Delespaul, P., & Krabbendam, L. (2009). A systematic review and meta-analysis of the psychosis continuum: Evidence for a psychosis proneness-persistence-impairment model of psychotic disorder. *Psychological Medicine, 39*(2), 179–195. https://doi.org/10.1017/S0033291708003814

Vieta, E., Salagre, E., Grande, I., Carvalho, A. F., Fernandes, B. S., Berk, M., Birmaher, B., Tohen, M., & Suppes, T. (2018). Early intervention in bipolar disorder. *The American Journal of Psychiatry, 175*(5), 411–426. https://doi.org/10.1176/appi.ajp.2017. 17090972

Weiner, L., Doignon-Camus, N., Bertschy, G., & Giersch, A. (2019). Thought and language disturbance in bipolar disorder quantified via process-oriented verbal fluency measures. *Scientific Reports, 9*(1), Article 14282. https://doi.org/10.1038/s41598-019-50818-5

Wilk, C. M., Gold, J. M., McMahon, R. P., Humber, K., Iannone, V. N., & Buchanan, R. W. (2005). No, it is not possible to be schizophrenic yet neuropsychologically normal. *Neuropsychology, 19*(6), 778–786. https://doi.org/10.1037/0894-4105.19.6.778

World Health Organization. (1992). *International statistical classification of diseases and related health problems* (10th ed.).

World Health Organization. (2019). *International statistical classification of diseases and related health problems* (11th ed.).

Yalincetin, B., Bora, E., Binbay, T., Ulas, H., Akdede, B. B., & Alptekin, K. (2017). Formal thought disorder in schizophrenia and bipolar disorder: A systematic review and meta-analysis. *Schizophrenia Research, 185*, 2–8. https://doi.org/10.1016/j.schres.2016.12.015

Yildiz, A., & Sachs, G. S. (2003). Age onset of psychotic versus non-psychotic bipolar illness in men and in women. *Journal of Affective Disorders, 74*(2), 197–201. https://doi.org/10. 1016/S0165-0327(02)00003-4

Zanelli, J., Reichenberg, A., Morgan, K., Fearon, P., Kravariti, E., Dazzan, P., Morgan, C., Zanelli, C., Demjaha, A., Jones, P. B., Doody, G. A., Kapur, S., & Murray, R. M. (2010). Specific and generalized neuropsychological deficits: A comparison of patients with various first-episode psychosis presentations. *The American Journal of Psychiatry, 167*(1), 78–85. https://doi.org/10.1176/appi.ajp.2009.09010118

17

Assessment of Manic-Depressive Personalities Within the Bipolar Spectrum

Odile Husain

Using a qualitative approach rooted in the European psychodynamic model of psychopathology and theoretical framework, I advocate for the existence of manic-depressive personality (MDP) as an identifiable type of psychic functioning. This model invites the reader to momentarily move away from the data-driven empiricism and specific psychometric methodology that dominate North American approaches to performance-based tests. The chapter includes a brief outline of the Lausanne School, a description of the journey that led from one specific response on the Rorschach to a research interest, and a presentation of the main results from two qualitative studies, the first carried out on a small group of patients with bipolar disorders (Chabot et al., 2003) and the second on a small group with MDP (Husain et al., 2006). I end the chapter with a structural approach to differential diagnosis.

THE LAUSANNE SCHOOL: HISTORY AND VIEWPOINTS

The Lausanne School is a French–Swiss group of personality assessors that was originally based in the city of Lausanne in the late 1970s. This group focused on the differential diagnosis of personality organizations (according

I would like to acknowledge the valuable contributions of Nicole Reeves, Fabrice Choquet, Marie Chabot, and Olivier Revaz to this research.

https://doi.org/10.1037/0000356-018
Psychological Assessment of Bipolar Spectrum Disorders, J. H. Kleiger and I. B. Weiner (Editors)

to the structural model of psychopathology proposed by Bergeret, 1974), based on phenomena observed on the Rorschach and the Thematic Apperception Test (TAT), rather than those derived from psychiatric observations and nosology. Currently, the method is referred to as Psychodynamic Analysis of Speech. In October 2021, members of the group decided to create a professional association and deemed it time to refer to their method as "the Lausanne School."

The group promotes a qualitative approach to analyzing patients' speech—including nonscorable responses—focusing both on frequent formulations and unique verbalizations (Barthes, 1980). The analysis uses a grid rather than a scoring system. The grid has six columns dedicated to object relations, boundaries, self and identity, anxiety, defense mechanisms, and thought processes (see Table 17.1 for an explanation of the grid's contents). The advantage of using the same grid for both tests is the ability to establish convergence of inferences.

For the Lausanne School, Bergeret's (1974) model of structural psychopathology provided the most useful explanatory fit with observations on tests. Fundamental concepts of his model (structure, character, normality, and decompensation) have been detailed elsewhere (Husain, 2015; Prudent et al., 2022). For Bergeret, there are three fundamental structures (psychotic; *état-limite*, not entirely the equivalent of borderline; and neurotic), and the differences between these are qualitative in nature and not quantitative. Each structure is defined by a type of object relation, a specific sense of self, the nature of the anxiety, defense mechanisms, and particularities of thought and language.

MANIC-DEPRESSIVE PERSONALITIES

In our initial years of publication, we focused primarily on differentiating different forms of psychotic functioning (Dreyfus et al., 1987, 1989; Husain, 1989; Husain & Rossel, 1998; Rousselle et al., 1990; Rousselle Gay-Crosier et al., 1989). For example, Racamier's (1966, 1980) work was paramount in our understanding of schizophrenia and paranoia. Both classical French psychiatry (Ey et al., 1978) and psychoanalytic psychopathology (Bergeret, 1974) identify a third form of psychosis or psychotic structure: manic-depressive psychosis. Unfortunately, this manic-depressive entity appears poorly defined, both in the field of psychoanalytic psychopathology and in the field of projective psychology in which issues of differential diagnosis with schizophrenia and bipolar, schizoaffective, and borderline personality disorders are complex (Singer & Brabender, 1993; Solovay et al., 1987; Weiner, 1966). Rorschach response characteristics such as "combinatory thinking, playful confabulations, and flippant remarks," are regularly mentioned and may convey a lack of integration between disparate aspects of self-experience and object representations (Kleiger, 2017).

TABLE 17.1. Grid for Psychodynamic Analysis of Speech (Method of the Lausanne School)

Object relations	Boundaries	Self and identity	Anxiety	Defense mechanisms	Thought processes
Level of self-object differentiation	Quality of boundaries	Integrity of the self	Nature of the anxiety	Type of defenses	Particularities of language
Relationship with the examiner	Inside-outside	Level of identity		Suppleness or rigidity of defenses	Reality testing
Nature of relations	Distance to the card	Self-representation		Effectiveness of defenses	Classical thought disorders
Parental images	Boundaries between classes	Affects, mood			Readability and coherence of speech
Identifications	Spatial criteria	Expression of drives			Reasoning
	Temporal criteria	Manifestations of the different agents of psychic functioning			Interpretive awareness
	Envelopes: 1st skin 2nd skin	All personality traits			Capacity for representation (distinction fantasy-reality)
					Constancy or degradation of thought processes

Note. Copyright 1992 by Odile Husain. Reprinted with permission.

From One Response to a Research Project on Manic-Depressive Personalities

Our interest in MDP started with an unusual response on Card IV of the Rorschach, given by a patient who was chronically depressed and repeatedly suicidal: "A raincoat all soaked with rain." The response became a *punctum*, a concept introduced by Barthes (1980) to describe an observation that captivates the viewer or listener as something both striking and meaningful. If we imagine the response as a prism, we could rotate it and examine its various facets and meanings: (a) a raincoat should be vastly impermeable, so the boundaries between clothing and rain have become porous; (b) the reference to "soaked" would make the weight of the coat different, conveying a sense of heaviness; (c) with that much rain, we could hypothesize that the ambiance is both gloomy and depressing; and (d) "soaked" also implies that the coat and the rainwater have become fused in a form of symbiosis.

With these points in mind, a group of five full-time clinicians working both in adult psychiatry and private practice decided to dig further. Two small qualitative research efforts unfolded over the next 10 years (Chabot et al., 2003; Husain et al., 2006). We first selected eight patients who had received a psychiatric diagnosis of bipolarity according to the *Diagnostic and Statistical Manual of Mental Disorders* (4th ed.; *DSM-IV*; American Psychiatric Association, 1994) and attempted to investigate whether these patients formed a homogenous group using the Rorschach and the TAT (Chabot et al., 2003). The group was structurally homogenous, in the sense that they all presented with an underlying psychotic form of functioning (fragmentation anxiety, paranoid anxiety, symbiotic object relation, thought disorders, and defenses such as denial of reality). However, beyond this structural homogeneity, there was much diversity—for some, thought disorders were paramount; for others, identity disorder was most prominent; and for yet others, persecutory ideation was at the forefront. Among the unifying factors was the observation that these patients with bipolar disorders, through verbs, nouns, adjectives, and adverbs, often introduce a reference to intensity. Back in 1820, Esquirol wrote that "everything makes on them a vivid impression, everything is forced, everything is exaggerated in their way of feeling, thinking and acting" (1820/1994, p. 62, my translation from French). He described this state as "a painful exaltation of sensitivity"; similarly, Bleuler (1922) commented that the patient with manic disorder "welcomes the outside world with bulimia and worries about it with excessive ardor." In the group of patients we selected, intensity was applied sometimes to affect, sometimes to the strength of percept, and sometimes to atmosphere and sensation.

The quest to find distinct characteristics of MDP was still on. We were struggling with an uneasy distinction between the search for a specific personality organization and the evidence of a disorder. As a disorder, "bipolarity," as it is called today, gives rise to abundant and sometimes confused debates about its conceptualization, given the existence of a significant symptomatic and evolutionary diversity (Chabot et al., 2003; see also the Introduction to this book).

Still, all of us have encountered countless patients who presented a history of recurring depressive conditions, often with suicidal attempts. Some showed signs of irritability and impulsivity. Their presentation was at times dramatic, but all of them exhibited clear signs of suffering for many years. When questioned, these patients recognized mood fluctuations, but they had been mostly diagnosed as having borderline personality disorder and prescribed antidepressants with either limited or no success (Phelps, 2016). None of these patients had received a bipolar disorder diagnosis or had a history along those lines. Could these be the patients with MDP we were looking for? The Rorschach and TAT had been administered to many such subjects during consultations. We selected the protocols of eight patients (identified in the text as P1–P8): two men and six women, aged 24 to 50. Five had been seen in private practice, while three had been assessed at an outpatient psychiatric clinic. Clinically, five of them had a depressive disorder, the other three seemed to have a more hypomanic presentation (Husain et al., 2006).

A first big-picture approach to their test data led to the following observations: object relations marked by a search for affective symbiosis (rather than a bodily or thought symbiosis), discrete fragmentation and persecution anxiety, a relatively constructed self infused with sensory and affective experience, manic defenses expressed through festive, playful, and joyful content, abundant speech with details seeking to communicate feelings and atmosphere, and a vocabulary that creates intensity.

It was at this point that the work of Akiskal (1999) and his research group (Cassano et al., 2002; Perugi & Akiskal, 2002) on the concept of "bipolar spectrum" or "soft bipolarity" came to our attention. These authors adopted the notion of temperament to describe a set of personalities struggling with an issue that is difficult to circumscribe and that resists the diagnostic criteria of the *DSM-IV* (American Psychiatric Association, 1994). The pertinence of their research appeared threefold: (a) reestablish the Kraepelinian vision of a manic-depressive continuum that gives a more coherent understanding of this entity; (b) insist on the lifespan approach, since the clinical history invariably points to the existence of a particular lifestyle; and (c) explain the symptomatic diversity of bipolar disorders that belong to three dimensions (mood, anxiety-sensitivity, and impulsivity; Perugi & Akiskal, 2002). The psychopathology of mood (i.e., the subliminal mood disorder throughout the lifespan) would constitute the foundation of soft bipolarity (Cassano et al., 2002). More recently, Phelps (2016) also recommended a spectrum approach to mood disorders, from major depression all the way to bipolar I. Bipolar spectrum disorders sit in the middle of this continuum. Phelps argued that "there are as many bipolar variations as there are patients—each person has a different mix of depression and manic experiences" (p. 2). Thus, in line with classical psychiatry, contemporary psychiatry understands bipolar disorders primarily as mood disorders

(Phelps, 2016), but it can be difficult to find the equivalents of mood disorders on tests such as the Rorschach and the TAT. For example, a person may have manic defenses on the Rorschach but not display mania or hypomania clinically, or vice-versa.

Moving away from Kretschmer's (1918/1963) concept of cyclicity to describe MDP, Bleuler (1922) identified the state of "syntony" as the common characteristic in different states of manic depression. *Syntony* refers to "vibrating in unison," or being similarly in tune. In other words, "the affectivity of a syntone person resonates with that of surrounding people and is in tune with external world conditions. At the same time, feelings of the moment all resonate internally. When the syntone patient is happy or sad, he is totally such and all other emotions are silenced" (Bleuler, 1922, p. 374, translated from German by Olivier Revaz). The concept describes the permanent way in which a person with MDP is in the world, a core organizer. As a result, Bleuler moved the emphasis from mood to affect and underlined the specific affective quality of manic depression. Patients with schizophrenia are not devoid of emotions, but they flee emotional stimulations, whereas those with manic depression actively seek them (Revaz, 2013).

To study this specific affective quality, the TAT seemed the correct tool, considering how the images can elicit relational scenarios and evoke affect. We analyzed the TAT protocols of our eight subjects (Husain et al., 2006) by systematically recording any reference to affect, any fragment of speech concerning affect, any manifestation of affect, keeping Bleuler's syntony in mind. Bouhsira and Parat (2005) referred to affect as a categorical term, grouping all subjective and qualitative aspects of emotional life. Affect can carry a pleasant or unpleasant connotation, can be defined or undefined, and can be coherent or incoherent, depending on the context.

Themes Dealing With Affect

Verbalizations concerning affect were divided into seven thematic categories, based on a consensus among four judges (Husain et al., 2006). The total number of formulations used for this group of MDPs was 318 observations. We then proceeded to rank these seven categories according to their relative importance (frequency), assigning them a rank from 1 to 7, with Rank 1 designating the theme with the highest occurrence. The seven themes are listed and a percentage is assigned to each. This percentage represents the proportion of formulations related to the given category out of the total number of comments (318). Note that the first three categories account for more than 75% of all collected observations.

1. Qualification of affect: 30.5%
2. Affective symbiosis: 29.87%
3. Presence of an emotional theme: 18.23%
4. Affective manifestation: 8.17%
5. Inconsistency of affect: 7.54%

6. Apparent emotional indifference: 3.14%
7. Reference to support: 2.51%

The main themes are described with several supporting examples. Identifying information associated with test responses has been eliminated or disguised to preserve confidentiality.

Qualification of Affect

Minkowski (1927/1997) recalled that syntony (i.e., the patient's attitude toward the ambiance) became for Bleuler an essential feature of differential diagnosis. Bleuler (1922) considered that what characterizes both "manic-depressive madness and corresponding temperaments" is not so much the intermittent or cyclical factor but this "particular affective quality." As a result, he noted that contact with reality is maintained and, despite their mental disorders, a good emotional contact is possible unlike in people suffering from schizophrenia, with whom "we have no emotional contact" (p. 374, translated from German by Olivier Revaz). The reference to affect appears as a constant concern in the TAT of our subjects. In the following examples, bolded words and phrases have been used to illustrate the themes being discussed.

> P5, T2 (P5 = Patient no. 5; T2 = TAT Picture 2): And then in the head of the pregnant woman, well she has, she is . . . we cannot say if she smiles or if she is, seems to rest. . . . Now the emotion it gives off is perhaps a little ambiguous . . . she seems happier rather than not happy. (Husain et al., 2006)

Most of the time, the patients try to identify the emotional state of the TAT characters. They seek affect everywhere and they insist on describing, qualifying, and refining the evoked affect. This is achieved in different ways, either by using several synonyms or by resorting to repetition. Sometimes, characters are described using contrasting affects (e.g., sad vs. happy), akin to the axes that Mormont (1983) described as "bipolar." Predominantly, MDPs manage to create an atmosphere of emotional intensity with their choice of words—qualifiers such as "fierce," "invasive," furious," and "curled up" and adverbs such as "always," "never," "very very," and "completely" are suggestive of intensity (Chabot et al., 2003).

> P7, T2: She looks at them and goes to study, she looks **sad**. In the evening she is **happy** to return to the land to see her parents. She looks **sad** . . . it's a **sad** story because that's not what the girl wanted to do. She leaves **with regret**. (Husain et al., 2006)

> P4, T1: . . . and this **great** violin was given as a gift to a little boy who is in awe of him . . . what he wants is to be able **to coax him, to work with him, to make him express everything that is in his being** through the music that will come out of the violin. (Husain et al., 2006)

Making the violin alive provides the child with company; the boy interacts with the instrument and is therefore not alone. The persistence of an animist stance, in Piagetian terms (Piaget, 1947; Piaget & Inhelder, 1966), might serve the purpose of denying loneliness and differs from the true confusion between animate and inanimate that we find in people with schizophrenia (Blatt & Wild, 1976).

> P5, T3: . . . it seems to me like a woman, who is squatting near an armchair and who is in a position of **very** intense pain, **very very** intense, she has a **lot** of pain, she is **very** sad. (Husain et al., 2006)

Clinically, it is not uncommon for these patients to describe themselves as confused regarding the nature of what they feel. We could hypothesize that this search for precision, this attempt at a hyper-definition of affect, serves to fight against what Zweig (1927) referred to in the title of his book as the *Confusion of Feelings* (translated from French by me). At times, this "confusion of feelings" appears to be clearly enjoyable. It is by design that we quote the title of this book by Zweig, who committed suicide with his wife in 1942, and whose life and literary style show many signs of MDP.

Despite these efforts at definition and delimitation, affect in patients with MDP arises with intensity and overflows. It has sometimes been said that their protective shield is weak; consequently, they passively experience flooding by affect. On the contrary, we have observed that the expression of affect is extremely present, even exacerbated. A hypothesis is that the sensation of affect might be actively sought. Excessive affect could then be understood as defensive overexcitement. Several of these patients reported a troubled childhood, with a depressed parent, often in the context of serious psychopathology or, in any case, with parents on whom patients with MDP had no impact. As adults, they are often romantically involved in seemingly sado-masochistic partnerships. Unlike people with borderline personality disorder, they do not seek domination and submissiveness per se, but rather a form of stimulation emanating from the harshness of the relationships and the psychic agitation generated. Such relations make them experience a "waltz of feelings" (Husain et al., 2006) and the emotional sensation of alternating sadness, anger, hatred, indignation, and despair animates these patients and gives them the feeling of being truly alive. Moreover, when their relationships are less chaotic, daily life with a partner leads to "mortal boredom" and an anxiety described as "unbearable." Relatedly, MDPs may complain about their mood-stabilizing medication because it renders their life banal and colorless.

We hypothesize that MDPs actively seek a "confusion of feelings" as a kind of emotional cacophony, intended to avoid hearing the sound of anxiety. In our previous work (Chabot et al., 2003), we suggested that if intensity is indeed a defense, then feeling everything intensely (sensation, affect, thought) could serve the purpose of fighting the anguish of feeling nothing (i.e., the anguish of emptiness and death).

Affect and Symbiosis

The expression "affective symbiosis" was coined by Wallon (1934/2002) to describe the stage of emotional sociability in babies a few months of age. The child's attitudes and mimicry (laughter, cries, smiles, grimaces, expressive postures) interact with the reactions of its entourage, creating a real emotional space with little differentiation between infant and adult (Bloch et al., 1997). This notion aptly describes the particular form of contact that MDPs establish with their environment.

These patients aspire to a kind of total affective union and synchrony between themselves and their relational objects. This is different from a typical symbiotic object relation encountered in performance tests of other psychotic structures where confusion and lack of differentiation between self and other are noted. MDPs appear better differentiated, but nevertheless in search of this union.

> P7, T4: A love story. The gentleman looks far ahead. He tells his lover what he sees in **their destiny**. The **lady laps up his words**, she can't think clearly. She looks with him to see **their projects, those are their projects**, otherwise she wouldn't be hooked like this to him. (Husain et al., 2006)

It is not uncommon for this affective closeness to be prolonged by a shared sensoriality.

> P8, T10: A man who hugs a woman and it brings him comfort . . . He **feels her warmth** . . . He **savors** it, it calms him, **fills** a void. The woman also **feels** that, that it fills him and fills a void. [The examiner asks about potential relationships between characters.] No, it would be a new relationship, it would have taken time before he could afford to **warm up** like that . . . that's what allows him to be filled by the **warmth** of that **contact**. (Husain et al., 2006)

The TAT protocols of our research subjects, Minkowski's (1927/1997) treatise, and the provocative book *The Sex Life of Catherine M.* (Millet, 2001) allowed us to connect the quest for "total union" and Bleuler's syntony, which he defined as "vibrating in unison with the ambiance." The word "ambiance," which appears in the French translation, is well chosen. Indeed, beyond their relationship with the object, MDPs eagerly seek continuity, or even contiguity, between self and the surrounding world. The phenomenon can be understood as a kind of symbiotic relationship, one that is more evolved than both the symbiosis of bodily identities found in schizophrenia and the symbiosis of systems of thought found in paranoia. Identities do not exist separately; they exist only in a relationship of continuity. This phenomenon potentially participates in the production of confabulations on the Rorschach, often described in manic functioning, as the subject creates links based on the contiguity of the blots.

Affective symbiosis manifests itself preferentially through relationships established between TAT characters, but it can also arise within the relationship with the examiner. Whereas patients with paranoia make sure that the other "thinks the same," those with MDP need the other to "feel the same." Such patients are endearing and communicative, both in their laughter and their sadness. In a way, the examiner would serve as an "auxiliary emotional self." When we extend the concept of object relation to Bleuler's "ambiance," it becomes apparent that other processes fall under the same category. MDPs can describe an emotional state in perfect harmony with the surroundings, a climate filled with sensations and "raw bodily experiences" to use the term by Aulagnier (1975). Rebourg's (1992) article titled "Mania or Sensory Exaltation" laid the groundwork for identifying the specificity of manic discourse on projective tests. She described the predominance of sensation at the expense of representation. Emphasis on light, heat, noise, texture, and odor can thus resonate with the state of happiness of the subject, while darkness and heaviness will resonate with affects of sadness and despair.

> P1, T16: A little girl sitting on a swing with her parents . . . . Also, the same little girl, older now, on a veranda with **wicker** furniture, the sea is not far away, everything is in **pastel colors**, then there is a guy with her, then there are children, then there is a lot of life, happiness, you **hear the sound** of the waves, especially **it smells of the sea**. (Husain et al., 2006)

In his text "The Manic Defense," Winnicott (1935/1969) mentioned individuals who illustrate the use of this defensive modality by exploiting all physical aspects of sexuality and sensuality. The hypersexuality of patients with manic disorders is known and mentioned by Akiskal (1999), who underlined that people with low-grade bipolar disorder often retain throughout their depressive phases a sexuality that is quite atypical of their depressive symptomatology. Other aspects of symbiosis are apparent in a certain representation of time. Indeed, some subjects propose a narrative with a theme of perpetuity: This can be an object, an affect or an attitude that survives across time, thus establishing a kind of immutability, a symbiosis between present and future.

> P4, T1: Once upon a time, there was a musical instrument created by a great musician called Stradivarius; he put all his soul into the making of the instrument . . . both the music and the instrument have taken on great value and they have been, they have been **passed down from generation to generation for centuries and centuries**. (Husain et al., 2006)

The durability of the instrument is part of a time dimension that is infinite and denies any idea of death. Indeed, the soul of Stradivarius continues to live beyond his death in his instrument and in his music, thus ensuring immortality.

Some stories might refer to "a new beginning," where the representation of time is cyclical rather than linear, a characteristic that is prominent in Flaubert's (1857/2001) classical novel *Madame Bovary* (Husain & Lepage, 2016). Speaking of melancholic "lethargy," Monette (1990) described how some of her patients aspire to a state of "perpetual rest," which defuses any potential excitement, any experience of pleasure, "out of loyalty to the psychically dead mother." This description fits with our observation of an unchanged and unchangeable temporality in MDP.

Affective symbiosis, harmony with the environment, durability of time—all these manifestations have in common a hypercathexis of linking, a complete contrast to the idea of "attacks on linking" expounded by Bion (1959). Although destructive attacks on links between objects can be evidenced in psychotic functioning, individuals with paranoid schizophrenia often display pathological interpretations by attributing excessive meaning and arbitrarily binding contents together. These exaggerated links lie outside the margins of social convention and are generally based on arbitrary and illogical reasoning (translated as FABCOMs and INCOMs on the Rorschach).

> Card I: I see hands up here, trying to clutch nothingness.

On the contrary, linking in MDPs remains understandable and appears less unrealistic.

> Card I: A butterfly creature mixed with a scarab. (P4)

Bearing in mind that according to Bergeret's (1974) model, fragmentation anxiety is always in play at all levels of psychotic functioning, we can hypothesize that this continuity of beings and things is also a particular form of defense against fragmentation.

The Presence of an Emotional Theme

At the level of content, we encountered themes of sadness, loss, fear, worry, and jealousy, but also several stories evoking comfort, joy, and fullness, often related to perfect romantic relationships. We noticed that object loss was rarely associated with a theme of rejection, as is the case in people with borderline personality disorder, particularly on Picture 4. Here is the story given by a woman with borderline personality disorder with important masochistic traits. The story emphasizes the loss of the other's love.

> T4: This is a man . . . who tries to leave this woman and she clings to him. She would like to hold him absolutely, obviously he has the upper hand; he does not care [The examiner asks how the story ends] . . . he doesn't love her anymore. I think, like all men, **he loved her once and then it can disappear from one day to another**. (Husain et al., 2006)

Here is another story of loss on Picture 10, given by a young woman from our MDP sample:

> P4, T10: A grandfather with his little girl. They are close. Her grandfather comforts her. One day, the grandfather will die, and the girl will feel the impact. She is very close to him; she loves him very much. (Husain et al., 2006)

The frequent association between separation and death noted in MDP differs from the object loss described by borderline personality disorders. For the former, loss itself is experienced as a psychic death; this is consistent with an identity whose integrity requires a "total union" with the other.

In the same way, the theme of maternal care is treated very differently in the following two stories, the first being provided by a patient with an infantile personality (borderline state) and the second by subject P7, a woman in our MDP group:

> T7: I see it as the maid of the little girl or the au pair or the housekeeper, a little girl who looks like **she's playing with a doll**, who looks bored, who doesn't know what to play, the housekeeper who looks at the baby and is telling a story. (Husain et al., 2006)

> P7, T7: A lady who lovingly tells her daughter **how she too will become a mother**, she seems to tell her that by using a book. A story of motherhood, taking care of your baby, it's important, we love him. The mother reads her a story. (Husain et al., 2006)

Whereas the first story presents the maternal figure as a utilitarian object (by assigning a subordinate function to her: "maid," "au pair," or "housekeeper"), the second story situates the child as an extension of the parent through the previously mentioned theme of continuity and perpetuity ("she too will become a mother"). What typifies MDPs is not the presence of affective connotations on TAT stories, since that can appear in many different personalities, but rather the insistence on this affective symbiosis.

The following minor themes require little elaboration, since each represents only a small percentage (from 2% to 8%) of the total observations. Nevertheless, we will review them briefly, in decreasing order of importance.

Affective Manifestation

Since we had decided to identify every phenomenon related to affect, it became important to record not only the discourse on affect but also its behavioral components. Laughter is by far the most frequent manifestation and generally functions as a manic defense. For example, P8 laughs as he evokes a murder and a tragic story on Picture 13. P2 cries in the context of an intense persecutory experience. However, these behavioral expressions of affect are far from frequent in our sample (8.17%), a finding that contradicts our initial expectation of MDP as always being emotionally on edge.

Incoherence of Affect

This was scored when the affect evoked did not fit the usual interpretation of the characters' emotional state or when the affect was unmotivated. Emmanuelli et al. (2005) were also attuned to this phenomenon and distinguished affects that were in tune with the picture from those that proved inadequate or inappropriate.

Apparent Emotional Indifference

In MDPs, affect is actively sought and treated with intensity. Yet, on a few occasions—and this is true for only two of the eight subjects in our sample—the TAT story has striking expressions of indifference.

> P8, T6: This is my brother Peter who announces his departure to my mother . . . she doesn't express her feelings. **She remains indifferent . . . she is not interested** in his adventure. (Husain et al., 2006)

Not surprisingly, these two subjects present with a more depressive, even melancholic, symptomatology. The person may report an emotional void, a clearly expressed absence of feeling, or an indifferent or "frozen" parent. Irony might be used in depicting situations likely to cause painful affects, such as a sentimental breakup. In fact, affect remains present, but muted, through veiled references to annoyance, bitterness, and disappointed expectations, which are all sources of suffering. These personalities always seek intense affective communion with the object. When the latter does not react, the indifference is experienced in a hostile and persecutory way. Interestingly, the outcome of these stories is that parent and child end up sharing the same indifference, the same absence of affective reaction, thus restoring a form of affective symbiosis.

Reference to Support

In a few rare cases, the theme of support emerges (i.e., the need or the ability to rely on the other), along with a concomitant anguish of object loss. Although this theme is shared by patients with borderline personality disorder, its rendering in those with MDP is generally accompanied by the previously mentioned specific intense affective quality.

DISCUSSION

Do MDPs exist, and are they expressed on a test such as the TAT? We believe so (Husain et al., 2006). The images are treated preferentially in an emotional way; affect is conveyed with insistence and intensity; and relationships with others and the surrounding world are colored with a specific form of symbiosis that constantly seeks the continuity of beings and things, in a fantasy of "total union." Bleuler's (1922) concept of syntony became the missing guiding thread in our understanding of MDPs.

The quest for harmony can be viewed as a process of unifying and linking. It ensures symbiosis, but it could also fight an underlying anxiety. In MDP, identity, although better constructed than in schizophrenia, cannot survive independently of the environment, as noncontiguity itself is experienced as deadly. It is by design that we evoke the theme of death, often brought up by these subjects, both on the Rorschach and the TAT. Hypothesizing an underlying anxiety of death makes it possible to ascribe a defensive function to the exacerbation of affect—the search for excitement enables patients to escape the threat of feeling nothing.

Winnicott's (1935/1969) use of the concept of "flight into reality" allows for some interesting overlap with Bleuler's syntony (Revaz, 2013). According to Winnicott, in their greedy contact with external reality, patients with manic disorder seek sensations that allow them to flee their internal reality. In fact, the hypercathexis of the surrounding atmosphere (external reality) does not exclude the exacerbation of internal sensations. Khan (1974) also referred to patients who display an astonishing greed for both external environment and internal fantasy: "They must always be absorbed, tortured, stimulated, otherwise they sink into apathy, into a kind of non-existence, of non-being" (Khan, 1974, p. 93, translated from French by me).

MDP Versus Bipolar Spectrum Disorders

The demonstration of MDP as an identifiable type of psychological functioning (Husain et al., 2006), nevertheless leaves an open question: What is the relationship between MDP and bipolarity? Between the first sample of eight patients with bipolar disorder (Chabot et al., 2003) and the second one of eight MDPs (Husain et al., 2006), there certainly was some overlap. For example, intensity in language and heightened emotional experience appear in both groups. We could hypothesize that bipolar disorders are the most likely decompensation of a person with MDP. However, our two groups are not superimposable: Those with bipolar disorders had a greater heterogeneity of functioning than those with MDP. This finding is not surprising, as subjects who are ultimately diagnosed as having "bipolar" disorder using the *DSM-IV* (American Psychiatric Association, 1994) or the *Diagnostic and Statistical Manual of Mental Disorders* (5th ed., text rev.; *DSM-5-TR*; American Psychiatric Association, 2022) often end up with multiple diagnoses over the years, and many are misdiagnosed as evidenced by their evolution. If concepts such as Akiskal's "soft bipolarity" (Cassano et al., 2002) and Phelps's (2016) "mood spectrum" were more widespread in psychiatry, then there would be better identification of these cases. And if personality assessments using the Rorschach and the TAT were more systematically requested, then precision would increase even more. Indeed, as a result of our qualitative studies (Chabot et al., 2003; Husain et al., 2006), several subjects of this sample of MDPs finally received a mood stabilizer that contributed to less chaotic functioning. Another consequence of these findings is that since the publication of our work, more and more assessors are in a position to correctly identify MDP and make appropriate recommendations.

Differential Diagnosis Around MDP in a Structural Approach

In a structural approach, differential diagnosis can also be established and may not converge with the psychiatric diagnosis based on symptoms. The use of our grid allows for inferences in several areas of functioning that enable fine distinctions between MDP and neighboring psychopathological conditions.

Bipolarity and Borderline Personality Disorder

On numerous occasions, subjects with MDP are labeled as having borderline personality disorder, possibly because of their exuberance and impulsive tendencies (see also Chapter 14 in this volume). The intensity of their exuberance is understood as a histrionic dramatization, whereas their relational mode is not aimed at manipulating others. Their impulsivity is equated with character disordered opposition. In fact, the challenge for MDPs is not the manipulation of others but the affective communion with others. This diagnostic confusion deprives patients with MDP of adequate understanding and help, "thereby missing the opportunity to make sense of the temperamental foundations of instability" in their lives (Perugi & Akiskal, 2002, p. 714). Phelps (2016) also underlined the distinction that experienced clinicians can make between borderlinity and bipolarity: "The transference energy is often intense, early, and trends toward rapidly overvaluing or devaluing providers" (pp. 40–41). The Lausanne School has also developed tools to make this distinction by studying subcategories of borderline personality disorder (Merceron et al., 1985, 1990; Rossel et al., 1991).

Bipolarity and Schizoaffective Disorder

Although most signs of an affective component are present, patients with schizoaffective disorder present with both qualitative and quantitative differences, such as more severe thought disorders, more signs of fragmentation anxiety and symbiosis, heightened paranoid anxiety, and clear dissociation of the self.

Bipolarity and Paranoia

This can be a difficult issue, as we have often encountered people with paranoia (equivalent to paranoid personality disorders) who have an affective component and MDPs who show signs of persecution. The character trait labelled as "der sensitive Beziehungswahn" (in German; "paranoia sensitive" in French), which dates back to Kretschmer (1918/1963), captured this combination of affect and paranoia but has totally disappeared from our current psychiatric nomenclature.

CONCLUSION

The notion of a bipolar spectrum appears as the best option to capture the diversity of both clinical bipolarity and structural manic depressivity. MDPs come in many different shades; they can present themselves as prototypes, but they can also occur with overlaps: an overlap with schizophrenia as in schizoaffective personality organization or an overlap with paranoia as in sensitive paranoia. It can also be hidden under borderline personality traits. The use of our grid helps in establishing a convergence between different areas of psychic functioning, thus enabling the psychologist to extract the core indicators of MDP. In the last 2 decades, more testing data have been recorded and analyzed and in closing, we propose a summary grid of the most common indicators of MDP (Husain, 2020) derived from both the Rorschach and the TAT (see Table 17.2).

TABLE 17.2. Manic-Depressive Personalities: Markers on the Rorschach and the TAT

Object relations	Boundaries	Self and identity	Anxiety	Defense mechanisms	Thought processes
Yearning for symbiosis, especially affective symbiosis: emphasis on contact, togetherness, harmony Fantasy of total union Confusion and lack of differentiation between self and other Perennity of the object Symbiosis in death Setting the object in its environment Lost object Nostalgia for the past Indifferent (parental) figures especially in melancholia Search for support Some persecutory or dominant/submissive relationships	Some boundary disturbances Perturbed distance to the blot	Some disorder of self-integrity and identity Prevalence of a sensory self with emphasis on the senses, the ambiance, and gyratory movements Split experience with contrasting poles: heavy/light, dark/light, full/empty, and happy/sad Responses of objects falling or associated with potential falls Alternating moods: upward and downward movements Depressive/melancholic quality (dark, ruined, and dead) Presence of affect Intensity especially of affect In search of the core Fantasy of eternal renewal Infantile traits Impulsivity Immobility Masochistic stance Disinhibition in the expression of drives	Discrete fragmentation anxiety Discrete persecutory anxiety Depressive anxiety (sense of collapsing) Death anxiety Object loss through death Anxiety of nonexistence Emptiness	Splitting Idealization Self-devaluation Omnipotence Projection of feelings Projection of intentions Manic defenses, manic denial Denial of the finitude of death Negation of aggressivity Acting out (often suicidal)	Speech marked by intensity via adverbs or "strong" words or repetition or gradation of words Confabulatory responses are often linked because of spatial contiguity Connecting independent responses Some disturbance in interpretive awareness Abundance of responses and speech when more manic Loose associations when more manic Agitation when more manic (e.g., gestures, miming, laughter) Dominance of melancholia: paucity of content, breaks in speech, many negations, prevalence of "not" and "nothing," and responses in the negative form

Note. Copyright 2020 by Odile Husain. Reprinted with permission.

REFERENCES

Akiskal, H. S. (1999). The clinical necessity of a return to Kraepelin's broad schema of manic depression. *The Psychiatric Clinics of North America, 22*(3), xi–xii. https://doi.org/10.1016/S0193-953X(05)70092-7

American Psychiatric Association. (1994). *Diagnostic and statistical manual of mental disorders* (4th ed.).

American Psychiatric Association. (2022). *Diagnostic and statistical manual of mental disorders: DSM-5-TR* (5th ed., text rev.).

Aulagnier, P. (1975). *La violence de l'interprétation* [The violence of interpretation]. PUF.

Barthes, R. (1980). *La chambre claire* [The bright room]. Gallimard.

Bergeret, J. (1974). *La personnalité normale et pathologique* [Normal and pathological personality]. Dunod.

Bion, W. R. (1959). Attacks on linking. *International Journal of Psychonanalysis, 40,* 5–6.

Blatt, S., & Wild, C. (1976). *Schizophrenia: A developmental analysis.* Academic Press.

Bleuler, E. (1922). Die probleme der schizoidie und der syntonie [The problem of schizoid states and syntony]. *Zeitschrift für die Gesamte Neurologie und Psychiatrie, 78*(1), 373–399. https://doi.org/10.1007/BF02867623

Bloch, H., Dépret, E., Gallo, A., Garnier, Ph., Gineste, M.-D., Leconte, P., Le Ny, J.-F., Postel, J., Reuchlin, M., & Casalis, D. (1997). *Dictionnaire fondamental de la psychologie* [Fundamental dictionary of psychology]. Larousse.

Bouhsira, J., & Parat, H. (2005). L'affect [Affect]. In J. Bouhsira & H. Parat (Eds.), *Monographies de psychanalyse de la revue française de psychanalyse* (pp. 7–9). PUF.

Cassano, G. B., Frank, E., Miniati, M., Rucci, P., Fagiolini, A., Pini, S., Shear, M. K., & Maser, J. D. (2002). Conceptual underpinnings and empirical support for the mood spectrum. *The Psychiatric Clinics of North America, 25*(4), 699–712. https://doi.org/10.1016/S0193-953X(02)00025-4

Chabot, M., Husain, O., Reeves, N., & Choquet, F. (2003). La maladie bipolaire au Rorschach et au TAT: Diversité ou homogénéité? [Bipolar illness on the Rorschach and the TAT: Diversity or homogeneity?]. *Psychologie Clinique et Projective, 9*(9), 255–283. https://doi.org/10.3917/pcp.009.0255

Dreyfus, A., Husain, O., & Rousselle, I. (1987). Schizophrénie et TAT: Quelques considérations sur les aspects formels [Schizophrenia and the TAT: Some considerations on formal aspects]. *Psychologie Française, 32*(3), 181–186.

Dreyfus, A., Husain, O., & Rousselle Gay Crosier, I. (1989). Schizophrénie simple et schizophrénie paranoïde à travers le Rorschach: Étude comparative [Simple schizophrenia and paranoid schizophrenia on the Rorschach: A comparative study]. *Psychologie Médicale, 21*(7), 831–841.

Emmanuelli, M., Pheulpin, M.-C., & Bruguière, P. (2005). Un destin des affects dans la dépression: L'émoussement affectif. Élaboration d'une méthodologie de recherche à partir des épreuves projectives [An outcome of affects in depression: Emotional blunting. Development of a research methodology using projective methods]. *Bulletin de Psychologie, 58*(2), 195–205. https://doi.org/10.3917/bupsy.476.0195

Esquirol, E. (1994). De la lypémanie ou mélancolie [Regarding lypemania or melancholia]. In J. Postel (Ed.), *La psychiatrie: Textes essentiels* (pp. 57–65). Larousse. (Original work published 1820)

Ey, H., Bernard, P., & Brisset, Ch. (1978). *Manuel de psychiatrie* [Manual of psychiatry] (5th ed.). Masson.

Flaubert, G. (2001). *Madame Bovary.* Gallimard. (Original work published 1857)

Husain, O. (1989). La linéarité du temps et sa non-intégration chez le schizophrène. Exemple d'application: Le TAT [The linearity of time and its non-integration in schizophrenics. An application: The TAT]. *Psychologie Médicale, 21*(7), 851–857.

Husain, O. (2015). From persecution to depression: A case of chronic depression—Associating the Rorschach, the TAT, and Winnicott. *Journal of Personality Assessment, 97*(3), 230–240. https://doi.org/10.1080/00223891.2015.1009081

Husain, O. (2020, September). *Manic-depressive personalities on projective tests* [Paper presentation]. The 2020 ISR Virtual Summer Seminars of the International Rorschach Society, on Zoom.

Husain, O., & Lepage, M. (2016). Une figure de l'organisation maniaco-dépressive : La mélancolie d'Emma Bovary [A figure of manic-depressive organization: The melancholy of Emma Bovary]. *Psychologie Clinique et Projective, 22,* 271–301. https://doi.org/10.3917/pcp.022.0271

Husain, O., Reeves, N., Choquet, F., Chabot, M., & Revaz, O. (2006). À la recherche d'une organisation maniaco-dépressive au TAT [In search of a manic-depressive organization on the TAT]. *Psychologie Clinique et Projective, 12,* 429–458. https://doi.org/10.3917/pcp.012.0429

Husain, O., & Rossel, F. (1998). Paranoïaques, défendez-vous ! Le magma paranoïde vous guette! [Paranoiacs, defend yourselves! The paranoid magma awaits you!] *Bulletin de Psychologie, 51*(1), 67–78. https://www.persee.fr/doc/bupsy_0007-4403_1998_num_51_433_14702

Khan, M. (1974). *Le soi caché* [The hidden self]. Gallimard.

Kleiger, J. H. (2017). *Rorschach assessment of psychotic phenomena.* Routledge. https://doi.org/10.4324/9781315271385

Kretschmer, E. (1963). *Paranoïa et sensibilité* [Paranoia and sensitivity]. PUF. (Original work published 1918)

Merceron, C., Husain, O., & Rossel, F. (1985). Aménagement particulier des états-limites: Les organisations perverses de la personnalité à travers le Rorschach [A specific type of borderline: Perverse personality organizations on the Rorschach]. *Psychologie Française, 30*(2), 202–212.

Merceron, C., Rossel, F., & Cedraschi, C. (1990). Réflexions sur la notion de faux-self: Deux niveaux de fonctionnement mis en évidence au Rorschach [Some thoughts on the notion of false-self: Two levels of functioning evidenced on the Rorschach]. *Revue de Psychologie Appliquée, 40*(2), 183–203.

Millet, C. (2001). *La vie sexuelle de Catherine M* [The sexual life of Catherine M]. Éditions du Seuil.

Minkowski, E. (1997). Schizoïdie et syntonie [Schizoid states and syntony]. In *La schizophrénie* (pp. 9–76). Payot & Rivages. (Original work published 1927)

Monette, L. (1990). Les fidèles de la mort [The faithful of death]. *Sante Mentale au Quebec, 15*(2), 212–220. https://doi.org/10.7202/031572ar

Mormont, C. (1983). Quelques expressions de la bipolarité maniaco-dépressive au Rorschach [Some expressions of manic-depressive bipolarity on the Rorschach]. *Les Feuillets Psychiatriques de Liège, 16,* 37–40.

Perugi, G., & Akiskal, H. S. (2002). The soft bipolar spectrum redefined: Focus on the cyclothymic, anxious-sensitive, impulse-dyscontrol, and binge-eating connection in bipolar II and related conditions. *The Psychiatric Clinics of North America, 25*(4), 713–737. https://doi.org/10.1016/S0193-953X(02)00023-0

Phelps, J. (2016). *A spectrum approach to mood disorders.* W. W. Norton.

Piaget, J. (1947). *La représentation du monde chez l'enfant* [The representation of the world in the child]. PUF.

Piaget, J., & Inhelder, B. (1966). *La psychologie de l'enfant* [Child psychology]. PUF.

Prudent, C., Kleiger, J. H., Husain, O., & De Tychey, C. (2022). On psychosis: An international comparative single case study of the Nancy French, Lausanne, and American Rorschach Approaches. *Rorschachiana, 43*(1), 42–69. https://doi.org/10.1027/1192-5604/a000151

Racamier, P.-C. (1966). Esquisse d'une clinique psychanalytique de la paranoïa [Sketching a psychoanalytic clinic of paranoia]. *Revue Française de Psychanalyse, 30*(1), 145–172.

Racamier, P.-C. (1980). *Les schizophrènes* [Schizophrenics]. Payot.

Rebourg, C. (1992). La manie ou l'exaltation sensorielle: La notion d'éprouvés corporels bruts au Rorschach [Mania or sensory exaltation: The notion of rough bodily experiences on the Rorschach]. *Psychologie Médicale, 24*(11), 1134–1136.

Revaz, O. (2013). La syntonie, notion-clé du « spectre » bipolaire? [Syntony, a key notion of the bipolar spectrum?]. *Psychologie Clinique et Projective, 19*, 75–89. https://doi.org/10.3917/pcp.019.0075

Rossel, F., Cedraschi, C., & Merceron, C. (1991). False-self: Personality or defence? Comparative study of two Rorschach protocols. *British Journal of Projective Psychology, 36*(1), 35–62.

Rousselle, I., Husain, O., & Dreyfus, A. (1990). Les prudents et les méfiants: Diversité de la paranoïa au Rorschach [The cautious and the suspicious: Diversity of paranoia on the Rorschach]. *Bulletin de Psychologie, 43*, 716–719. https://www.persee.fr/doc/bupsy_0007-4403_1990_num_43_396_13188

Rousselle Gay-Crosier, I., Dreyfus, A., & Husain, O. (1989). Le statut du réel et de la représentation chez le paranoïaque à travers le Rorschach et le TAT [The status of reality and representation in paranoia on the Rorschach]. *Psychologie Médicale, 21*(7), 887–890.

Singer, H. K., & Brabender, V. (1993). The use of the Rorschach to differentiate unipolar and bipolar disorders. *Journal of Personality Assessment, 60*(2), 333–345. https://doi.org/10.1207/s15327752jpa6002_10

Solovay, M. R., Shenton, M. E., & Holzman, P. S. (1987). Comparative studies of thought disorders. I. Mania and schizophrenia. *Archives of General Psychiatry, 44*(1), 13–20. https://doi.org/10.1001/archpsyc.1987.01800130015003

Wallon, H. (2002). *L'évolution psychologique de l'enfant* [The psychological evolution of the child]. Armand Colin. (Original work published 1934)

Weiner, I. B. (1966). *Psychodiagnosis in schizophrenia*. Wiley.

Winnicott, D. W. (1969). La défense maniaque [Manic defense]. In *De la pédiatrie à la psychanalyse* (pp. 15–32). Payot. (Original work published 1935)

Zweig, S. (1927). *La confusion des sentiments* [The confusion of feelings]. Librairie Générale Française.

18

Assessment of Bipolar Spectrum Disorders Within a Multicultural Context

Linda Fleming McGhee

The assessment of bipolar spectrum disorders (BSDs) is complex, multidimensional, and nuanced. The human element of the diagnostic process is central to our analysis of psychopathology. The life experience of a person who presents themselves in clinical and community settings is shaped by the groups with whom they affiliate, the identities they assume, and the characteristics that society foists upon them. How do these affiliations, identities, and characteristics play out in the lives and functioning of those we assess for BSDs?

Culture has many meanings that encapsulate these connections. It plays a part in how we live our lives. If we are members of marginalized cultures and communities, we likely move through the world differently and face the associated hardships and systematic handicaps. Being a part of certain cultures may make people in those cultures more susceptible to mental illness, specifically mood disorders such as BSDs. Underlying the analysis of lived experience is the impact of trauma connected to such membership and how clinicians analyze and incorporate trauma in our assessments (see Chapter 15 in this volume).

It is not just the patients we diagnose and assess who must be analyzed. The clinician, their culture, upbringing, and training also come into play. Thus, the lived experiences of the patient and the clinician meet in the assessment room. Moreover, this meeting is filtered through the backdrop of a biopsychosocial

https://doi.org/10.1037/0000356-019
Psychological Assessment of Bipolar Spectrum Disorders, J. H. Kleiger and I. B. Weiner (Editors)

lens. It also incorporates the history of this country and perceptions of the past. Diagnoses are not made in a vacuum, but are made and filtered by the society that houses clinicians and patients alike. A society contains systems and institutions that treat people differently based on certain aspects of culture, including race, gender, and sexuality.

Although many aspects of multiculturalism have not been researched or thoroughly investigated, we will follow the literature on women; LGBTQIA people; and racial groups, mainly Black/African Americans, Latinos/Latinas/Hispanics, and Asians/Asian Americans.

The focus is on how being a member of these cultures affects mental health and how culture influences the diagnostic, assessment, and treatment process of BSDs. The impacts potentially include misdiagnosis, a misalignment of psychopharmacological treatment, and undercutting the quality of treatment, often already compromised in marginalized communities. Of course, the study of culture has been the subject of research, but there are still many areas that require further inquiry. We explore those areas as well. Ultimately, we hope to guide clinicians to optimize assessment by thinking about their clients and themselves through the cultural lens.

There is a dearth of research on various racial and ethnic communities and bipolar disorders, including indigenous populations and ethnic and racial populations outside of the United States. Thus, while these cultures are vitally important to our discussion of BSDs, they are not covered here due to the paucity of data and research.

SPECIAL CONSIDERATIONS FOR ASSESSING WOMEN

Most of the scant research on bipolar disorders and gender (as opposed to transgender, highlighted later) uses the terms "women and men" and "male and female." The researchers often do not define the terms. In addition, our ideas about gender and sex are changing and older research can easily become outdated. It is usually not clear whether they are referring to sex or gender. *Sex* typically refers to the biological aspects of maleness or femaleness. *Gender* implies the psychological, behavioral, social, and cultural aspects of being male or female (i.e., masculinity or femininity; American Psychological Association [APA], n.d.).

Moreover, gender or sex are traditionally categorized in early research as binary choices. The state of our theoretical understanding of gender and sex has and is evolving rapidly. For this chapter, we use common terms in the relevant literature for gender and sex.

Although women are statistically in the majority, historically, they are often marginalized in many aspects of society. They do not receive focus in terms of research generally and the diagnosis of psychopathology specifically. The vast majority of research shows either an equal or nearly equal prevalence of BSDs in men and women (Hendrick et al., 2000). The one exception is that the fifth edition of the *Diagnostic and Statistical Manual of Mental Disorders* (*DSM-5*) reported a slightly higher prevalence of men diagnosed with bipolar disorder than women (American Psychiatric Association, 2013). Few consistent gender differences were found in key bipolar variables, including symptoms, rates of depressive episodes, age and polarity of onset, the severity of the illness, response to treatment, and suicidality (Diflorio & Jones, 2010). However, there is a consistent finding that women are overrepresented in bipolar II, even though there is no meaningful difference between genders in total bipolar diagnoses (Hendrick et al., 2000).

Women in reproductive stages are vulnerable to BSDs. After giving birth, they are more likely to be diagnosed with a bipolar disorder and face a greater likelihood of experiencing a recurrence of symptoms in postpartum and perimenopausal stages (Leibenluft, 1996; Miller et al., 2015). Women of color with bipolar disorders experience more pregnancy complications (Toffey et al., 2018). Research also indicates that women are more prone to hypomania, rapid cycling, and mixed bipolar episodes. Hospitalization for mania is also more likely for women than men. Salient gender differences are found in patterns of comorbidity (Diflorio & Jones, 2010). Men diagnosed as bipolar are significantly more likely than women with a similar diagnosis to have a comorbid substance use disorder. However, compared with the general population of women, women with bipolar disorder had 4 times the rate of alcohol use disorders and they were 7 times more likely to have substance abuse disorders (Hendrick et al., 2000).

While there is no appreciable discrepancy between the prevalence rate for men and women, there is some disparity in bipolar diagnoses among women. One such disparity is misdiagnosis between bipolar disorder and other illnesses, primarily borderline personality disorder and, to a lesser extent, posttraumatic stress disorder (see Chapters 14 and 15 in this volume). Women are approximately 3 times more likely to be diagnosed with borderline personality disorder than men. Several factors are at play, including the overlap in symptoms, clinician error, clinical bias, and lack of adequate training and experience in making differential diagnoses (Becker & Lamb, 1994).

As outlined in the text revison of *DSM-5* (*DSM-5-TR*; American Psychiatric Association, 2022), there is considerable symptomatic overlap between bipolar and borderline disorders, particularly in hypomania and depressive bouts, which makes differential diagnosis difficult (Green, 2020). Difficulties differentiating between the diagnosis of mood disorders and borderline personality disorders persisted even when men and women presented with similar symptoms, according to Becker and Lamb (1994). Their study found that women were more likely to be diagnosed with borderline personality disorder than a mood disorder. Findings such as these indicate that, diagnostic difficulty notwithstanding, clinician bias plays some role in assessing mood disorders (Becker & Lamb, 1994).

SPECIAL CONSIDERATIONS FOR ASSESSING LGBTQIA CLIENTS

LGBTQIA stands for lesbian, gay, bisexual, transgender, queer/questioning (one's sexual or gender identity), intersex, and asexual/aromantic/agender (Gold, 2019). Like the acronym, much of the research is also aggregated by the broad category of LGBTQIA or provides unclear categorization, making it difficult to ascertain the complex and disparate life experiences. The more recent categories of intersex and asexual/aromantic/agender have not been the subject of substantial research, particularly in relation to the diagnosis of BSDs. Conceptualizing LGBTQIA as characteristics that can exist on a continuum with varying degrees of interest and identity is often unexplored in the research literature.

The LGBTQIA communities are generally more vulnerable to mental illness and face a higher rate of mood disorders and substance use disorders. LGBTQIA communities are 1.5 to 2.6 times more likely to develop a mood disorder, including bipolar disorders (Husain-Krautter, 2017).

One vein of research utilizing neuroimaging found that nonheterosexual people (as defined by the Kinsey scale as individuals who do not endorse all heterosexual feelings; i.e., they endorse some homosexual feelings) are more likely to have a psychiatric illness (Abé et al., 2018; Kidd et al., 2016; Kinsey et al., 1948). In contrast with the Kinsey scale, the current conceptualization of sexual orientation allows one to identify as heterosexual even if one endorses homosexual feelings.

Abé et al. (2018) found that many (61%) female clients who were diagnosed with bipolar disorders or attention-deficit/hyperactivity disorder reported nonheterosexual sexual orientation. They found that nonheterosexual female patients (nHEW) had significantly larger cortical volumes in medial occipital brain regions than the exclusively heterosexual female group (HEW). The Abé study also used a heterosexual versus nonheterosexual model in which any homosexual feeling designates one as homosexual. Neuroimaging is a burgeoning area of research that will require repetition and larger sample sizes in order to gain traction as a predictor of psychopathology.

LGBTQIA populations have been found to experience a considerably greater prevalence of depression and depressive episodes (adjusted odds ratio [OR] = 1.80) and suicide attempts (OR = 2.21) relative to the general population (Kidd et al., 2016). People who identify as bisexual and gay at the younger and older ends of the age spectrum are more vulnerable to mood disorders (Semlyen et al., 2016). In a widespread study called the Trevor Project, the 2019 National Survey on LGBTQ Youth Mental Health found that 39% of LGBTQ youth seriously contemplated suicide in the prior year, while 71% of LGBTQ youth reported feeling sad or hopeless (The Trevor Project, 2019).

There are theories about factors influencing the correlation between psychological disorders and sexual orientation or gender. One school of thought suggests that shared underlying characteristics (such as hormonal factors, genetic traits, and personality markers) connect sexual orientation and mental illness (Abé et al., 2018). Zietsch et al. (2012) posited that shared genetic traits across same-sex sexual orientation and affective disorders are the basis for the connection. Some studies suggest genetic or early developmental events, such as infection in the birth canal or exposure to certain drugs (Husain-Krautter, 2017). Research also points to certain environmental factors, such as emotional abuse, as playing a role in the development of bipolar disorders. Gay people may be more likely to experience environmental risk factors for trauma, other mental health issues, and physical health issues. Lack of access to mental health care may also contribute to poor treatment outcomes in this population (Abé et al., 2018; Husain-Krautter, 2017).

A central theory is that the stress or trauma associated with being a part of the LGBTQIA communities can lead to the development of psychopathology, including BSDs. Members of sexual minority cultures are often targeted, victimized, and stigmatized (Abé et al., 2018). Hardships or discrimination also likely impact psychopathology. Thus, the LGBTQIA communities are more subject to stress and trauma. If such trauma is severe, chronic, and untreated, it can lead to the development of psychopathology. Lee and his co-researchers reported an increased prevalence of mood disorders in gay women who had experienced discrimination as opposed to those women who had not. They also found that gay men who had experienced discrimi-nation (57.4% of the study participants) reported higher odds of drug and cannabis use disorders compared to gay men who reported that they had never experienced discrimination (Lee et al., 2016). At least part of this increased prevalence rate is related to prolonged and chronic minority stress. Hendricks and Testa (2012) applied Meyer's minority stress model to trans-gender people (Meyer & Frost, 2013). This model addresses the likelihood that individuals will experience mental health challenges when they experi-ence both proximal and distal challenges. Research conducted by Nadal and his fellow researchers (Nadal et al., 2015) focused on microaggressions directed toward individuals in the LGBTQIA community and the impacts of such microaggressions on mental health functioning. Nadal et al. also highlighted individuals at the intersections of race, gender, sexuality, ethnic-ity, and religion. They found that the impact of being in multiple groups exacerbates stressors (Hendricks & Testa, 2012; Nadal et al., 2015, 2016). The myriad of environmental factors faced in the LGBTQIA communities also impacted the cognitive processes associated with rumination and emotional dysregulation (Abé et al., 2018).

Assessing Transgender Clients

Consistent with the other LGBTQIA findings, transgender individuals are more susceptible to mood disorders, bipolar disorders, and schizophrenia than the general population (Hendricks & Testa, 2012). Though the research on trans-gender populations is limited, the rate of suicide attempts among transgender and gender nonconforming adults was substantially higher than that of the general population (41% of transgender/gender nonconforming vs. 4.6% of the general population had lifetime suicide attempts; Kidd et al., 2016).

SPECIAL CONSIDERATIONS FOR ASSESSING INDIVIDUALS OF DIFFERENT RACES AND ETHNICITIES

Blacks/African Americans/Black Americans

The terms "African American" and "Black" are used interchangeably in the literature. While these terms often overlap, they are not synonymous, as not all African Americans are Black and not all Black people are Americans. These terms are combined in our discussion.

Historically, the prevailing wisdom in the mental health community was that Black/African American people had lower rates of affective disorders than Whites/European Americans. Even in modern times, studies consistently find racial differences with respect to the diagnosis, treatment, and medication of mood disorders. This belief system is in part rooted in systemic racism. In *Race and Psychiatry*, Thomas and Sillen trace this diagnostic and treatment misalignment to clinician belief that Blacks/African Americans possessed a "state of primitive mentality" (see also Perzichilli, 2020). Moreover, throughout the history of psychology, the symbolic use of language around darkness and blackness of skin drives the negative connections with darkness of character, venality, and psychopathology. This is consistent with numerous attempts in the history of psychology to distinguish between the races and to prove the superiority of White people over Black people in a specialty often called scientific racism. While the history of race and racism is beyond the scope of this chapter, there is a plethora of research that highlights this unfortunate history (Perzichilli, 2020).

Historically, psychology posited that Black/African American people did not have as many mood disorders because most were deprived of self-esteem, material possessions, and status, and, as such, they did not have what was required to experience a "loss" which is a precipitator of depression (Thomas & Sillen, 1972). In early psychoanalytic writings in the United States, Evarts (1914) argued that Black/African Americans were equated to primitive and inferior beings, prone to psychosis and incapable of emotional regulation. O'Malley (1914) argued that mental disorders in Blacks/African Americans were a compensatory defense against living in a higher order civilization that was beyond their capacity to navigate successfully. He concluded that Black/African American patients did not have depression, as mood disorders suggested evolutionary advancement, which Black/African American patients lacked.

In most studies, Black/African American people were diagnosed with bipolar disorders at a lower rate than Whites/European Americans. Research indicates the range of the diagnostic error and found that Black/African American people were diagnosed with bipolar disorders at one-fourth the rate of Whites/European Americans (Akinhanmi et al., 2018). Astonishingly, G. Johnson et al. (1968)

reviewed 3 years of admissions records to Bellevue Psychiatric Hospital and did not find one case of a Black/African American patient being diagnosed with manic depression. Moreover, research suggests that Blacks/African Americans were vulnerable to inaccurate assessment of symptoms and, as a result, were given poor care, consisting of less intensive treatment than Whites/European Americans (G. Johnson et al., 1968).

Therefore, the assessment and diagnostic process of Black/African American people with bipolar disorders often culminates in a misdiagnosis. Typically, the incorrect diagnosis is either psychotic-based disorders, such as schizophrenia or unipolar depression (Akinhanmi et al., 2018; Bell & Mehta, 1980). As bipolar disorders are often underdiagnosed, schizophrenia appears to be overdiagnosed in Black/African American populations. Depending on the study, the rate of diagnosis ranges from 25% to 100% higher than for Whites/European Americans (Akinhanmi et al., 2018; Bell & Mehta, 1980). Researchers reviewed medical records and compared rates of misdiagnosis of 76 individuals who had bipolar disorders. They found that a greater proportion of Blacks/African American and Hispanics/Latinos/Latinas were previously misdiagnosed with schizophrenia as compared with White/European American patients (misdiagnosis rates were 85.7% for Blacks/African Americans, 83.3% for Hispanics, and 51.4% for Whites/European Americans; Mukherjee et al., 1983).

Findings from research led by Blow suggest that race-specific clinician interpretation accounted for the differences in diagnosis (Blow et al., 2004). Strakowski et al. (2003) found a proportionate number of 79 Black/African Americans and Whites/European Americans received a bipolar disorder diagnosis when the diagnosticians did not have ethnicity data attached to files (39 Black/African Americans and 40 White/European Americans). The researcher deemed that the patient's race and sex were the primary factors surrounding the schizophrenia diagnosis. The use of an expert panel that reviewed diagnostic criteria (as opposed to clinical diagnosis and structured interview) appeared to yield a more accurate diagnosis (Strakowski et al., 2003).

Age was a factor in misdiagnosis in a study of veterans. Older Blacks/African Americans in the Veterans Administration system were more likely to be diagnosed with schizophrenia (67%) than younger Blacks/African Americans (34%), older Whites/European Americans (38%), and younger Whites/European Americans (27%; Kilbourne et al., 2004).

There are many reasons why clinicians often misdiagnose Blacks/African Americans. Institutional and individual biases partially account for over and misdiagnosis. A National Institute for Mental Health study led by Taube (1971) found a strong correlation between race and a diagnosis of schizophrenia as opposed to affective disorder. But, when independent diagnoses were made by the study's clinicians, no relationship between race and diagnosis was found. In other words, when a careful assessment of symptoms took place, the overdiagnosis of schizophrenia in the Black/African American population disappeared (Akinhanmi et al., 2018; Bell & Mehta, 1980). Generally, Black/African American people have lower access to care and face stigmas in seeking care. Thus, they often present for treatment later. Later presentation for treatment increases the likelihood that mania would drive the presentation for treatment, which in turn makes correct diagnosis more difficult. Mania at later stages may include delusions, often associated with psychotic disorders (Akinhanmi et al., 2018).

The impact of diagnosing a psychotic-based disorder instead of the accurate diagnosis of a bipolar disorder is far-reaching and tragic. Lack of accuracy prevents prompt treatment of manic symptoms, and studies show that the delay negatively impacts the trajectory and prognosis of Black/African American people who are so misdiagnosed. K. R. Johnson and Johnson (2014) posited that the overdiagnosis of schizophrenia as opposed to bipolar disorders is the result of a failure to understand and identify mania as a construct that is distinct from psychotic-based symptoms.

K. R. Johnson and Johnson (2014) also found that language barriers of Black/African American people immigrating from other countries might impede clinicians' understanding of symptoms. Some symptoms proffered by Blacks/African Americans might be misinterpreted as psychopathology rather than a reaction to sociocultural factors. For example, a persecutory delusion classified as a psychotic symptom may be considered anxiety around social and environmental phenomena. These misattributions could fuel misdiagnosis and ineffective treatment. One study suggests that training clinicians with culturally competent treatment regimens in populations of different sociocultural backgrounds may help address racial bias and aid in yielding more appropriate treatment recommendations (Bazargan et al., 2021).

Inaccurate diagnosis restricts access to optimal evidence-based psychotherapies for individuals suffering from bipolar disorders (Akinhanmi et al., 2018). Often when diagnosed incorrectly, the diagnosis sticks. So, when a Black/African American client is referred to outpatient services after being hospitalized, for example, an inaccurate diagnosis is likely to follow the client to his next treatment destination, perpetuating the misalignment between diagnosis and treatment. Clearly, inaccurate diagnoses often mean a poorer prognosis (Akinhanmi et al., 2018; Bell & Mehta, 1980). Therefore, misdiagnosis often leads to ineffective treatment, including psychopharmacological medication. An incorrect diagnosis of unipolar depression (when a bipolar disorder is the correct diagnosis) often means that the client is treated with antidepressants, which could result in treatment failure, as antidepressants would likely increase the likelihood of drug-induced mood destabilization or mania. Misdiagnosis of schizophrenia restricts the ability to treat a true bipolar disorder with lithium or mood-stabilizing anticonvulsants. Recent research found that even a lower dose of lithium proved to have positive results (Akinhanmi et al., 2018). However, Black/African American patients are less likely to receive lithium and newer generations of mood disorder drugs, such as selective serotonin reuptake inhibitors (SSRIs), and are significantly more likely to receive first-generation antipsychotics. The ramification of such drug misalignments also implicates susceptibility to physical and psychological symptoms and side effects. There are concerns about the safety and toxicity of these commonly used psychotropic medications, the increased risk of diabetes, and the increased risk of suicidal ideation from the use of SSRIs (Akinhanmi et al., 2018).

It is a perception among clinicians that Black/African American patients are less likely to be medication compliant, and there is some evidence to support this supposition. However, Fleck et al. (2005) found that medication adherence was low for both Blacks/African Americans and Whites/European Americans However, clinicians failed to consider the reasons for Black/European American patients' fears of medications, including fear of addiction and medication as a symbol of illness. Differing reasons for not adhering to medication protocols may be culturally influenced. Black/African American patients' negative feelings about self, which stem from having to take medication, may account for some of the disparity in the nonadherence rate for Blacks/African Americans and Whites/European Americans.

Blacks/African Americans also have less access to quality medical care and do not utilize health care services generally as much as Whites/European Americans. The patient advocacy group Depression Bipolar Support Alliance conducted two membership surveys 10 years apart (1994 and 2004) and found that Blacks/African Americans experienced lengthy delays (in some cases over 10 years) in receiving an accurate diagnosis (Akinhanmi et al., 2018; Hirschfeld et al., 2003).

The other tragic consequence of poor diagnosis is the issue of life expectancy. Serious mental illness has long been associated with lower life expectancy. Late diagnosis combined with economic impoverishment means that Black/African American people (as with other races) often have decreased life expectancy due to the reality of bipolar disorders and severe mental illness. In the case of Black/African American people and bipolarity, the shortened life span could range from 2 to 10 years (Akinhanmi et al., 2018). Poor access to services also negatively impacts life expectancy. Thus, unfortunately, incorrect initial misdiagnosis or delay in receiving the correct diagnosis leads to delayed appropriate treatment, which often leads to poorer prognosis and reduced life expectancy (Akinhanmi et al., 2018; Bell & Mehta, 1980; K. R. Johnson & Johnson, 2014).

Research indicates that clinician bias also contributes to assessment and diagnostic and treatment disparities (Akinhanmi et al., 2018). Studies reviewed by McGuire and Miranda (2008) found that mental health care providers may allow implicit bias and stereotypes of minority groups to impact their diagnoses and treatment recommendations.

A community-based study looked at the bias question with results suggesting that clinician biases are more likely to explain problems in misdiagnosis than fundamental differences in the presentation of bipolar disorders across racial/ethnic groups. Other clinical factors help to explain the discrepancy in diagnosis, including the stage of mania at the time of treatment, the hospital setting where the diagnosis is made, symptom presentation, and clinical interpretation of symptom presentation (Akinhanmi et al., 2018; Mukherjee et al., 1983).

The Epidemiologic Catchment Area Study was a landmark piece of research that utilized a highly structured diagnostic interview that nonclinicians administered in community settings in five U.S. metropolitan areas (Preedy & Watson, 2010). The study had a total of 20,000 patient-participants. They found that there was no clinically significant difference in rates of bipolar disorders by race (Akinhanmi et al., 2018; Regier et al., 1993). One of the lessons learned from this research is that the structured clinical interview is important in removing biases and discrepant diagnoses by reducing clinical interpretative differences.

Latinos/Latinas/Hispanics

In general, geography or language is used to distinguish between Latino/Latina and Hispanic. Latino or Latina refers to (almost) anyone born in or with ancestors from Latin America and living in the United States. Hispanic is generally accepted as a narrower term that includes people only from Spanish-speaking Latin America, including countries/territories of the Caribbean or Spain itself (Simón, 2018). In this discussion, the term used by researchers is used in our analysis. Although more gender-neutral, Latinx is not used here because surveys show that most people who identify with Latino or Hispanic communities have not heard of the term or do not prefer it (Pew Research Center, 2020).

Research shows clear disparities in treatment for mental illness compared to White/European American counterparts. Hispanics were less likely to see a professional and less likely to receive medication. In a study led by Minsky, Hispanics were more likely to be diagnosed with major depressive disorder, even when they showed behavioral and psychotic symptoms (Minsky et al., 2003).

Even when factoring out differences in social and demographic factors, and symptom profile, ethnicity significantly predicted treatment participation and whether a mood stabilizer figured prominently in the treatment protocol. In one study led by Salcedo et al. (2017), there were no Hispanics diagnosed with BSDs who were taking mood stabilizers, as opposed to White/European American patients who were prescribed mood stabilizers at a rate of 21%. In fact, Hispanics were less likely to be prescribed medication to alleviate emotional distress (Salcedo et al., 2017).

Researchers offer various theories for the disparities in psychotropic treatment and service utilization. Insurance was a factor. Theorists suggest that Hispanics are nearly 3 times less likely to have health insurance than Whites/European Americans. Studies show that statistically, even when racial and ethics minority communities have insurance, they are still reluctant to seek mental health care. Thus, it does not appear that insurance coverage explains Hispanic-White/European American diagnostic and medication disparities for BSDs (Salcedo et al., 2017).

Another marker that might explain the difference in pharmacological treatment involves the theory of acculturation or the process by which individuals adopt a new culture. Language is often used as a proxy for measuring acculturation. In one study, Latinos/Latinas who preferred speaking in Spanish were 50% less likely to seek mental health services than Whites/European Americans. In a larger study, this trend was contingent upon diagnosis. A long-term study of

Latino/Latina patients with serious mental illness in California revealed that Spanish-speaking Latino/Latina patients were less likely to utilize services for depression than Latinos/Latinas who preferred speaking English. English- and Spanish-speaking Latino/Latina patients were equally likely to seek and utilize mental health services for bipolar disorders and schizophrenia (Folsom et al., 2007). This research is the only study analyzing treatment results for Latinos/Latinas based on the impact of acculturation variables and the treatment of bipolar disorders. Moreover, the use of language as the sole marker of acculturation is limited. For one, the effects of language are confounded by a lack of knowledge about health care needs in single-language groups. Further studies would need to use another measure of acculturation, including the adoption of American culture and whether one is native-born (Salcedo et al., 2017).

In one study, Hispanics were shown to prefer assistance for mental illness from physicians and members of their family rather than from mental health professionals (Salcedo et al., 2017). Not seeking care through traditional mental health providers may, in part, be due to fear of the stigma surrounding mental health diagnosis, particularly among foreign-born Hispanics (Gonzalez et al., 2007). The fear of stigma is related to findings that Hispanics are less likely to connect mood-related symptoms to biological causes, and thus, make it less likely that Hispanic clients would engage in conventional medical treatment (Salcedo et al., 2017).

Asians/Asian Americans

Research into Asians/Asian Americans and bipolar disorders is very scarce. One large study reviewed participating systems with 11 private, not-for-profit health care organizations constituting the Mental Health Research Network (MHRN). The MHRN had a combined 7,523,956 patients aged 18 years or older who received care in 2011. The diagnosis rate for bipolar disorders for Asian Americans was less than 3 times that of Blacks/African Americans and less than 5 times that of Whites/European Americans. Across combined mental health conditions, after adjusting for health care sites, only Asians/Asian Americans had lower rates of utilizing psychotherapy in comparison with non-Hispanic Whites/European Americans (Coleman et al., 2016). Hwang and her coresearchers found that Asian/Asian Americans and Latinos/Latinas as compared with White/European American patients had a significantly higher diagnostic rate of bipolar I disorder (58.8% and 60.0% vs. 37.2%, respectively; Hwang et al., 2010).

HOW CLINICIANS CAN IMPROVE BIPOLAR ASSESSMENTS OF MULTICULTURAL POPULATIONS

Given all the concerns expressed about our assessment of diverse population groups highlighted previously, how can clinicians improve their diagnostic and assessment capabilities and outcomes when considering a diagnosis of BSD or any other mental health condition? The intent to change is critical. Setting the intention and then obtaining the requisite training in multiculturalism and all other salient and related topics is essential. This includes training in bias; racial and gender identity; sexual orientation; and trauma, which can easily be mistaken for a BSD. Testing instruments should also be studied, including those that might aid in more accurate diagnoses and those instruments that over-pathologize diverse populations. Clinicians should also direct their attention toward building strong dyads with diverse populations that include partnering with clients and reducing the power differential in the service of optimizing assessment goals. Race, gender, and sexuality can be fraught with tension and are often uncomfortable for clinicians to discuss. Therefore, these topics are easy to avoid. However, competent care requires us to sit with our discomfort and risk mistakes in order to serve diverse populations equitably.

We should seek a balance of structural and cultural competency. Structural competency is how social, economic, and political conditions produce inequalities and cultural competency is the focus on improving clinical bias and client relationships. COVID-19 has had particularly traumatic impacts on marginalized communities and diverse cultures, and these traumas should be queried and incorporated into the process of assessment. Finally, traumas based on marginalization, discrimination, and oppression need to be incorporated fully into our thinking about trauma and our assessments of diverse populations.

The APA offers guidance to help us along the way. The *Ethical Principles of Psychologists and Code of Conduct* (APA, 2017) covers assessment, human relations, and education and training. The Council of National Psychological Associations for the Advancement of Ethnic Minority Interests (2016) has also published *Testing and Assessment With Persons & Communities of Color*, which incorporates a strength-based approach to assessment. Finally, the APA also has a plethora of resources to aid in the assessment of LGBTQIA communities, including the *APA Guidelines for Psychological Practice With Sexual Minority Persons* (American Psychological Association, APA Task Force on Psychological Practice With Sexual Minority Persons, 2021; see also Boroughs et al., 2015).

REFERENCES

Abé, C., Rahman, Q., Långström, N., Rydén, E., Ingvar, M., & Landén, M. (2018). Cortical brain structure and sexual orientation in adult females with bipolar disorder or attention deficit hyperactivity disorder. *Brain and Behavior, 8*(7), Article e00998. https://doi.org/10.1002/brb3.998

Akinhanmi, M. O., Biernacka, J. M., Strakowski, S. M., McElroy, S. L., Balls Berry, J. E., Merikangas, K. R., Assari, S., McInnis, M. G., Schulze, T. G., LeBoyer, M., Tamminga, C., Patten, C., & Frye, M. A. (2018). Racial disparities in bipolar disorder treatment and research: A call to action. *Bipolar Disorders, 20*(6), 506–514. https://doi.org/10.1111/bdi.12638

American Psychiatric Association. (2013). *Diagnostic and statistical manual of mental disorders* (5th ed.).

American Psychiatric Association. (2022). *Diagnostic and statistical manual of mental disorders: DSM-5-TR* (5th ed., text rev.).

American Psychological Association. (n.d.). Gender. In *APA dictionary of psychology.* https://dictionary.apa.org/gender

American Psychological Association. (2017). *Ethical principles of psychologists and code of conduct* (2002, amended effective June 1, 2010, and January 1, 2017). https://www.apa.org/ethics/code/

American Psychological Association, APA Task Force on Psychological Practice With Sexual Minority Persons. (2021). *Guidelines for psychological practice with sexual minority persons.* https://www.apa.org/about/policy/psychological-sexual-minority-persons.pdf

Bazargan, M., Cobb, S., & Assari, S. (2021). Discrimination and medical mistrust in a racially and ethnically diverse sample of California adults. *Annals of Family Medicine, 19*(1), 4–15. https://doi.org/10.1370/afm.2632

Becker, D., & Lamb, S. (1994). Sex bias in the diagnosis of borderline personality disorder and posttraumatic stress disorder. *Professional Psychology: Research and Practice, 25*(1), 55–61. https://doi.org/10.1037/0735-7028.25.1.55

Bell, C. C., & Mehta, H. (1980). The misdiagnosis of Black patients with manic depressive illness. *Journal of the National Medical Association, 72*(2), 141–145.

Blow, F. C., Zeber, J. E., McCarthy, J. F., Valenstein, M., Gillon, L., & Bingham, C. R. (2004). Ethnicity and diagnostic patterns in veterans with psychoses. *Social Psychiatry and Psychiatric Epidemiology, 39*(10), 841–851. https://doi.org/10.1007/s00127-004-0824-7

Boroughs, M. S., Andres Bedoya, C., O'Cleirigh, C., & Safren, S. A. (2015). Toward defining, measuring, and evaluating LGBT cultural competence for psychologists. *Clinical Psychology: Science and Practice, 22*(2), 151–171. https://doi.org/10.1111/cpsp.12098

Coleman, K. J., Stewart, C., Waitzfelder, B. E., Zeber, J. E., Morales, L. S., Ahmed, A. T., Ahmedani, B. K., Beck, A., Copeland, L. A., Cummings, J. R., Hunkeler, E. M., Lindberg, N. M., Lynch, F., Lu, C. Y., Owen-Smith, A. A., Trinacty, C. M., Whitebird, R. R., & Simon, G. E. (2016). Racial-ethnic differences in psychiatric diagnoses and treatment across 11 health care systems in the Mental Health Research Network. *Psychiatric Services, 67*(7), 749–757. https://doi.org/10.1176/appi.ps.201500217

Council of National Psychological Associations for the Advancement of Ethnic Minority Interests. (2016). *Testing and assessment with persons & communities of color.* American Psychological Association. https://www.apa.org/pi/oema/resources/cnpaaemi-pubs

Diflorio, A., & Jones, I. (2010). Is sex important? Gender differences in bipolar disorder. *International Review of Psychiatry, 22*(5), 437–452. https://doi.org/10.3109/09540261.2010.514601

Evarts, A. B. (1914). Dementia praecox in the colored race. *Psychoanalytic Review, 1*(4), 388–403.

Fleck, D. E., Keck, P. E., Jr., Corey, K. B., & Strakowski, S. M. (2005). Factors associated with medication adherence in African American and White patients with bipolar disorder. *The Journal of Clinical Psychiatry, 66*(5), 646–652. https://doi.org/10.4088/JCP.v66n0517

Folsom, D. P., Gilmer, T., Barrio, C., Moore, D. J., Bucardo, J., Lindamer, L. A., Garcia, P., Hawthorne, W., Hough, R., Patterson, T., & Jeste, D. V. (2007). A longitudinal study of the use of mental health services by persons with serious mental illness: Do Spanish-speaking Latinos differ from English-speaking Latinos and Caucasians? *The American Journal of Psychiatry, 164*(8), 1173–1180. https://doi.org/10.1176/appi.ajp.2007.06071239

Gold, M. (June 7, 2019). The ABCs of L.G.B.T.Q.I.A.+. *New York Times.* https://www.nytimes.com/2018/06/21/style/lgbtq-gender-language.html

Gonzalez, J. M., Perlick, D. A., Miklowitz, D. J., Kaczynski, R., Hernandez, M., Rosenheck, R. A., Culver, J. L., Ostacher, M. J., Bowden, C. L., & the STEP-BD Family Experience Study Group. (2007). Factors associated with stigma among caregivers of patients with bipolar disorder in the STEP-BD study. *Psychiatric Services, 58*(1), 41–48. https://doi.org/10.1176/ps.2007.58.1.41

Green, S. M. (2020). Exploring gender differences between bipolar disorder and border-line personality disorder in responses on the Personality Assessment Inventory (PAI). *Dissertations*, 513. https://digitalcommons.nl.edu/diss/513

Hendrick, V., Altshuler, L. L., Gitlin, M. J., Delrahim, S., & Hammen, C. (2000). Gender and bipolar illness. *The Journal of Clinical Psychiatry, 61*(5), 393–396. https://doi.org/10.4088/JCP.v61n0514

Hendricks, M. L., & Testa, R. J. (2012). A conceptual framework for clinical work with transgender and gender nonconforming clients: An adaptation of the minority stress model. *Professional Psychology: Research and Practice, 43*(5), 460–467. https://doi.org/10.1037/a0029597

Hirschfeld, R. M., Lewis, L., & Vornik, L. A. (2003). Perceptions and impact of bipolar disorder: How far have we really come? Results of the national depressive and manic-depressive association 2000 survey of individuals with bipolar disorder. *The Journal of Clinical Psychiatry, 64*(2), 161–174. https://doi.org/10.4088/JCP.v64n0209

Husain-Krautter, S. (2017). A brief discussion on mood disorders in the LGBT population. *The American Journal of Psychiatry Residents' Journal, 12*(5), 10–11. https://doi.org/10.1176/appi.ajp-rj.2017.120505

Hwang, S. H. I., Childers, M. E., Wang, P. W., Nam, J. Y., Keller, K. L., Hill, S. J., & Ketter, T. A. (2010). Higher prevalence of bipolar I disorder among Asian and Latino compared to Caucasian patients receiving treatment. *Asia-Pacific Psychiatry, 2*(3), 156–165. https://doi.org/10.1111/j.1758-5872.2010.00080.x

Johnson, G., Gershon, S., & Hekimian, L. J. (1968). Controlled evaluation of lithium and chlorpromazine in the treatment of manic states: An interim report. *Comprehensive Psychiatry, 9*(6), 563–573. https://doi.org/10.1016/S0010-440X(68)80053-7

Johnson, K. R., & Johnson, S. L. (2014). Inadequate treatment of Black Americans with bipolar disorder. *Psychiatric Services, 65*(2), 255–258. https://doi.org/10.1176/appi.ps.201200590

Kidd, S. A., Howison, M., Pilling, M., Ross, L. E., & McKenzie, K. (2016). Severe mental illness in LGBT populations: A scoping review. *Psychiatric Services, 67*(7), 779–783. https://doi.org/10.1176/appi.ps.201500209

Kilbourne, A. M., Haas, G. L., Mulsant, B. H., Bauer, M. S., & Pincus, H. A. (2004). Concurrent psychiatric diagnoses by age and race among persons with bipolar disorder. *Psychiatric Services, 55*(8), 931–933. https://doi.org/10.1176/appi.ps.55.8.931

Kinsey, A. C., Pomeroy, W. R., & Martin, C. (1948). *Sexual behavior in the human male.* Indiana University Press.

Lee, J. H., Gamarel, K. E., Bryant, K. J., Zaller, N. D., & Operario, D. (2016). Discrimination, mental health, and substance use disorders among sexual minority populations. *LGBT Health, 3*(4), 258–265. https://doi.org/10.1089/lgbt.2015.0135

Leibenluft, E. (1996). Women with bipolar illness: Clinical and research issues. *The American Journal of Psychiatry, 153*(2), 163–173. https://doi.org/10.1176/ajp.153.2.163

McGuire, T. & Miranda, J. (2008). New evidence regarding racial and ethnic disparities in mental health: Policy implications. *Health Affairs, 27*(2), 393–403. https://doi.org/10.1377/hlthaff.27.2.393

Meyer, I. H., & Frost, D. M. (2013). Minority stress and the health of sexual minorities. In C. J. Patterson & A. R. D'Augelli (Eds.), *Handbook of psychology and sexual orientation* (pp. 252–266). Oxford University Press.

Miller, L. J., Ghadiali, N. Y., Larusso, E. M., Wahlen, K. J., Avni-Barron, O., Mittal, L., & Greene, J. A. (2015). Bipolar disorder in women. *Health Care for Women International, 36*(4), 475–498. https://doi.org/10.1080/07399332.2014.962138

Minsky, S., Vega, W., Miskimen, T., Gara, M., & Escobar, J. (2003). Diagnostic patterns in Latino, African American, and European American psychiatric patients. *Archives of General Psychiatry, 60*(6), 637–644. https://doi.org/10.1001/archpsyc.60.6.637

Mukherjee, S., Shukla, S., Woodle, J., Rosen, A. M., & Olarte, S. (1983). Misdiagnosis of schizophrenia in bipolar patients: A multiethnic comparison. *The American Journal of Psychiatry, 140*(12), 1571–1574. https://doi.org/10.1176/ajp.140.12.1571

Nadal, K. L., Davidoff, K. C., Davis, L. S., Wong, Y., Marshall, D., & McKenzie, V. (2015). A qualitative approach to intersectional microaggressions: Understanding influences of race, ethnicity, gender, sexuality, and religion. *Qualitative Psychology, 2*(2), 147–163. https://doi.org/10.1037/qup0000026

Nadal, K. L., Whitman, C. N., Davis, L. S., Erazo, T., & Davidoff, K. C. (2016). Microaggressions toward lesbian, gay, bisexual, transgender, queer, and genderqueer people: A review of the literature. *Journal of Sex Research, 53*(4–5), 488–508. https://doi.org/10.1080/00224499.2016.1142495

O'Malley, M. (1914). Psychosis in the colored race. *Journal of Insanity, 71*, 309–336.

Perzichilli, T. (2020). The historical roots of racial disparities in the mental health system. *Counseling Today.* https://ct.counseling.org/2020/05/the-historical-roots-of-racial-disparities-in-the-mental-health-system/

Pew Research Center. (2020). *About one-in-four U.S. Hispanics have heard of Latinx, but just 3% use it.* https://www.pewresearch.org/hispanic/2020/08/11/about-one-in-four-u-s-hispanics-have-heard-of-latinx-but-just-3-use-it

Preedy, V. R., & Watson, R. R. (Eds.). (2010). Epidemiologic Catchment Area Study. In *Handbook of disease burdens and quality of life measures* (pp. 35–47). Springer. https://doi.org/10.1007/978-0-387-78665-0_5601

Regier, D. A., Farmer, M. E., Rae, D. S., Myers, J. K., Kramer, M., Robins, L. N., George, L. K., Karno, M., & Locke, B. Z. (1993). One-month prevalence of mental disorders in the United States and sociodemographic characteristics: The Epidemiologic Catchment Area study. *Acta Psychiatrica Scandinavica, 88*(1), 35–47. https://doi.org/10.1111/j.1600-0447.1993.tb03411.x

Salcedo, S., McMaster, K. J., & Johnson, S. L. (2017). Disparities in treatment and service utilization among Hispanics and non-Hispanic whites with bipolar disorder. *Journal of Racial and Ethnic Health Disparities, 4*(3), 354–363. https://doi.org/10.1007/s40615-016-0236-x

Semlyen, J., King, M., Varney, J., & Hagger-Johnson, G. (2016). Sexual orientation and symptoms of common mental disorder or low wellbeing: Combined meta-analysis of 12 UK population health surveys. *BMC Psychiatry, 16*(1), Article 67. https://doi.org/10.1186/s12888-016-0767-z

Simón, Y. (2018, September 14). Hispanic vs. Latino vs. Latinx: A brief history of how these words originated. *Remezcla.com.* https://remezcla.com/features/culture/latino-vs-hispanic-vs-latinx-how-these-words-originated/

Strakowski, S. M., Keck, P. E., Jr., Arnold, L. M., Collins, J., Wilson, R. M., Fleck, D. E., Corey, K. B., Amicone, J., & Adebimpe, V. R. (2003). Ethnicity and diagnosis in patients with affective disorders. *The Journal of Clinical Psychiatry, 64*(7), 747–754. https://doi.org/10.4088/JCP.v64n0702

Taube, C. (1971). *Admission rates to state and county mental hospitals by age, sex, and color, United States, 1969* (Statistical Note 41, pp. 1–7). Department of Health, Education, and Welfare, National Institute of Mental Health, Biometry Branch.

Thomas, A., & Sillen, S. (1972). *Racism and psychiatry.* Brunner/Mazel.

Toffey, D. E., Chatroux, L. R., & Caughey, A. B. (2018). Racial disparities in maternal and neonatal outcomes among pregnant women with bipolar disorder. *Obstetrics and Gynecology, 131*(1), Article 170. https://doi.org/10.1097/01.AOG.0000533164.22660.4f

The Trevor Project. (2019). *National survey on LGBTQ mental health.*

Zietsch, B. P., Verweij, K. J., Heath, A. C., Madden, P. A., Martin, N. G., Nelson, E. C., & Lynskey, M. T. (2012). Do shared etiological factors contribute to the relationship between sexual orientation and depression? *Psychological Medicine, 42*(3), 521–532. https://doi.org/10.1017/S0033291711001577

V

CASE ILLUSTRATIONS

19

Assessment of Bipolar Spectrum Disorders in an Adolescent

A Multimethod Case Example

James H. Kleiger

Cyla is a 14-year-old middle-class girl of Lebanese descent in her freshman year at a private high school.[1] Her therapist of 2 years, Dr. C., referred her for a psychological evaluation to rule out a bipolar or dissociative identity disorder. Dr. C. became concerned when Cyla arrived for a session in what Dr. C. thought was a hypomanic state. During the session, Cyla reportedly paced back and forth, spoke rapidly, and talked about the voice she sometimes heard in her head. Although Dr. C. viewed Cyla as an emotionally labile girl with a history of trauma, depression, and suicidal ideation, she had not previously appeared hypomanic. She was a good student and a talented musician, who dreamed of becoming a renowned concert cellist. Dr. C. described her as a bright and insightful girl with no history of experimenting with drugs or alcohol. Much of the focus in their sessions had involved her history of early emotional abuse and bullying at school. Dr. C. recalled that in the session prior to this referral, Cyla had been talking about her stepmother's "abusive behavior."

In addition to her therapist, Cyla was also seeing a child and adolescent psychiatrist who had begun managing her medication following her discharge from a university psychiatric facility, where she had been hospitalized briefly

---

[1] The identity of this individual has been heavily disguised to protect their privacy.

https://doi.org/10.1037/0000356-020
Psychological Assessment of Bipolar Spectrum Disorders, J. H. Kleiger and I. B. Weiner (Editors)

for suicidal ideation 6 months prior to the present evaluation. She had been discharged with a diagnosis of major depression and placed on venlafaxine. The psychiatrist questioned Cyla's diagnosis and wondered whether there were any indications of borderline personality or an underlying bipolar disorder. He was awaiting input from the psychological evaluation before considering any change in her medication.

Cyla's biological parents, both of whom were interviewed separately by the therapist, consented to the evaluation and said they hoped it would help understand her moodiness, anxiety, and intrusive thoughts. They acknowledged her early history of abuse, bullying victimization, ongoing conflicts between parents, binge-eating, and sleeping problems. They hoped that an evaluation would help with a differential diagnosis and pharmacological decision making. Cyla indicated that she wanted answers about what was going on with her mind. When asked to elaborate, she said she had done some research and wondered if she might have a borderline personality, dissociative identity disorder, or a bipolar or psychotic disorder. She also indicated that there were chronic strains in her family relationships.

The present evaluation included clinical interviews and the Wechsler Intelligence Scale for Children, Fifth Edition (WISC-V; Wechsler, 2014), the Minnesota Multiphasic Personality Inventory–Adolescent–Restructured Form (MMPI-A-RF-A; Archer et al., 2016), the Millon Adolescent Clinical Inventory, Second Edition (MACI-II; Millon & Tringone, 2020), and the Rorschach Performance Assessment System (R-PAS; Meyer et al., 2011). Additionally, Cyla's parents completed the Parent General Behavior Inventory (P-GBI; Youngstrom et al., 2008).

CASE HISTORY

Cyla's father was Lebanese and her mother was White. Her parents met and married while they were college students, and had been married for 5 years when Cyla was born. The father worked as a musician and the mother owned a small novelty shop. They described a stormy marriage, with frequent fights that sometimes escalated to physical violence. The father frequently used cocaine and cannabis, and he said he was often depressed and moody. The mother was more emotionally volatile than her husband and was quickly aroused to anger. She reported drinking heavily most evenings, while the father was out playing music with friends. Cyla recalled early instances of her mother having "screaming fits" that led to verbally abusive behavior when she was intoxicated. The mother acknowledged that she had a "red hot" temper and was quick to find fault. The father was aware of the mother's verbal abuse but reportedly looked the other way and did not intervene on Cyla's behalf.

Both parents acknowledged having extramarital affairs, and they divorced when Cyla turned 7. They shared legal custody of Cyla, but she lived with her father and saw her mother only on weekends. Two years after the divorce, Cyla's father married a woman with a 2-year-old son, and 2 years after that they had a son together. When Cyla turned 12, her mother moved to a neighboring state and occasionally visited her during the summer months.

During separate interviews, both of Cyla's parents acknowledged that they had exposed her to a high level of household conflict. Her mother in particular expressed remorse about her emotional abuse of her daughter prior to the divorce. Neither parent described the other as having been physically abusive; however, they wondered if Cyla had been sexually molested by a male babysitter when she was 6.

Developmental History

Cyla's mother's pregnancy was uncomplicated, but when some fetal distress appeared during labor, Cyla was delivered by emergency C-section. Her umbilical cord was wrapped around her neck, and she was moved temporally to a neonatal intensive care unit (NICU). Her birth weight was 6 pounds 3 ounces, but her initial APGAR scores were low. Once she was placed in the NICU, her condition stabilized and her scores rose to the normal range.

Cyla's parents reported that she met early developmental milestones during the expected time frames. Unfortunately, however, Cyla's first year was difficult for her and for her parents. Her mother described her as having been an intense, colicky infant who never seemed to sleep and was inconsolable. She felt frustrated that, no matter what she did, her baby continued to cry. This colic persisted for Cyla's first 12 months. When she finally quieted, she clung to her mother, who said she felt trapped and held prisoner by her infant daughter.

Cyla's toilet training was reportedly a struggle, which further exacerbated the strain on parent–child bonding. Between ages 2 and 5, both parents remembered, Cyla had numerous fears and became panicky when they dropped her off for daycare. Except for an instance in which she bit another child, she reportedly kept to herself and spent all of her time at a toy piano. During these preschool years, parental conflict and violence in the home continued to increase.

Social History

Cyla exhibited no behavioral problems in elementary school. Always quiet and reserved, Cyla developed a few friendships with classmates. Teachers shared several episodes of bullying during recess when a group of girls began taunting her. She became more interested in music and began taking guitar lessons after school. After her mother moved out, Cyla reportedly became more withdrawn, spending much of her time singing and practicing guitar or studying in her room. When she turned 10, she announced that she would move to Nashville and get a Grammy. Her interest in music became a passion and preoccupation. Her father appeared to identify with her dreams of musical achievement. Her mother, while acknowledging Cyla's musical talent, was not convinced that she "had what it takes" to become a rock star.

Cyla also described a checkered history of peer relationships. Severe bullying dated back to elementary school. Prior to beginning middle school, the taunting occasionally turned into sexual assault, including uninvited touching and groping. She indicated that even recently, she had a confrontation with a classmate who teased her about the size of her breasts.

Cyla reached menarche just before she entered middle school. She developed more quickly than others and began drawing negative attention from male and female peers. Her father received several reports from the middle school counselor that Cyla had been sexually harassed by peers. After an incident of sexual groping by male peers, she was transferred to a parochial school, where the bullying continued. In the summer before eighth grade, she was sexually assaulted by two male classmates, while other students watched without intervening. The assault consisted of unwanted groping, as one boy held Cyla and the other pulled up her skirt.

Medical History

Cyla had repeated episodes of otitis media and multiple respiratory infections during early childhood. She suffered a concussion after she fell off playground equipment. There were no reported neurological sequellae in the months that followed.

When a teacher spotted suspicious scratches on Cyla's legs and arms, the school urged her father to have her evaluated. She began seeing Dr. C. in the fifth grade. The following year, she became depressed and moody and began having nightmares. Cyla reportedly became enraged when she felt her brothers had entered her room and she threatened to kill one of them. Dr. C. arranged for an emergency evaluation when she could not provide assurance that she would not act on her homicidal or suicidal impulses. Cyla was hospitalized for 2 weeks and discharged with a diagnosis of major depression with mixed features and an eating disorder. Prior to discharge, she was started on Prozac but reportedly became agitated and hyper the day after. Her medication was switched to venlafaxine at the time of discharge.

Family mental health history on her father's side included alcoholism and depression in his mother. Her paternal grandfather was said to have had a severe temper and mood swings. Her maternal grandmother had been psychiatrically hospitalized and diagnosed with a bipolar disorder.

INTERVIEW INFORMATION

In preliminary interviews with Cyla's parents and stepmother, I explored the extent to which her father's ethnic background and cultural practices had played a role in Cyla's development and identity. All agreed that her Middle Eastern heritage played a negligible role in her life. Her father's parents were Muslim, but he denied identification or affiliation with the Islamic faith or cultural practices. Parents both regarded their daughter as a White middle-class girl. When her parents were together, they brought Cyla to an Episcopal church for Sunday

School. After they separated, Cyla stopped attending church. At the time of the evaluation, she did not identify with any religious or cultural group.

Cyla was a delightful adolescent, who arrived for her testing sessions with her stepmother. She was dressed in a colorful sweater with a series of stringed instruments on the front and back. Her boots were bright pink. Cyla had a pierced eyebrow and a small silver nose stud. Her shortly cropped dark hair had a prominent blue streak.

She was highly verbal, eagerly answered questions, and was willing to elaborate spontaneously. Her thoughts were organized and coherent. There was no indication that she was responding to internal stimuli. Cyla's affect was animated and full-ranging. She spoke enthusiastically about her involvement in a band and described how she was rehearsing for a musical festival. She spoke more rapidly when talking about her upcoming concerts. When we began formal testing procedures, she became less verbal and animated.

Cyla described her mood as "full of ups and downs." She said that she feels sad and tired for a day or so. Something will happen to make her feel worthless and all she can do is go home and lie on her bed. However, the next day, her mood reportedly "shoots up" and she feels excited and happy. She denied current suicidal ideation or impulses to cut herself.

Cyla's passion for performing was reflected in her affect and demeanor. When she was talking about writing songs and playing guitar, her speech quickened and her affect brightened. She said she "lived" for her performances and for her dream of moving to Nashville and eventually receiving a Grammy award. She said that the main reason she would never kill herself is that she had a plan of becoming a celebrated musician and songwriter. When I wondered how it would be if she did not move to Nashville or receive a Grammy but was still recognized as a talented performer, Cyla shot back, "Well, then I would kill myself, but that won't happen because I know I'll make it in Nashville!"

Speaking openly about her history of trauma, feeling of neglect, and bullying and sexually assaultive incidents at school, Cyla went into great detail regarding angry feelings toward her parents and perpetrators. She referred to her mother by her first name, criticized her for being a horrible parent, but then added that she had a "good heart."

In sixth grade, Cyla began hearing a voice whisper to her through the walls of her room. She made out the words, "You're worthless, you slut. You should die." This figure, whom she named "Specter," reportedly appeared in her room a year later. Over time, he materialized on a daily basis. At times, she saw him standing in the corner. Sometimes, she only heard his voice inside her head. Over time, she described his presence as intrusive thoughts that urged her to take violent action. Cyla began being fearful at night and told her father and stepmother about hearing a voice. The parents initially dismissed this report and attributed it to her active imagination and spending too much time on YouTube. Later they told Dr. C., who had already been talking with Cyla about Specter. For the next year, she reportedly had some sort of contact with this figure on a daily basis. Cyla explained how Specter began threatening her less and accusing her instead of being weak for letting others hurt her. The threatening quality of these messages shifted, as did her feelings about them. She became less anxious and felt ambivalent about Specter. Cyla explained that "He has always been with me. He is like a constant companion."

With the help of her therapist, Cyla said she came to understand that Specter was something she imagined. She described him as a part of her mind. However, later in the interview, her certainty wavered as she talked about not knowing whether he was real or not. She reported becoming anxious when she felt compelled to act on his commands to hurt others, such as her friends or brothers.

Test Results

Wechsler Intelligence Scale for Children, Fifth Edition, Similarities Subtest

Cyla obtained a Full Scale WISC-VIQ of 101 (53rd percentile), which placed her in the Average range of intellectual functioning. Her Index scores were highly consistent, all falling between the 42nd and 66th percentiles. Apart from assessing cognitive-intellectual abilities and processing efficiency, verbal subtests provide speech samples that reveal qualities of thought organization (Kleiger, 2021). Similarities, in particular, is an open-ended subtest, which not only assesses verbal concept identification, organization, and logic, but may also reveal a respondent's ability to focus on essential ideas and filter extraneous associations. Several of Cyla's responses presented in Exhibit 19.1 contained loose and idiosyncratic associations that revealed an expansive and poorly filtered ideational style, infused with affective associations that went well beyond the Similarities task. For test security purposes, the actual items are not reproduced; however, you can see how Cyla responded to the numbered items. As one can see, she began with a conceptual-level response, which she then expanded and embellished with inappropriate affective themes. Beyond the infusion of affect into her responses, Cyla demonstrated significant difficulty filtering and regulating her ideas.

EXHIBIT 19.1

Examples of Responses to WISC-V Similarities Subtest

Response to Item 9

"Both are very strong emotions. Both are fueled by something deeper inside you that comes from you or is triggered by an event. Both are temporary."

Response to Item 16

"Both are strong; both are dangerous. They can be quite beautiful. They're found naturally occurring in nature, but have horror movies that take place in them. Both can be very old."

Response to Item 23

"Both are larger than all of us. Both can kill you. Both are being researched but still not super well understood. Both hold many secrets."

Note. WISC-V = Wechsler Intelligence Scale for Children, Fifth Edition.

Millon Adolescent Clinical Inventory, Second Edition (MACI-II)

The Millon Adolescent Clinical Inventory, Second Edition (MACI-II; Millon & Tringone, 2020) is a 160-item adolescent personality inventory with scales assessing personality patterns, expressed concerns, and clinical syndromes. Base Rate (BR) scores, an alternative to *T* scores, reflect prevalence rates for the clinical phenomena being measured. A BR of 75–84 represents problematic features of a personality pattern or clinical syndrome, and a BR of ≥85 suggests the presence of the disorder (see Chapter 5 in this volume). Key scale elevations in Cyla's Profile Summary are presented in Table 19.1. Her highest elevations on Personality Patterns scales were Borderline Tendency (BR 95), Dramatizing (BR 85), and Discontented (BR 75) and her highest Clinical Syndrome scales were Suicidal Tendency (BR 84), Posttraumatic Stress (BR 96), Depressive Affect (BR 89), Disrupted Mood Dysregulation (BR 88), Binge-Eating Patterns (82), and Reality Distortion (BR 76). Collectively, Cyla's elevated scales reflected patterns of dramatic attention-seeking, mood lability, and self-dissatisfaction of borderline-level severity. Symptomatically, her profile suggested depressive and dysregulated mood with symptoms associated with exposure to trauma. Finally, there is an indication that she may experience unusual thoughts and occasionally have difficulties distinguishing reality from fantasy.

Minnesota Multiphasic Personality Inventory–Adolescent– Restructured Form

The Minnesota Multiphasic Personality Inventory–Adolescent–Restructured Form (MMPI-A-RF; Archer et al., 2016) includes (a) Higher Order, (b) Restructured Clinical, (c) Somatic/Cognitive and Internalizing scales, (d) Externalizing and Interpersonal scales, and (e) Personality Psychopathology Five (PSY-5) scales. Cyla's substantive Higher-Order scales (*T* score ≥65) included EID (Emotional/Internalizing Dysfunction, *T* score 67) and Thought Dysfunction (THD, 76). Elevated Restructured Clinical scales included RCd (Demoralization, 65), RC6 (Ideas of Persecution, 65), RC8 (Aberrant Experiences, 78), and RC9 (Hypomanic Activation, 70). PSY-5 Scales showed a significant elevation on PSYC-r (Psychoticism–Revised). Cyla's elevated scales documented a blending of depressive and hypomanic features, along with

TABLE 19.1 MACI-II Scales (BR > 75)

Scale	BR score
Dramatizing	85
Discontented	75
Borderline Tendency	95
Binge-Eating Patterns	82
Depressive Affect	89
Suicidal Tendency	84
Disruptive Mood Dysregulation	90
Posttraumatic Stress	95
Reality Distortion	76

Note. BR = base rate; MACI-II = Millon Adolescent Clinical Inventory, Second Edition.

TABLE 19.2 MMPI-A-RF (*T* Score > 65)

Scale	*T* score
EID	67
THD	76
RCd	65
RC6	65
RC8	78
RC9	70
STW (Stress & Worry)	75
AXY (Anxiety)	72
PSYC-r	71

Note. MMPI-A-RF = Minnesota Multiphasic Personality Inventory–Adolescent–Restructured Form; EID = Emotional/Internalizing Dysfunction; THD = Thought Dysfunction; RCd = Reconstructed Scales–Demoralization; PSYC-r = Psychoticism–Revised.

atypical experiences and reality distortion. Only clinically significant scales (*T* score ≥65) are presented in Table 19.2.

Rating Scales (Bipolarity Index and P-GBI Scale)

Two screening measures focused specifically on clinical features of bipolar spectrum disorders (see Chapter 7 in this volume). Parents' Total Score on the 10-item version of the P-GBI (Youngstrom et al., 2008) placed Cyla in the High Risk range for the diagnosis of bipolar spectrum disorders. Representative items with parental ratings appear in Exhibit 19.2.

The Bipolarity Index (Aiken et al., 2015) is a clinician-rated measure of key clinical aspects of bipolarity, rated across five domains (see Chapter 7 in this

---

EXHIBIT 19.2

P-GBI Sample Responses

1. Is your child's mood or energy shifted rapidly back-and-forth from happy to sad or high to low? (Often)

2. Has your child had periods of extreme happiness and intense energy lasting several days or more when she also felt much more anxious or tense than usual? (Often)

3. Have there been times several days or more when, although your child was feeling unusually happy and intensely energetic that she also had to struggle very hard to control inner feelings of rage and an urge to smash or destroy things? (Often)

4. Has your child had periods of extreme happiness and intense energy when, for several days or more, it took her over an hour to get to sleep at night? (Often)

5. Have you found that your child's feelings or energy are generally up or down, but rarely in the middle? (Often)

6. Has your child had periods, lasting several days or more, when she felt depressed or irritable, and other period of several days or more when she felt extremely high, L8, and overflowing with energy? (Often)

7. Have there been periods when, although your child was feeling unusually happy and intensely energetic, almost everything got on her nerves and made her irritable or angry? (Often)

Note. P-GBI = Parent General Behavior Inventory. Parent's responses are given in parenthesis.

volume). Scores $\geq$ 50 have shown adequate sensitivity and specificity for identifying bipolar disorders. A review of clinical characteristics, family history, age of onset, course of illness, and response to treatment yielded a score of 55. Scorable items are presented in Exhibit 19.3.

Rorschach Performance Assessment System

Exhibits 19.4 and 19.5 present samples of Cyla's Rorschach responses and clinically significant Page 1 and selected Page 2 R-PAS Summary Scores (Meyer et al., 2011). Several Engagement and Cog. Processing variables were clinically significant. Cyla's high Complexity score, along with her elevated Sy, Blend, and Human Movement variables, reflect her high level of mental energy and cognitive-organizational activity as she responded to the standard Rorschach question "What might this be?"

Cyla's human movement and weighted color–potentially problematic determinants was within the Average range (standard score 105, Cplx. Adj, 111), which at first glance would suggest that she possessed adequate internal resources to cope with psychosocial stress. However, the quality of her M and C responses contradicted this inference. Of her nine Ms, four were form quality, indicating that deliberate thought is not an adaptive resource. Likewise, of Cyla's eight color responses, six were either color form (CF) or pure C, again suggesting that emotional coping is not a source of ego strength.

Variables in the Perception and Thinking Domain were highly problematic. Ego Impairment Index–3 and thought and perception composite were greater than 4 *SD*s above the mean. WSumCog, SevCog, and all measures of perceptual accuracy were clinically significant. Taken together, Cyla's scores indicate that, in open-ended, impromptu processing and problem-solving situations, she has difficulty thinking logically and forming accurate impressions. More specifically,

---

EXHIBIT 19.3

The Bipolarity Index (Scores by Domain)

Episode Characteristics (DSM-5-TR *Symptoms*)
- Hypomania, cyclothymia, or manic after antidepressant (within 12 weeks). 10

Family History
- First-degree relative with depressions and behavioral evidence suggesting BD. 15

Age of Onset (First Depression)
- Less than 15 or between 20 and 30. 15

Course of Illness and Associated Features
- More than three prior episodes of depression or Borderline PD; anxiety (including PTSD and OCD); eating disorder; history of ADHD. 5

Response to Treatment
- Worsening dysphoria or mixed during antidepressant Rx. 10

Note. DSM-5-TR = Diagnostic and Statistical Manual of Mental Disorders, Fifth Edition, Text Revision; BD = bipolar disorder; PD = personality disorder; OCD = obsessive-compulsive disorder.

EXHIBIT 19.4

Sample of Cyla's Rorschach Responses

Card I

1. RP: Looks like 2 ravens (D2), see the head, beak and body.
   CP: (ERR) Angels are on the side (D1) holding something in the middle

    D2 A 2 u F ODL

3. RP: A wolf
   CP: (ERR) the face, ears, eyes, and nose

    W Si Ad o F AGC

Card II

5. RP: 2 bloody dogs kissing
   CP: (ERR) One dog, there and there (D1) and you can see their noses on each other
   (bloody?) Can see the red on them and around (D2 & 3)

    W A,Bl Sy 2 o P FMa, CF MOR ODL

6. RP: Or . . . maybe 2 bloody dogs fighting over their prize.
   CP: (ERR) The same dogs but instead of kissing, maybe this up here (D2) is what they want,
   the guts of a dead animal. They're growling because they both want it (guts of a dead
   animal?) the shape and color.

    W A, Ad, An, Bl Sy 2 u P FMa, FC AGM, MOR, MAP

7. RP: Or maybe it's a man's face. Like his eyes, nose, beard and moustache, and his mouth is
   bleeding and can see his sunken eyes.
   CP: (ERR) Eyes look sad and all the black part is the beard and moustache, and the nose is
   poking through. It's either his tongue bleeding or his mouth is bloody (sunken eyes?)
   the shape and coloring looks very sad and tired and in the white makes it look like the
   eyes are sunken.

    W A, An, Bl Sy o Mp, ma, CF, V MOR ODL

8. RP: Or going back to the dogs, it looks like 2 hands are ripping a woman's face in the top
   half and the dogs were waiting to catch and eat the blood and stuff.
   CP: (ERR) The eyes up here and the hands at the sides and the red between them looks like
   blood spurting apart (Remember 2 maybe 3 responses)

    W Hd, A, Bl Sy—Ma, FMa, ma, C FAB2 AGM, MOR, MAP ODL Pu

Card III

9. RP: Looks like 2 dancers having a good time (D9).
   CP: (ERR) There they are on the sides. (Good time?) Those look like happy colors, right?

    D9 H Sy o P Ma, C

Card IV

10. RP: It's a crazy monster that's either puking or spewing something out of its mouth down
    on someone.
    CP: (ERR) This at the top looks like light hair and these are the feet and the person below is
    covered in stuff from the giant's mouth (What makes it look like stuff from the giant's
    mouth?) It's lighter and dark there.

    W (H), NC Sy—Ma, Y AGM, AGC, MOR, MAP ODL

12. RP: A forest that's being destroyed by a flood.
    CP: (ERR) You can see these are trees and this is the source of the water crashing through
    the dam and flooding everything (trees?) shape and it looks like there is a depth in the
    water (depth in the water?) the different shades of gray.

    W NC Sy, Vg ma, V u Ex, Fi AGM, MOR, MAP

Card V

14. RP: I could say a bat but that's boring. I'm gonna say 2 happy dolphins jumping out of the
    water.
    CP: (ERR) Here are the dolphins and the rippling stuff are the waves splashing (happy
    dolphins?) I think dolphins always look happy

    V W A, NC Sy 2 u FMa, ma

(continues)

EXHIBIT 19.4

Sample of Cyla's Rorschach Responses (*Continued*)

Card VI

16. RP: Like a space rocket bursting up.
    CP: (ERR) Space ship is up here (D3) and the smoke is all around. Kinda gives the feeling of smoke, the darker and lighter is the smoke
        W Fi, NC Sy u ma, Y

Card VII

20. These look like 2 identical people who are about to kiss so it makes me think of a person looking in a mirror and wanting to kiss themselves.
    CP: (ERR) They look like they're puckering their lips, just the face (D1) and the hair is sticking up.
        D1 Hd Sy o P Ma, r ODL

Card VIII

23. RP: . . . This had a happy circus vibe. Looks like these are either tigers or some kind of animal walking on something and pulling on something maybe in a circus.
    CP: (ERR) These look like tigers. The colors are so bright, like you see in a circus
        W A, NC Sy 2 o P FMa, C

25. RP: Also looks like someone who is being torn apart physically, like torn in half
    CP: (ERR) Hands are tied up and legs spread so far that it's ripping them in half and the people are laughing at them and up here are angels. The whole thing gives me the vibe of heaven and hell, and the person is being torn in half and the people are laughing (Heaven and hell?). Perfect colors for it.
        Dd 99 H, (H), NC Sy—Ma, C FAB2 AGM, MOR, MAP

Card IX

26. RP: Like a waterfall.
    CP: (ERR) This looks like a pretty waterfall coming down. (Pretty waterfall?) It's so colorful flowing down.
        Dd99 NC u ma, CF

Card X

28. RP: This is like a person who is dressed in crazy clothing. Maybe it's an eccentric with a long face and big eyelashes. The fur around the neck and a blue bra, green cowboy pants, and fluffy blue parts around it.
    CP: (ERR) Here is the face and eyes, the fur is around. The coat, it's pink and there are 2 blue fluffy pompoms (fluffy) it's shaped like that
        Dd99 H, Cg, Sx Sy—CF

29. RP: It also looks like a mass slaughter of innocent people. Well maybe not innocent but looks like a mass slaughter.
    CP: (ERR) It's all of it. The red is all the blood.
        W H, Bl Sy—CF AGC, MOR, MAP

Note. RP = Response Phase; CP = Clarification Phase; FMa = animal movement active; ODL = oral dependent language; AGC = aggressive content; CF = color form; MOR = morbid content; FC = form color; AGM = aggressive movement; MAP = mutuality of autonomy pathology; FAB = fabulized combination; NC = not classified; ERR = examiner repeats response. Examiner's queries are in parentheses.

when left on her own to make sense of unfamiliar stimulus situations, Cyla may have great difficulty testing reality and distinguishing fantasy from external reality. Additionally, both the nature of her logic and the content of her thoughts reveal highly regressive trends.

Extremely elevated Stress and Distress variables include inanimate movement (m), Y, morbid content (MOR), and suicide concern composite (SC-Comp)

EXHIBIT 19.5

Clinically Significant R-PAS Summary Scores and Profiles—Pages 1 and 2

Page 1 (SS ≥ 110)

Engagement and Cog. Processing (Complexity Adjusted)

Variable	SS	Cplx. Adj	Stress and distress		
Complexity	131	—	YTVC'	104	75
R	117	97	m	143	25
Blend	128	106	MOR	146	146
Sy	134	112	SC-Comp	115	101
M	125	106	**Self and Other Representation MC**		
(CF + C)/SumC	113	113	ODL%	112	102
Perception and Thinking Problems			MAP/MAHP	123	136
EII-3	143	143	PHR/GPHR	132	132
TP-Comp	142	142	M- (4)	136	136
WSumCog	127	121	AGC	120	116
SevCog	123	123	*Page 2 (SS ≤ 115)*		
FQ-%	143	134	WSumC	128	110
WD-%	118	113	C	130	130
FQo%	77	2	CritCont%	141	137
P	111	77	V-Comp	122	100
			AGM	146	146

Note. R-PAS = Rorschach Performance Assessment System; SS = standard score; YTVC' = diffuse shading, texture, vista, achromatic color; MOR = morbid content; SC-Comp = suicide concern composite; MC = human movement and color; CF = color form; ODL = oral dependent language; MAP = mutuality of autonomy pathology; MAHP = mutuality of autonomy health and pathology; EII-3 = Ego Impairment Index-3; PHR = poor human representation; GPHR = good human representation; TP-Comp = thought and perception composite; AGC = aggressive content; FQ = form quality; WD = whole and common detail; AGM = aggressive movement.

scores. Collectively, Cyla's scores indicate both acute stress and instability, along with marked depressive inclinations. Elevated MOR and SC-Comp strongly support the presence of severe depression and the risk of self-destructive behavior. Additionally, elevated color variables (CF + C/SumC, WSumC, and C) indicate a propensity for intense, dramatic, and unfiltered affectivity, with the potential for emotional flooding.

Clinically significant Self and Other Representation variables were oral dependent language% (112), mutuality of autonomy pathology (MAP)/mutuality of autonomy health and pathology (123), poor human representation (PHR)/good human representation (132), M- (136), and aggressive content (120). Page 2 elevations included CritCont% (141), V-Comp (122), and aggressive movement (146). Cyla's scores indicate significant relational difficulties, conflicts between strong dependency needs and aggressive impulses, interpersonal wariness, and mistrust. Elevated M- and PHR reflect problems understanding others' thoughts and feelings. The high number of MAP responses suggests internalized aggressive, abusive, and sadistic representations of self and other relationships. Together with her elevated CritCont%, there are indications that much of Cyla's severe psychopathology may be rooted in trauma.

ANALYSIS OF CYLA'S ASSESSMENT RESULTS

Major findings include the psychological residue of trauma, mood dysregulation, unstable sense of self, and reality distortion. Based on interviews with Cyla and her parents, multicultural issues did not seem to play a significant role in understanding Cyla's struggles. Several diagnoses fit the clinical picture, history, and psychological testing; however, making a differential diagnosis is complicated by developmental factors, symptom overlap, and comorbidity. All of this makes the diagnostic picture fluid and evolving, which necessitates fine-tuning and possible revision over time. Specifically, trauma-related, bipolar spectrum, and borderline personality disorders all share a great deal of symptom overlap but may also be concurrent conditions (see also Chapters 14 and 15 in this volume).

Developmental Trauma Disorder (Trauma- and Stressor-Related Disorder)

A diagnosis of complex trauma disorder reflects Cyla's ongoing history of neglect, exposure to intense parental conflict, and repeated episodes of childhood bullying, all of which can lead to affect dysregulation, disrupted attachment, unstable sense of self, and reality distortions. A trauma-based disorder has a great deal of explanatory utility and fits well with the data.

Bipolar Spectrum Disorder (Cyclothymia)

In addition to a complex developmental trauma, there is evidence of a comorbid disorder along the mood spectrum that is not sufficiently explained by posttraumatic stress disorder (PTSD) alone. Furthermore, major depression is also not consistent with the scope of Cyla's symptoms and behavior. A key element in Cyla's difficulties has to do with mood instability with subthreshold and short-duration depressive and hypomanic episodes that cycle rapidly (within hours to days). Her parents and therapist have observed increased talkativeness, flight of ideas, and exuberance oscillating with depression. The testing revealed a tendency toward expansive, over-inclusive reasoning in unstructured situations. Neither bipolar I nor II fits best with the available information. Mood swings are present, but fall short of the criteria for either hypomanic or major depressive episodes, especially in terms of the sustained presence of such features. In terms of criteria for hypomanic episodes, Cyla does not have a history of reduced need for sleep or excessive involvement in risky activities. Parents also refuted the presence of grandiosity or distractibility. Finally, Cyla became activated after she was prescribed Prozac.

Reality Distortion

Although the presence of psychotic-like symptoms is not sufficient to diagnose a primary psychotic disorder, Cyla's hearing and seeing Specter reflects hallucinatory reality distortion, which, according to Cyla, "makes it hard to separate what's real from an illusion." This weakness in reality testing and logic was represented in several testing measures. Cyla's reality distortions did not represent a primary psychosis and were not mood-congruent features of bipolar spectrum disorders, but, instead, were understood as symptoms of her severe trauma history.

Beyond acknowledging the chronic presence of this symptom, testing showed a significant vulnerability in Cyla's psychological functioning under unstructured, open-ended conditions. When left on her own to perceive and make sense of situations characterized by uncertainty and impromptu decision making, Cyla is prone to distort perceptions and reach inaccurate conclusions about herself and others. Perceptual distortion and illogical reasoning led to the projection of her internal experiences onto others (including her imagined alter ego), which lays the groundwork for the misperception of others' thoughts and feelings about her.

Cyla's chronic hallucinatory experiences are a prominent feature that has created a great deal of distress and ambivalence. Although Specter is present on a daily basis, she noticed him more when feeling either high or low, which suggests a mood-congruent component of her hallucinatory experience. On a positive note, Cyla demonstrated insight into the nature of this psychotic-like presence, which she said was a part of herself and, as such, a product of her own thoughts and feelings. According to Cyla, "I know he's not real. Logically, I know he's created from my head and is a personification of my feelings and thoughts." This reported insight indicated that Cyla was not delusional, and hence not in an active psychotic state.

Cyla's hallucinatory symptom can also be understood in the context of trauma and dissociation. Childhood histories of abuse and neglect are associated with the possible presence of hallucinatory phenomena, which in some respects encapsulate the re-experiencing of intrusive trauma affects and images (see also Chapter 15 in this volume).

Cyla and her parents agreed that her patterns of binging and purging were extremely problematic. She gave in to urges to overeat or binge in an attempt to regulate her stressful negative emotions. Although providing temporary relief, binging and purging evoked guilt and shame, which further fueled her self-criticism.

Finally, there is compelling evidence of an evolving borderline personality. However, making a personality disorder diagnosis is premature for an adolescent, especially in the presence of complex trauma disorder. At the same time, borderline features were present and not inconsistent with trauma and bipolar spectrum conditions. Developmental trauma and mood instability affect personality development, specifically in terms of affect management, sense of self, and attachment patterns. Without substantial treatment, a borderline personality disorder could congeal into a comorbid problem.

Given Cyla's multiple symptoms and the fluid nature of her diagnoses, she will need to be closely followed, and a range of psychotherapy and pharmacology options will need to be considered. Psychotherapy should be broad-based and include individual, group, and family components. Medication trials, including mood stabilizers, and eventually atypical antipsychotic medication, may target symptoms of mood instability, depression, and reality distortions.

REFERENCES

Aiken, C. B., Weisler, R. H., & Sachs, G. S. (2015). The Bipolarity Index: A clinician-rated measure of diagnostic confidence. *Journal of Affective Disorders, 177*, 59–64. https://doi.org/10.1016/j.jad.2015.02.004

Archer, R. P., Handel, R. W., Ben-Porath, Y. S., & Tellegen, A. (2016). *Minnesota Multiphasic Personality Inventory–Adolescent Restructured Form*. Regents of the University of Minnesota.

Kleiger, J. H. (2021). Assessing disordered thought and perception with an adolescent: A multimethod case example. In I. B. Weiner & J. H. Kleiger (Eds.), *Psychological assessment of disordered thinking and perception* (pp. 305–321). American Psychological Association. https://doi.org/10.1037/0000245-018

Meyer, G. J., Viglione, D. J., Mihura, J. L., Erard, R. E., & Erdberg, P. (2011). *Rorschach Performance Assessment System: Administration, coding, interpretation, and technical manual*. Rorschach Performance Assessment System.

Millon, T., & Tringone, R. (2020). *Millon Adolescent Clinical Inventory* (2nd ed.). DICANDRIEN.

Wechsler, D. (2014). *Wechsler Intelligence Scale for Children–Fifth edition*. PsycCORP.

Youngstrom, E. A., Frazier, T. W., Demeter, C., Calabrese, J. R., & Findling, R. L. (2008). Developing a 10-item mania scale from the Parent General Behavior Inventory for children and adolescents. *The Journal of Clinical Psychiatry, 69*(5), 831–839. https://doi.org/10.4088/JCP.v69n0517

20

Assessment of Bipolar Spectrum Disorders in an Adult

A Multimethod Case Example

Irving B. Weiner

Ms. BR is a single 26-year-old White woman who was born into a middle-class family in a medium size town in middle America and grew up with her parents and a sister 2 years younger than her. Her father was an accountant and her mother a high school mathematics teacher. Information about BR's developmental years was obtained from her and from her mother, who was consulted while BR was hospitalized, which is discussed later.[1]

BR developed normally during her early childhood without any health or behavioral problems. It was observed in a preschool class, however, that she seldom interacted with other children and spent much of her time by herself. This distancing continued into elementary school, according to her mother, with BR becoming increasingly shy and socially isolated. This isolation was exacerbated by her missing many days of school because of bouts of fatigue that were diagnosed by the family doctor as symptomatic of mononucleosis. When she was in the fifth grade, BR's one good friend moved away, and for some months afterward, she was markedly sad and withdrawn. She fared little better in her junior and senior high school years, during which she was physically healthy but

---

[1] The identity of the person in this case illustration has been disguised to protect their privacy.

https://doi.org/10.1037/0000356-021
Psychological Assessment of Bipolar Spectrum Disorders, J. H. Kleiger and I. B. Weiner (Editors)

troubled by peer rejection, loneliness, feelings of emptiness, low self-esteem, and worries about the future.

At age 15, BR was diagnosed with depression and began weekly meetings with a therapist, whose treatment included medication with Zoloft. Two years later, she had a severe manic episode, at which time she was hospitalized, diagnosed with bipolar disorder Type 1, and placed on a regimen of lithium and Lamictal to stabilize her moods. During these difficult years, she had the benefit of two sources of psychological strength. First, she had a close and loving relationship with her parents and sister. Her mother described her as having been an "affectionate and empathic" child. Second, she was a bright and able student. Her full-scale WAIS IQ was measured in the present evaluation at 116, with a very superior verbal IQ of 130. In high school, she received mainly As and Bs in her courses, took honors and advanced placement classes, and as a senior was accepted for admission to a nearby branch of a state university.

As a college student, BR continued to live at home and commuted to campus for her classes. She was no longer troubled by psychologically painful peer interactions and left her adolescent turmoil largely behind. However, she did remain socially isolated and did not form any close friendships with her college classmates. She went on occasional dates, as she had done in high school, but she rarely saw the same boy more than once. Influenced by her parents' interest in numbers, she took a part-time job in which she was tasked with accessing websites and recording data from them. She continued to get along well with her parents and sister, was content with otherwise leading a solitary life, and became engrossed in her studies, which included a major in economics. After receiving her bachelor's degree, she was employed as a data analyst at an insurance company. She enjoyed her work and performed well in it, and for a few uneventful years she continued to live at home and had little in the way of a social life.

Then, for unknown reasons, she stopped taking her medication and uncharacteristically began to engage in frequent and indiscriminate heterosexual activity. This promiscuity culminated at age 26, when she was hospitalized with a second manic episode marked by an elated mood, racing thoughts, pressured speech, and a grandiose sense of self. With the resumption of her medication, these manic symptoms subsided over the next 2 weeks, and she was considered ready for discharge from the hospital. An evaluation at this time included a psychological assessment that yielded the following test results on the Personality Assessment Inventory (PAI; Morey, 2003), the Rorschach Inkblot Method (Rorschach; Weiner, 2003), and the Thematic Apperception Test (TAT; Teglasi, 2013).

PERSONALITY ASSESSMENT INVENTORY

BR's PAI full-scale and subscale scores appear in Exhibits 20.1 and 20.2. As shown in Exhibit 20.1, two of the four validity scales are slightly elevated, with Information (INF) at 63 and Negative Impression (NIM) at 62. The other two

EXHIBIT 20.1

Personality Assessment Inventory Scale Scores

Scale	T score
ICN (Inconsistency)	49
INF (Infrequency)	63
NIM (Negative Impression)	62
PIM (Positive Impression)	36
SOM (Somatic Complaints)	68
ANX (Anxiety)	71
ARD (Anxiety-Related Disorders)	60
DEP (Depression)	67
MAN (Mania)	42
PAR (Paranoia)	40
SCZ (Schizophrenia)	51
BOR (Borderline)	70
ANT (Antisocial Features)	54
ALC (Alcohol Problems)	47
DRG (Drug Problems)	50
AGG (Aggression)	49
SUI (Suicidal Ideation)	51
STR (Stress)	50
NON (Nonsupport)	53
RXR (Treatment Rejection)	31
DOM (Dominance)	53
WRM (Warmth)	46

validity scales are low, however, with Inconsistency (ICN) at 49 and Positive Impression (PIM) at 36. Taken together, these values warrant proceeding with a clinical interpretation of the record.

In the Clinical and the Treatment Consideration scales, four elevations stand out: Anxiety (ANX) at 71, Borderline (BOR) at 70, Depression (DEP) at 67, and Somatic (SOM) at 68. Although she has apparently recovered from or is perhaps in denial of her manic episode, as suggested by her low Mania (MAN) of 42, these four elevations indicate that she remains upset, concerned about her health, and in need of continued treatment. Her therapist should be made aware in this regard of the suicide potential suggested by her score of 60 on the Self-Harm (SOM-H) subscale (Exhibit 20.3).

Among other remnants of her previously diagnosed bipolar disorder Type 1, BR has an elevated score of 69 on the Affective Instability (BOR-A) subscale, which usually identifies a continuing susceptibility to mood swings. Moreover, her PAI indications of depression are accompanied by an elevated score of 67 on the Stimulus-Seeking (ANT-S) subscale, which points to the heightened level of energy and activity that characterizes mania (Exhibit 20.4).

EXHIBIT 20.2

Personality Assessment Inventory Subscale Scores

Subscale	*T* score
SOM-C (Conversion)	51
SOM-S (Somatization)	62
SOM-H (Health Concerns)	80
ANX-C (Cognitive)	78
ANX-A (Affective)	68
ANX-P (Physiological)	61
ARD-0 (Obsessive-Compulsive)	65
ARD-P (Phobias)	59
ARD-T (Traumatic Stress)	48
DEP-C (Cognitive)	75
DEP-A (Affective)	58
DEP-P (Physiological)	60
MAN-A (Activity Level)	57
MAN-G (Grandiosity)	33
MAN-I (Irritability)	46
PAR-H (Hypervigilance)	42
PAR-P (Persecution)	42
PAR-R (Resentment)	41
SCZ-P (Psychotic Experiences)	43
SCZ-S (Social Detachment)	56
Scz-T (Thought Disorder)	52
BOR-A (Affective Instability)	69
BOR-I (Identity Problems)	68
BOR-N (Negative Relationships)	59
BOR-S (Self-Harm)	68
ANT-A (Antisocial Behaviors)	48
ANT-E (Egocentricity)	45
ANT-S (Stimulus-Seeking)	67
AGG-A (Aggressive Attitude)	45
AGG-V (Verbal Aggression)	51
AGG-P (Physical Aggression)	52

RORSCHACH INKBLOT METHOD

As shown in Exhibit 20.5 (Structural Summary), BR produced a valid Rorschach protocol of 29 responses with no card rejections. Contrary to expectations, given her history of one of the bipolar spectrum disorders and her recent manic episode, her protocol is notable more for its indications of personality strengths than for evidence of psychological disorder. The indications of personality strengths include normal range scores of 0 on the Perceptual Thinking Index (PTI), 3 on the Depression Index (DEPI), 2 on the Coping Deficit Index (CDI), Negative on

EXHIBIT 20.3

Rorschach Responses With Location Choice

Card I

1. Some type of mutated moth . . . like I've been watching too much X-Men on TV (WS). The whole thing. The way the ink goes side to side looks like wings. (Mutated?) It doesn't look like a normal moth. It has gaps that look like holes. I've had enough moths fly in my face to know what a normal one looks like.

2. A dancer.
   It looks like a dancer being reflected on herself. It's the whole thing, with the hands here (D1), and a fabric flowing off her body. (Fabric flowing?) The dancer is the middle part, and the section on the side looks like it's being blown out (Dd24).

3. Looks like some sort of weird kite. They make kites in weird shapes a lot.
   All of it, looks like a manta ray kite. I don't know if they make them. (Weird?) It's not a normal kite shape. I think of a normal kite shaped like a diamond or box.

Card II

4. A pair of wombats high-fiving. [Note: wombat is a small, 4-legged furry animal resembling a beaver or possum]
   The whole, no, the black part (D6). It's wombat shaped, and they're doing a high-five.

5. [inverts card] . . . a pelvis (D6).
   It looks like a pelvic bone, the way it's shaped.

6. [card inverted] And the red things coming down here (D2) could be femurs.
   Well, the shape is like two legs.

7. A uterus (DS5o).
   The blank space in the middle looks like diagrams you see of the uterus. (Diagrams?) Just the way it's inside the black areas and the way it's shaped looks like diagrams you see in a health magazine.

Card III

8. An ultrasound (D1 & D3).
   Looks like a picture that women post online when they're having a baby and have an ultrasound. You can see the baby in the middle and outside is the uterine walls (Where do you see the baby?) It's the pink part (D3), babies are supposed to be pink when they're doing well, but not when they're blue. It (D3) kind of looks like a kidney bean, and babies are shaped that way on an ultrasound, if they're small enough. (What suggests an ultrasound?). The contrast of black and white.

9. A cow with a bow on its forehead.
   The cow face is a couple of lighter areas in black that look like eyes, and a defined edge to the white that makes it look like a white patch on the cow's face, and the part here looks like a nose (D7), two curved pieces attached to a piece in the middle, so it looks like a bow (D3), but I don't know how it's staying there. There's not much to attach it to in that part of a cow's face.

10. A vase.
    Looking at this part again (D1 & D3). The sweep looks like the neck of a vase, one of the vases you see in a museum. The way the ink is on the card makes it look printed the way you put a design on it.

Card IV

11. A final boss in a video game (D7). I
    It's like you were looking up at some giant dude that's about to stomp on you, kind of like the perspective you see on video games, like when you're about to fight the final boss.

(continues)

EXHIBIT 20.3

Rorschach Responses With Location Choice (*Continued*)

12. It looks like a picture of a wendigo (W).
    (Wendigo?). It's a mythical creature from native American Indian folklore. I'm looking at this spot in particular (Dd25), because wendigos are supposed to have gaunt faces. It's shaped like how you see cow skulls in museums. [Note: In the myth wendigos are cannibalistic creatures that haunt forests in the northern United States and Canada looking for people to eat.]

13. It also looks like some odd-shaped mountain.
    Looking at the whole, the sides look like a mountain slope. Not a regular mountain, because it's got some caves at its base. (Caves?) The negative space at the bottom of the picture, down here it looks like openings, there's light in them (DdS24).

Card V

14. A butterfly.
    It looks like a swallowtail butterfly. Looking at the whole thing, because there's an antenna and tail and wings.

15. The bat symbol.
    The Batman symbol. It looks like a bat except . . . it's a bat shape, but it has a split (D6), so it's not entirely a bat symbol.

16. It looks like a crab claw reflected on itself.
    It's as if the crab was curious and approaching the mirror, and the claw was the first part that came in front.

Card VI

17. [inverts card] mmm . . . A maple leaf.
    The stem, and at the top it's vaguely maple-leaf shaped.

18. It looks like one of those fur rugs too. My uncle has one of those.
    Like one of those fur rugs where you skin the animal and put it on the floor. This is the tail and limbs here, and it doesn't have a head. It looks like the head is cut off. (What suggests a fur rug?) The shape of it. It looks like you see in photos. Most rugs are not rectangular or oval, only fur ones are strangely shaped.

19. It also kind of looks like some weird mutated string instrument. I'm not sure what kind of sound you'd get out of a shape like that.
    There's a neck and knobs to tune the strings, and this is the body of the instrument. (How do you mean weird and mutated?) You never see one like this, most are curved and round, you never see one with angles like these.

Card VII

20. A necklace.
    It looks like it's going up around someone's neck, and these stones are big ones.

21. A woman looking in the mirror (W).
    This looks like a face and that looks like a hairdo coming off the top of her head. Since it's a reflection I thought she'd be looking in a mirror, maybe doing her hair or something.

22. A caterpillar.
    These are segments of a caterpillar's body, chunks.

Card VIII

23. [Holds sideways] A bear crossing a river.
    This is the bear and these look like rocks or logs, a fallen tree, roots coming up, so it's climbing on stones to keep dry. It suggests water to me because its symmetrical, and the other half would be a reflection.

(continues)

EXHIBIT 20.3

Rorschach Responses With Location Choice (*Continued*)

24. Some sort of fighter jet.
   This would be the cockpit area (D4). It looks almost like Star Trek. I guess it's towing something (D2).

25. [Inverts card]. A deflated hot air balloon.
   This part is like it was at one point round, but now it's not (D2). This is the basket (D5), it's swinging back and forth. (Suggests?). The colors and the design printed on it. This part looks like it's collapsing, and other parts are billowing down. (Collapsing?). It's not round, it's lumpy.

Card IX

26. It looks like a mantis shrimp.
   It looks like a shrimp's nose and mouth and antenna, very colored shrimp (D3), hiding out in a coral reef (D1), like in the ocean, and poking its head out to see if the coast is clear, whether there are any predators around. A very colorful shrimp on coral reefs. [Note: A mantis shrimp is a carnivorous sea creature with sharp appendages that can cause cuts and scratches when handled without care.]

27. That thing at the bottom looks like more crabs.

Card X

28. The Eiffel tower (D1).
   The top bit and the base, it gets wider and curved.

29. Looks like crabs out here (D7).
   On the sides, look alike.

Note. Examiner's queries are in parentheses.

the Hypervigilance Index (HVI), and 0.03 on the Ego Impairment Index (EII-2). These findings indicate that she is currently capable for the most part of perceiving people and objects accurately (XA% = .79), thinking logically about relationships between events (WSum6 = 11), maintaining a balance between reality-based and fantasy-based thinking (RFS-P = 0.41), and managing daily demands without becoming unduly distressed by them (CDI = 2). It may well be that the coping resources identified by these normal range scores made it possible for her to work effectively as a college student and for the past 2 years in her career as a data analyst, despite remaining socially isolated during these times (Exhibit 20.6).

Nevertheless, although she appears for the most part to have recovered from her recent manic episode, her Rorschach responses include some lingering traces of both manic and depressive tendencies, some instances of cognitive slippage, and some guidelines for her continued treatment. Informative in these respects is a comparison of BR's Rorschach summary scores with the Composite International Reference Values (CIRV) for the Rorschach. As reported by Meyer et al. (2007), the CIRV are based on Rorschach records obtained from 4,704 nonpatient adults in 21 samples from 17 countries in North and South America, Europe, and Asia whose protocols were administered and coded in accordance with the Comprehensive System.

EXHIBIT 20.4

Rorschach Sequence of Scores

Card I
1. WSo Fo A 3.5 PER
2. W+ ma.Fro H,Cg 4 .0
3. Wo Fu ID 1.0

Card II
4. D + 6 Mau (2) A 3.0 INCOM1
5. Do6 Fo An
6. Do2 F-Hd
7. DS5o Fu An,Art

Card III
8. D + (1&3) FC- H,SC 4.0 DR1
9. DdS + F- Ad,Cg 4.0 INCOM1
10. DdSo Fu Art

Card IV
11. Do7 Mp.FDo H
12. Wo Fu (A) 2.0
13. WS + Fu Ls 5.0

Card V
14. Wo Fo A P 1.0
15. Wo Fo Art 1.0 PSV
16. W + Mp.Fru Ad 2.5 INCOM1

Card VI
17. Wo Fu Bt 2.5
18. Wo Fo Ad P 2.5
19. Wo Fu Sc 2.5

Card VII
20. Wo Fu Cg 2.5
21. D + 6 Ma.Fro Hd P 3.0
22. Wo F- Ad 2.5

Card VIII
23. W + FMa.Fro A,Na P 4.5
24. D + 6 ma- Sc 3.0
25. D + 2&5 ma.FCu ID 3.0

Card IX
26. D + 2&3 Ma.FC- A,Bt 2.5 INCOM1
27. Do6 Fu (2) A

Card X
28. Do11 Fo Ls
29. Do7 Fo (2) A

Manic Tendencies

Lingering traces of manic tendencies appear in BR's Rorschach productivity and indications of grandiosity. With respect to her productivity, she gives a longer-than-average record, with her 29 responses exceeding the CIRV average *R*

EXHIBIT 20.5

Rorschach Structural Summary

Thinking (ideation)	Cognitive functioning	Perception (mediation)	Affect	Interpersonal
R = 29	L = 1.90*			
EB = 5:1.5	EA = 6.5	EBPer = 3.3	FC:CF + C = 3:0*	COP = 1 AG = 1
eb = 4:0	es = 4	D = 0	Pure C = 0	GHR:PHR = 3:5
	Adjes = 2	AdjD = +1*	Const. index = 0:1.5	a:p = 7:2
			Afr = 0.32*	Fd = 0
FM = 1	SumC' = 0	SumT = 0*	S = 5*	SumT = 0*
m = 3	SumV = 0	SumY = 0	Complex.	Human
			index = 7:29	content = 5
			CP = 0	Pure H = 3
				PER = 1
				Isolation
				index = 0.21

Thinking (ideation)	Cognitive functioning	Perception (mediation)	Attention (processing)	Self-perception
a:p = 7:2	Sum6 = 5	XA% = .79	Zf = 21	Egoc. index = 0.52*
Ma:Mp = 3:2	Lv2 = 0	WDA% = .81	W:D:Dd = 14:13:2*	Fr + rF = 4*
INTELL = 3	WSum6 = 11	X–% = .21	W:M = 14:5	Sum V = 0
MOR = 0	M– = 1	S– = 1	Zd = –10.5*	FD = 1
	Mnone = 0	P = 4	PSV = 1	An + Xy = 2
		X+% = .38	DQ+ = 11	MOR = 0
		Xu% = .41*	DQv = 0	H:(H) + Hd + (Hd) = 3:2
PTI = 0	DEPI = 3	CDI = 2	S-CON = 4	HVI = No OBS = No
FM + m = 4	Col-Shd = 0			
RFS-P = 0.41	RFS-S = 2.53	EII-2 = –0.03	AdjDMD = 1	

Note. PTI = Perceptual Thinking Index; DEPI = Depression Index; CDI = Coping Deficit Index; HVI = Negative on the Hypervigilance Index; EII-2 = Ego Impairment Index.

of 22.31. Also of note are her five Blends, which is above the CIRV average of four, and her sometimes free-flowing, fanciful, and upbeat elaboration of her responses, as in the "wombats high-fiving" in response II.4. These Rorschach characteristics do not warrant an inference of mania, but they do identify an extent of energy and task involvement that would characterize manic tendencies.

As for grandiosity, BR's three reflections—a dancer "being reflected on herself" in response I.2, a crab approaching a mirror and "reflected on itself" in response V.16, and a woman "looking in a mirror and doing her hair" in response VII.21—far exceed normative expectations. The CIRV show the average frequency of reflection responses as just 0.41, which means that the majority of nonpatients do not give any reflection responses. As would be expected in light of her three reflections, BR's Egocentricity Index of .52 exceeds the CIRV mean of .38. Her numerous reflections and elevated Egocentricity Index point to above-average self-centeredness, self-admiration, and self-assurance. Such grandiosity

---

EXHIBIT 20.6

Thematic Apperception Test Responses

Card 1

It was Wednesday afternoon, and John had to sit down and play the violin again. He was tired from the day at school and always resented his mother for forcing him to practice this instrument. He gazed at the television screen and decided . . . he . . . would reward himself with TV, and he then practiced for 20 minutes.

Card 3BM

Tom . . . It was Thursday, and Tom had a long week of school and therefore he was exhausted. He realized that he needed to complete an essay that he hadn't started. He decided he would need to do it. He felt annoyed and tired and wanted to complain, but he knew he'll have to muster all his energy to finish. For starting, he decided to take a quick power nap. This way he'd have more energy to write the essay.

Card 5

It was Saturday afternoon, and Anna's mother decided she would peer in and check on Anna and her friends. She opened the door and was astonished that she found her daughter and her friends smoking cigarettes in the house, and she gasped and was shocked that her daughter engaged in such unsafe unhealthy behavior and proceeded to tell Anna that she would be punished. (How did Anna feel about this?) She was taken aback, embarrassed, and bothered by this lack of privacy.

Card 13MF

[laughs to herself] It was Saturday morning and Henry got out of bed after a night of drinking and partying. He was sleepy and groggy and realized he had brought a woman home with him. It made him feel startled and sad that he'd have to leave her because he knew he wasn't interested in starting a relationship. The woman was asleep, and he didn't even know her name.

---

is a defining feature of mania, and it is usually a stable personality characteristic. BR's test data accordingly suggest a continuing susceptibility to manic episodes at times of stress and call for ongoing supportive management aimed at moderating her unrealistic and probably maladaptive sense of superiority.

Depressive Tendencies

Lingering traces of depression in BR's responses include indications of interpersonal detachment, concerns about being safe in a dangerous world, and a downside perspective on events. A key finding in this regard is her affective ratio (AFR) of .32, which is far below the CIRV average of .53 and tends to indicate such features of depression as an aversion to becoming emotionally involved with other people and discomfort in situations that call for an exchange of feelings. This finding is consistent with her developmental history of social isolation, and it might also account for her selecting a career as a data analyst in which she would be working with numbers, not with people, and would be engaged more in solitary than in collaborative endeavors.

Notable with respect to such interpersonal adversity is her saying in response IV.10 that "It's like looking up at some giant dude that's about to stomp on you." Concerns about safety are captured as well by her percepts of such fearsome creatures as, in response IV.12, a "wendigo" (which is a mythological humanoid purported to be cannibalistic) and in response IX.26, a "mantis shrimp" (which is a carnivorous marine creature). Notable in illustrating a downside perspective on events is the impression in response VIII.25 of a hot air balloon that is "deflated" and "collapsing."

In addition to these indications of continuing manic and depressive tendencies, BR's responses suggest a preoccupation with the reproductive system. Notable in this regard are the pelvic bone in response II.5, the diagram of a uterus in response II.7, and the ultrasound of a pregnant woman with the baby visible in response III.8. In her continuing treatment, it would be advisable for BR's therapist to explore her apparent concerns about conception and pregnancy, to seek to modify any erroneous or troubling beliefs she may have about them, and to determine what role these concerns may have played in her past and present sexual activity.

Cognitive Slippage

BR's WSUM6 of 11 is somewhat larger than the CIRV average of 7.63 and identifies occasional cognitive slippage, consisting in this instance of one Deviant Response (DR) and four Incongruous Combinations (INCOMs). The DR appears in the previously noted response III.8, in which she adds to her percept of a baby in the ultrasound of a pregnant woman the extraneous information that "babies are supposed to be pink when they're doing well, but not when they're blue." The INCOMs are the wombats high-fiving on response II.4, the cow with a bow on its forehead on response III.9, the curious crab approaching a mirror on response V.16, and the shrimp hiding and looking out for predators on response IX.26. Research has indicated in this regard that manic patients can generally be expected to show more signs of cognitive slippage on the Rorschach than depressed patients, perhaps due in part to their giving longer and more complex responses (Singer & Brabender, 1993).

THEMATIC APPERCEPTION TEST

In Cards 1 and 3BM in BR's TAT, the characters John and Tom are faced with the necessity of completing unwelcome tasks—practicing the violin in Card 1 and writing an essay in Card 3BM. John is "tired from the day in school," and Tom is "exhausted" and needs to "muster all of his energy" to complete his task. These stories suggest that BR was becoming weary with the testing process and finding it difficult to sustain her participation in it. Along with her fatigue, she may have been upset by her story on Card 5, in which Anna is unhappy with her mother's invasion of her privacy and is threatened with being punished for her alleged misbehavior. BR may accordingly have come to regard the testing as an unwelcome intrusion into her thoughts and feelings, and to anticipate unwelcome consequences should her fatigue prevent her from cooperating fully with the examination process.

In light of these possibilities, it was decided to spare BR any further distress by ending the TAT administration and the testing session after showing her just one more TAT card, which was 13MF. In the 13MF story she told, Henry awakens from a night of drinking and partying to find a woman asleep in his bed. But the story is not really about Henry but about the sleeping woman, whose situation mirrors the emptiness of BR's indiscriminate sexuality. She has allowed herself to be seduced by a man who "wasn't interest in starting a relationship" and who "didn't even know her name."

SUMMARY

Ms. BR is a 26-year-old single woman, a college graduate employed as a data analyst, who has a history of diagnosed bipolar disorder Type 1 and has recently had her second manic episode. Her psychological testing with the PAI, the Rorschach Inkblot Method (Rorschach), and the TAT indicate that she had for the most part recovered from her recent manic episode, with most of her test scores falling in the normal range. She nevertheless shows some lingering traces of both mania and depression, and there is some risk of further episodes of disorder that might include harming herself. She should receive continued treatment to monitor her emotional state, address her interpersonal adversity, and explore her apparent concerns about sexuality and the reproductive process.

REFERENCES

Meyer, G. J., Erdberg, P., & Shaffer, T. W. (2007). Toward international normative reference data for the comprehensive system. *Journal of Personality Assessment, 89*(Suppl. 1), S201–S216. https://doi.org/10.1080/00223890701629342

Morey, L. C. (2003). *Essentials of PAI assessment.* Wiley.

Singer, H. K., & Brabender, V. (1993). The use of the Rorschach to differentiate unipolar and bipolar disorders. *Journal of Personality Assessment, 60*(2), 333–345. https://doi.org/10.1207/s15327752jpa6002_10

Teglasi, H. (2013). *Essentials of TAT assessment.* Wiley.

Weiner, I. B. (2003). *Principles of Rorschach interpretation.* Lawrence Erlbaum. https://doi.org/10.4324/9781410607799

INDEX

ABOUT THE EDITORS

James H. Kleiger, PsyD, ABAP, ABPP, is an assessment psychologist psychologist, psychoanalyst, and writer in Olney, Maryland. Formerly the director of postdoctoral psychology training at the Menninger Clinic and a past president of the Baltimore Washington Society for Psychoanalysis, Dr. Kleiger is board certified in clinical and assessment psychology and is a fellow of the Society for Personality Assessment.

Dr. Kleiger has published numerous papers and book chapters and is the author of *Disordered Thinking and the Rorschach* (1999), *Assessing Psychosis: A Clinician's Guide* (2015, coauthored by Ali Khadivi), and *Rorschach Assessment of Psychotic Phenomena* (2017). Dr. Kleiger is the coeditor with Dr. Weiner of *Psychological Assessment of Disordered Thinking and Perception,* published in 2021 by the American Psychological Association (APA). His debut novel, *The 11th Inkblot,* was published in 2020.

Irving B. Weiner, PhD, ABPP, is a retired professor of psychiatry and behavioral neurosciences at the University of South Florida. He has diplomas in clinical and forensic psychology and is a fellow of APA and the Association of Psychological Science. Dr. Weiner has been president of the Society for Personality Assessment, APA Division 12 (Society of Clinical Psychology), APA Division 5 (Quantitative and Qualitative Methods), and the International Rorschach Society.

Dr. Weiner has written assessment books including *Psychodiagnosis in Schizophrenia* (1966), *Principles of Rorschach Interpretation* (1998, 2003), *Handbook of Personality Assessment* (2008, 2017), and *Rorschach Assessment of Senior Adults* (2019).

His edited books include *Clinical Methods in Psychology* (1976, 1983) and four editions of the *Handbook of Forensic Psychology* (1987, 1999, 2008, 2017). He has been editor of the *Journal of Personality Assessment* and editor-in-chief of Wiley's 12-volume *Handbook of Psychology* (2003, 2013).